T0259350

The Impact of Obesity and Nutrition on Chronic Liver Diseases

Editor

ZOBAIR M. YOUNOSSI

CLINICS IN LIVER DISEASE

www.liver.theclinics.com

Consulting Editor
NORMAN GITLIN

February 2014 • Volume 18 • Number 1

ELSEVIER

1600 John F. Kennedy Boulevard • Suite 1800 • Philadelphia, Pennsylvania, 19103-2899

http://www.theclinics.com

CLINICS IN LIVER DISEASE Volume 18, Number 1
February 2014 ISSN 1089-3261, ISBN-13: 978-0-323-26664-2

Editor: Kerry Holland
Developmental Editor: Susan Showalter

Clinics in Liver Disease (ISSN 1089-3261) is published quarterly by Elsevier Inc., 360 Park Avenue South, New York, NY 10010-1710. Months of issue are February, May, August, and November. Business and Editorial Offices: 1600 John F. Kennedy Blvd., Ste. 1800, Philadelphia, PA 19103-2899. Customer Service Office: 3251 Riverport Lane, Maryland Heights, MO 63043. Periodicals postage paid at New York, NY and additional mailing offices. Subscription prices are $295.00 per year (U.S. individuals), $145.00 per year (U.S. student/resident), $401.00 per year (U.S. institutions), $395.00 per year (foreign individuals), $200.00 per year (foreign student/ resident), $498.00 per year (foreign instituitions), $340.00 per year (Canadian individuals), $200.00 per year (Canadian student/resident), and $498.00 per year (Canadian institutions). Foreign air speed delivery is included in all *Clinics* subscription prices. All prices are subject to change without notice. **POSTMASTER:** Send address changes to *Clinics in Liver Disease*, Elsevier Health Sciences Division, Subscription Customer Service, 3251 Riverport Lane, Maryland Heights, MO 63043. **Customer Service: Telephone: 1-800-654-2452 (U.S. and Canada); 314-447-8871 (outside U.S. and Canada). Fax: 314-447-8029. E-mail: journalscustomer service-usa@elsevier.com (for print support); journalsonlinesupport-usa@elsevier.com (for online support).**

Reprints. For copies of 100 or more of articles in this publication, please contact the Commercial Reprints Department, Elsevier Inc., 360 Park Avenue South, New York, NY 10010-1710. Tel.: 212-633-3874; Fax: 212-633-3820; E-mail: reprints@elsevier.com.

Clinics in Liver Disease is covered in *MEDLINE/PubMed (Index Medicus)*, Science Citation Index Expanded, Journal Citation Reports/Science Edition, and Current Contents/Clinical Medicine.

Printed and bound by CPI Group (UK) Ltd, Croydon, CR0 4YY

Transferred to digital print 2013

Contributors

CONSULTING EDITOR

NORMAN GITLIN, MD, FRCP (LONDON), FRCPE (EDINBURGH), FACG, FACP
Formerly, Professor of Medicine, Chief of Hepatology, Emory University; Currently, Consultant, Atlanta Gastroenterology Associates, Atlanta, Georgia

EDITOR

ZOBAIR M. YOUNOSSI, MD, MPH, FACG, FACP, AGAF
Chairman, Department of Medicine, Inova Fairfax Hospital; Vice President for Research, Inova Health System; Professor of Medicine, VCU-Inova Campus; Betty and Guy Beatty Center for Integrated Research, Falls Church, Virginia, USA

AUTHORS

FRANCISCO BARRERA, MD
Storr Liver Unit, Westmead Millennium Institute, Westmead Hospital, University of Sydney, Sydney, New South Wales, Australia; Department of Gastroenterology, Pontificia Universidad Católica de Chile, Santiago, Chile

AYBIKE BIRERDINC, PhD
Research Assistant Professor, Betty and Guy Beatty Center for Integrated Research, Center for Liver Disease, Inova Health System, Falls Church; Center for the Study of Chronic Metabolic Diseases, School of Systems Biology, George Mason University, Fairfax, Virginia

KERRI N. BOUTELLE, PhD
Professor of Pediatrics and Psychiatry, Departments of Pediatrics and Psychiatry, University of California, San Diego, La Jolla; Division of Pediatric Gastroenterology, Hepatology, and Nutrition, Rady Children's Hospital, San Diego, California

ELISABETTA BUGIANESI, MD, PhD
Division of Gastroenterology and Hepatology, Department of Medical Sciences, University of Torino, Torino, Italy

YOGESH KUMAR CHAWLA, MBBS, MD, DM, FACG
Head, Department of Hepatology; Director, Post Graduate Institute of Medical Education and Research, Chandigarh, India

DIAN J. CHIANG, MD, MPH
Department of Gastroenterology and Hepatology, Digestive Disease Institute, Cleveland Clinic, Cleveland, Ohio

KATHLEEN E. COREY, MD, MPH
Gastrointestinal Unit, Weight Center, Massachusetts General Hospital; Instructor in Medicine, Harvard Medical School, Boston, Massachusetts

JOHN B. DIXON, PhD, MBBS, FRACGP, FRCP Edin
NHMRC Senior Research Fellow and Head, Clinical Obesity Research, Baker IDI Heart & Diabetes Institute, Melbourne, Victoria; Adjunct Professor, Primary Care Research Unit, Monash University, Melbourne, Australia

JEAN-FRANÇOIS DUFOUR, MD
University Clinic for Visceral Surgery and Medicine, University of Bern, Inselspital, Freiburgstrasse; Hepatology, Department of Clinical Research, University of Bern, Bern, Switzerland

AJAY DUSEJA, MBBS, MD, DM, FACG
Department of Hepatology, Post Graduate Institute of Medical Education and Research, Chandigarh, India

ARIEL E. FELDSTEIN, MD
Professor of Pediatrics; Chief, Division of Pediatric Gastroenterology, Hepatology, and Nutrition, Rady Children's Hospital, San Diego; Division of Pediatric Gastroenterology, Hepatology, and Nutrition, University of California, San Diego, La Jolla, California

JACOB GEORGE, PhD, FRACP
Storr Liver Unit, Westmead Millennium Institute, Westmead Hospital, University of Sydney, Sydney, New South Wales, Australia

LYNN H. GERBER, MD
Director of Research, Department of Medicine, Inova Fairfax Hospital, Virginia

ZACHARY D. GOODMAN, MD, PhD
Center for Liver Diseases, Inova Fairfax Hospital, Falls Church, Virginia

NICOLAS GOOSSENS, MD, MSc
Clinical Fellow, Division of Gastroenterology and Hepatology, Geneva University Hospital, Geneva, Switzerland

STEPHEN A. HARRISON, MD
Division of Gastroenterology and Hepatology, Department of Medicine, San Antonio Military Medical Center, San Antonio, Texas

WASSEM JUAKIEM, MD
Department of Medicine, San Antonio Military Medical Center, San Antonio, Texas

LEE M. KAPLAN, MD, PhD
Gastrointestinal Unit, Weight Center, Obesity, Metabolism and Nutrition Institute, Massachusetts General Hospital; Director, Obesity, Metabolism and Nutrition Institute; Associate Professor of Medicine, Harvard Medical School, Boston, Massachusetts

VIGNAN MANNE, MD
Department of Surgery, University of California, Los Angeles, Los Angeles, California

GIULIO MARCHESINI, MD
Professor of Clinical Dietetics; Head, Unit of Metabolic Disease & Clinical Dietetics, S. Orsola-Malpighi Hospital, Alma Mater Studiorum University, Bologna, Italy

NATALIA MAZZELLA, MD
Unit of Metabolic Diseases & Clinical Dietetics; Resident, Post-graduate School of Nutrition, S. Orsola-Malpighi Hospital, Alma Mater Studiorum University, Bologna, Italy

ARIANNA MAZZOTTI, MD
Unit of Metabolic Diseases & Clinical Dietetics; Resident, Post-graduate School of
Nutrition, S. Orsola-Malpighi Hospital, Alma Mater Studiorum University, Bologna, Italy

ARTHUR J. MCCULLOUGH, MD
Department of Gastroenterology and Hepatology, Digestive Disease Institute, Cleveland
Clinic, Cleveland, Ohio

CHRISTINE MCGOWN, MS
Center for the Study of Chronic Metabolic Diseases, George Mason University, Fairfax,
Virginia

ROHINI MEHTA, PhD
Research Scientist I, Betty and Guy Beatty Center for Integrated Research, Center for
Liver Disease, Inova Health System, Falls Church, Virginia

FRANCESCO NEGRO, MD
Professor, Divisions of Gastroenterology and Hepatology, and Clinical Pathology, Geneva
University Hospital, Geneva, Switzerland

RALUCA PAIS, MD, PhD
Université Pierre et Marie Curie, Assistance Publique Hôpitaux de Paris, Hôpital
Pitié-Salpêtrière, Paris, France

DANA PATTON-KU, MD
Division of Pediatric Gastroenterology, Hepatology, and Nutrition, Rady Children's
Hospital, San Diego; Division of Pediatric Gastroenterology, Hepatology, and Nutrition,
University of California, San Diego, La Jolla, California

LISA PAWLOSKI, PhD
Professor, George Mason University, Fairfax, Virginia

HUGO PERAZZO, MD
Hepatology Department, Liver Center, Groupe Hospitalier Pitié-Salpêtrière (GHPS),
Assistance Publique Hôpitaux de Paris; Pierre et Marie Curie University (Paris 6), Paris,
France

THIERRY POYNARD, MD, PhD
Hepatology Department, Liver Center, Groupe Hospitalier Pitié-Salpêtrière (GHPS),
Assistance Publique Hôpitaux de Paris; Pierre et Marie Curie University (Paris 6); Institute
of Cardiometabolism and Nutrition, Paris, France

VLAD RATZIU, MD, PhD
Pierre et Marie Curie University, Assistance Publique Hôpitaux de Paris, Hôpital
Pitié-Salpêtrière, Paris, France

LAURA M. RICCIARDI, MD
Assistant, Unit of Metabolic Diseases & Clinical Dietetics, S. Orsola-Malpighi Hospital,
Bologna, Italy

ELENA RUSU, MD, PhD
Institutul Clinic Fundeni, Bucharest, Romania

SAMMY SAAB, MD, MPH, AGAF
Departments of Surgery and Medicine, University of California, Los Angeles, Los Angeles,
California

DAWN M. TORRES, MD
Division of Gastroenterology, Department of Medicine, Walter Reed National Military Medical Center, Bethesda, Maryland

ESTER VANNI, MD, PhD
Division of Gastroenterology and Hepatology, Department of Medical Sciences, University of Torino, Torino, Italy

ALI WEINSTEIN, PhD
Associate Professor, George Mason University, Fairfax, Virginia

YUSUF YILMAZ, MD
Department of Gastroenterology, School of Medicine, Marmara University, Pendik; Institute of Gastroenterology, Marmara University, Maltepe, Istanbul, Turkey

ZOBAIR M. YOUNOSSI, MD, MPH, FACG, FACP, AGAF
Chairman, Department of Medicine, Inova Fairfax Hospital; Vice President for Research, Inova Health System; Professor of Medicine, VCU-Inova Campus; Betty and Guy Beatty Center for Integrated Research, Falls Church, Virginia, USA

Contents

also a considerable risk factor for the development of numerous other chronic diseases, such as insulin resistance, type 2 diabetes, heart disease and nonalcoholic fatty liver disease. The epidemic proportions of obesity and its numerous comorbidities are bringing into focus the highly complex and metabolically active adipose tissue. Adipose tissue is increasingly being considered as a functional endocrine organ. This article discusses the endocrine effects of adipose tissue during obesity and the systemic impact of this signaling.

There are trillions of microorganisms in the human intestine collectively called gut microbiota. Obesity may be affected by the gut microbiota through energy harvesting and fat storage by the bacteria. Small intestinal bacterial overgrowth is also responsible for endotoxemia, systemic inflammation, and its consequences including obesity and nonalcoholic fatty liver disease (NAFLD). Relationship between gut microbiota and NAFLD is also dependent on altered choline and bile acid metabolism and endogenous alcohol production by gut bacteria. Further evidence linking gut microbiota with obesity and NAFLD comes from studies showing usefulness of probiotics in animals and patients with NAFLD. This article reviews the relationship among gut microbiota, obesity, and NAFLD.

TREATMENT

The article is intended to provide an overview of the strengths and limits of controlled trials of pharmacologic treatment of nonalcoholic fatty liver disease. No drug has so far been approved, although validated on histologic outcomes. Several new drugs are under scrutiny, acting with different mechanisms along the chain of events from fatty liver to fibrosis, cirrhosis, and hepatocellular carcinoma. The article investigates which drug, if any, should be preferred for a tailored intervention in individual patients, according to age, comorbidities, and disease severity, and if treatment should be continued lifelong, to prevent disease progression and long-term occurrence of cirrhosis.

During the last few decades, the prevalence of obesity, insulin resistance and non-alcoholic fatty liver disease (NAFLD) have dramatically increased. Nutrition and modern lifestyle habits are intimately involved in this epidemiological change. Although lifestyle intervention can theoretically revert the metabolic disturbances and prevent the long-term complications of NAFLD, its efficacy is diminished in clinical practice by poor implementation and reduced adherence to lifestyle intervention programs. In this article we summarize the main elements of dietary interventions for NAFLD, describe practical strategies to optimize efficacy and review potential nutritional strategies under development that hopefully will improve outcomes in the future.

Nonalcoholic fatty liver disease (NAFLD) is frequently concomitant with obesity. This article discusses factors that influence health and functional outcomes of people who develop NAFLD, including increased burden of illness, whole body function, performance, and perception of self-efficacy. Changes in macronutrients, amount of calories consumed, and decreased physical activity all negatively influence patient outcome. The benefits of exercise in this population are also discussed. To be effective, exercise must be performed, regularly and in conjunction with dietary and other behavioral change. Therefore, a lifelong commitment to exercise, activity, and diet are needed if NAFLD is to be successfully treated.

Most patients with severe complex obesity presenting for bariatric-metabolic surgery have nonalcoholic fatty liver disease (NAFLD). NAFLD is associated with central obesity, insulin resistance, type 2 diabetes, hypertension, and obesity-related dyslipidemia. Weight loss should be a primary therapy for NAFLD. However, evidence supporting intentional weight loss as a therapy for NAFLD is limited. Bariatric-metabolic surgery provides the most reliable method of achieving substantial sustained weight loss and the most commonly used procedures are associated with reduced steatosis and lobular inflammatory changes, but there are mixed reports regarding fibrosis. Surgery should complement treatment of obesity-related comorbidity, but not replace established therapy.

OBESITY, NUTRITION, AND OTHER LIVER DISEASES

The metabolic syndrome and the hepatitis C virus (HCV) infection are 2 global health care challenges with a complex interaction. Insulin resistance, a central component of the metabolic syndrome, is epidemiologically and pathophysiologically intrinsically linked to HCV infection. Insulin resistance and diabetes affect clinical outcomes in patients with liver disease related to HCV, namely, incidence of hepatocellular carcinoma, liver-related mortality, fibrosis progression rate, response to antiviral therapy, and possibly the incidence of cardiovascular events. Viral and metabolic steatosis and its interactions with HCV and the metabolic syndrome are discussed. Management and the need for further research conclude the article.

Alcoholic liver disease (ALD) remains a major cause of chronic liver diseases and liver failure. Population-based prospective studies and patient cohort studies have demonstrated that obesity and the metabolic syndrome exacerbate progression of ALD and increase hepatocellular carcinoma (HCC) incidence and mortality. Emerging evidence also suggests a synergism between alcohol and obesity in mortality and HCC incidence. Recognition of these increased risks and detection of early-stage liver disease may offer the opportunity to address these modifiable risk factors and prevent disease progression in these patients.

Steatosis and insulin resistance (IR) are no more frequent in chronic hepatitis B (CHB) than in the general population. Although experimental studies suggest that the HBx protein induces liver fat, human studies have shown that steatosis and IR are related to coexistent metabolic risk factors, thus epidemiologically linked rather than virally induced. Diabetes and obesity are associated with advanced fibrosis and increased risk of hepatocellular carcinoma in CHB. Despite abundant experimental data showing that fatty liver is more susceptible to liver injury, drug-induced liver disease seems no more frequent in NAFLD patients, except, possibly, a higher incidence but not severity of acetaminophen hepatotoxicity.

SPECIAL TOPICS

Nutrition has not been a primary focus of many medical conditions despite its importance in the development and the severity of these diseases. This is certainly the case with nutrition and end-stage liver disease despite the well-established association of nutritional deficiencies and increased rates of complications and mortality in cirrhosis. This review provides an overview of nutrition in chronic liver disease with an emphasis on its pathogenesis as well as ways to assess nutritional status and intervene in an effort to improve nutrition.

Obesity is an established risk factor for many types of cancers, particularly for hepatocellular carcinoma (HCC), owing to its carcinogenic potential and the association with nonalcoholic fatty liver disease (NAFLD). HCC may develop in cirrhotic and noncirrhotic livers with NAFLD, particularly in the presence of multiple metabolic risk factors such as obesity and diabetes. This issue is alarming because the population potentially at higher risk is greatly increasing. This review summarizes current evidence linking obesity and liver cancer, and discusses recent advances on the mechanisms underlying this relationship.

Undernutrition and obesity are at opposite ends of a spectrum that has an enormous impact on all aspects of liver diseases. The myriad effects of the opposing ends of the nutrition spectrum have led to a wealth of research aimed at elucidating the exact mechanisms of how they cause liver damage. In this article, the role of the liver in nutrient and energy metabolism is discussed, as well as the known and possible effects of specific nutrient deficiencies and obesity.

In this article, several aspects of childhood obesity are discussed, including epidemiology, associated metabolic complications, management strategies, and therapy with particular attention to the impact of obesity on the liver, resulting in nonalcoholic or metabolic fatty liver disease. The deleterious effects of obesity on the liver and health overall can be significantly impacted by a culture that fosters sustained nutritional improvement and regular physical activity. The current evidence is summarized supporting pharmacologic, behavioral, and dietary interventions for the management of obesity and fatty liver disease in children.

A complex interaction among metabolic factors, adipose tissue lipolysis, oxidative stress, and insulin resistance results in a deleterious process that may link nonalcoholic fatty liver disease (NAFLD) with severe cardiovascular (CV) outcomes. Patients with NAFLD are at higher risk of atherosclerosis, new onset of CV events, and overall mortality. The strong association between NAFLD and CV disease should affect clinical practice, with screening and surveillance of patients with NAFLD. This review discusses the data linking these major diseases.

Nonalcoholic fatty liver disease (NAFLD) is a complex disease. The considerable variability in the natural history of the disease suggests an important role for genetic variants in the disease development and progression. There is evidence based on genome-wide association studies and/or candidate gene studies that genetic polymorphisms underlying insulin signaling, lipid metabolism, oxidative stress, fibrogenesis, and inflammation can predispose individuals to NAFLD. This review highlights some of the genetic variants in NAFLD.

CLINICS IN LIVER DISEASE

Preface

Obesity and Liver Disease

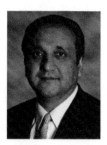

Zobair M. Younossi, MD, MPH, FACG, FACP, AGAF
Editor

In recent decades, obesity has reached epidemic proportions in the United States and Western countries. Obesity and its complications have been shown to have tremendous impact on clinical, economic, societal, and patient-reported outcomes. Due to this wide ranging impact of obesity, it was recently recognized by the American Medical Association as a "disease."

In particular, obesity affects the liver in a number of ways. Obesity is the most important risk factor for what is becoming the most common cause of liver disease, nonalcoholic fatty liver disease (NAFLD). In addition, obesity and type 2 diabetes can affect other chronic liver diseases such as hepatitis C, hepatitis B, alcoholic liver disease, and drug-induced liver disease. Visceral obesity and associated white adipose tissue are the likely sources of the inflammatory adipocytokines, which potentially play an important role in the pathogenesis of obesity-related complications, including NAFLD.

Although the increasing prevalence of obesity seems to be related to the individual's caloric intake, there is increasing evidence that obesity and its complications are consequences of complex interactions between environmental factors (food sources), personal habits or choices (calorie intake, activity, alcohol intake, and tobacco use), and an individual's genetic predisposition.

In this issue of *Clinics in Liver Disease*, several internationally renowned experts present topics related to obesity, nutrition, and liver disease. In the first article, the epidemiology of obesity and its association with liver disease are covered. The following two articles focus on the roles that visceral adipose tissue and microbiota potentially play in the pathogenesis of obesity-related liver disease. The next article focuses on the hepatic pathology seen in patients with obesity-related liver disease and those with malnutrition. The next five articles are focused on NAFLD and provide in-depth data on the natural history and treatment strategies for patients with NAFLD. The next six articles deal with the impact of obesity on other liver diseases and on special populations including children and liver-transplant recipients. The final article provides the most updated information regarding genomics and genetic targets that

Clin Liver Dis 18 (2014) xiii–xiv
http://dx.doi.org/10.1016/j.cld.2013.09.020
liver.theclinics.com

may provide better prognostic and diagnostic biomarkers and more personalized treatment targets for patients with NAFLD.

Cutting-edge information provided in this issue of *Clinics in Liver Disease* will help readers gain better understanding of the natural history and pathogenesis of primary and secondary liver diseases associated with obesity. As the information about obesity-related liver disease expands, clinicians will be able to provide more targeted therapeutic options for these patients and develop more accurate diagnostic and prognostic biomarkers.

Zobair M. Younossi, MD, MPH, FACG, FACP, AGAF
Department of Medicine, Inova Fairfax Hospital
Inova Health System
VCU-Inova Campus
Beatty Center for Integrated Research
3300 Gallows Road
Falls Church, VA 22042, USA

E-mail address:
Zobair.Younossi@inova.org

Obesity and Liver Disease
The Epidemic of the Twenty-First Century

Kathleen E. Corey, MD, MPH[a], Lee M. Kaplan, MD, PhD[b,*]

KEYWORDS

- Obesity • Nonalcoholic fatty liver disease • Nonalcoholic steatohepatitis • Cirrhosis
- Weight loss • Fat mass • Energy balance

KEY POINTS

- More than one-third of American adults have obesity, a disease that is growing rapidly in all parts of the world.
- Powerful environmental changes associated with modern society largely account for the obesity epidemic.
- Obesity results from the establishment and defense of an elevated fat mass that is maintained through abnormal energy homeostasis.
- Obesity is a heterogeneous disorder with multiple pathophysiological mechanisms and a variable response to each available therapy.
- Effective treatment of nonalcoholic fatty liver disease starts with treatment of the underlying obesity.

INTRODUCTION

Obesity, defined as the state of having excess body fat, is an epidemic and still-growing health problem across the world. Data from the 2009–2010 National Health and Nutrition Examination Survey reveal that 36% of Americans have obesity.[1] Globally, more than 400 million people have this disorder.[2] Obesity is associated with more than 65 demonstrated comorbidities, including diabetes mellitus, cardiovascular disease, and several forms of cancer; because of these sequelae, it is associated with a substantially increased all-cause mortality.[3,4] Moreover, obesity accounts for an estimated $163 to $300 billion in additional health care costs annually, accounting for up to 10% of overall health care costs in this country.[5]

Despite studies that correlate obesity with numerous societal changes and individual behaviors, full understanding of its pathogenesis and rising prevalence remains

[a] Gastrointestinal Unit, Weight Center, Massachusetts General Hospital, Harvard Medical School, 55 Fruit Street, Boston, MA 02114, USA; [b] Gastrointestinal Unit, Weight Center, Obesity, Metabolism and Nutrition Institute, Massachusetts General Hospital, Harvard Medical School, 149 13th Street, Room 8219, Charlestown, MA 02129, USA
* Corresponding author.
E-mail address: LMKaplan@partners.org

Clin Liver Dis 18 (2014) 1–18
http://dx.doi.org/10.1016/j.cld.2013.09.019
1089-3261/14/$ – see front matter © 2014 Elsevier Inc. All rights reserved.

liver.theclinics.com

elusive. Countless shifts in our environment over the past century likely contribute to obesity development.[6] These shifts include alterations in routine physical activity and muscle function, the chemical composition of our diets, and a variety of external stressors, each of which likely plays an important contributing role. Furthermore, obesity seems to be a symptom of multiple related disorders, each with distinct phenotypes, clinical characteristics, and proximate causes. This heterogeneity likely contributes to the difficulty in identifying broadly effective preventative and long-term treatment strategies and suggests that treatment plans individualized to disease subtypes will be required.

The recent increase in the prevalence of nonalcoholic fatty liver disease (NAFLD), now the most common cause of liver disease in the United States, is in large part a result of the obesity epidemic. This issue of *Clinics in Liver Disease* is devoted to addressing all aspects of NAFLD. To frame this important discussion, the authors begin with a review of the prevalence, comorbid conditions, and pathogenesis of obesity, a major underlying cause of NAFLD. The authors conclude their discussion with a review of the therapeutic options that can serve to treat obesity and, thereby, contribute to the effective treatment of NAFLD.

CHALLENGES IN OBESITY

Obesity treatment is challenging for myriad reasons. First, although obesity is largely considered one disease, the term *obesity* actually encompasses multiple disorders with distinct causes and treatments. The regulation of energy balance and body fat storage is complex, involving multiple central and peripheral, biochemical, metabolic, and signaling pathways; a disturbance in any of these pathways can disrupt normal physiologic regulation. Obesity can, thus, be viewed as analogous to cancer. No single pathway is responsible for the development of the many different types and subtypes of cancer, and no single therapy is successful in treating all cancers. Obesity can similarly be viewed as a heterogeneous disease, with varying mechanisms that contribute to its development, requiring individually tailored treatment after a thorough clinical evaluation.

Additional challenges to the effective treatment of obesity are the powerful and widespread environmental influences inherent to modern society that promote the development and maintenance of the obese state (**Table 1**). These environmental influences include profound changes in the chemical composition of ingested nutrients, including an increased prevalence of calorie-dense, highly processed, and often homogeneous foods. Our service-based economy, labor-saving devices, the increased speed and volume of communication and decision making, frequent disruption of sleep and circadian rhythms, and a variety of other cultural and economic factors add to the obesogenic environment. These forces act on a genetically and developmentally determined human biology that is frequently unable to resist these powerful influences. Added to these forces is the increasingly widespread use of medications

Table 1 Environmental influences on obesity	
Macroenvironmental	**Microenvironmental**
Nature of available food supply	Ingested food: chemical content and eating patterns
24-h day	Labor-saving devices: reduced need for exercise
Economic stress	Personal stress
Speed of life	Weight-promoting medications

that promote weight gain, including for complications of obesity itself (eg, diabetes, hypertension) and other diseases of modern society, such as psychological and in-flammatory disorders. Obesity, thus, reflects the perfect storm of numerous coopera-tive changes in the environment acting on a biology that evolved in a different era.

PREVALENCE OF OBESITY

More than a third of Americans currently suffer from obesity; an equal number are overweight, a designation that, although indicating a weight disorder of lesser inten-sity, is still associated with a significantly increased risk of potentially debilitating metabolic disease.[1] After increasing 2- to 3-fold over the past 40 years, the rate of growth seems to have abated in the past decade. Although the prevalence of obesity overall has begun to stabilize, however, the average weight of the population con-tinues to increase; the prevalence of the most severe classes of obesity continues to increase rapidly (Fig. 1).[7] Thus, despite early signs of hope, it is difficult to argue that we have yet made substantial progress in tackling this disease.

OBESITY-RELATED MORBIDITY AND MORTALITY

Obesity results in a wide variety of health-related complications and affects nearly all or-gan systems. Obesity-related complications can be conveniently considered in 6 cate-gories, including metabolic, structural (anatomic), inflammatory, degenerative, neoplastic, and psychological (Table 2). Metabolic complications include diabetes mel-litus, NAFLD, dyslipidemia, gallstones, thrombogenesis (from plasminogen activator inhibitor-1 deficiency), and various forms of infertility. Structural effects of obesity include gastroesophageal reflux disease, pseudotumor cerebri, arthritis in weight-bearing joints, obstructive sleep apnea (OSA), and injuries resulting from mechanical falls.[8] Obesity also contributes to the development of autoimmune and inflammatory dis-ease, including asthma, hypothyroidism, psoriasis, arthritis in non–weight-bearing joints, pancreatitis, and nonalcoholic steatohepatitis (NASH).[9] Obesity-associated degenerative disorders include several longer-term sequelae of acute manifestations, such as atherosclerotic cardiovascular disease, other complications of type 2 diabetes, pulmonary hypertension from OSA, and NASH-associated cirrhosis.[10,11] They also

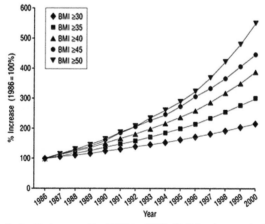

Fig. 1. Prevalence of obesity by severity, 1986 to 2000. BMI, body mass index. (*From* Sturm R. Increases in clinically severe obesity in the United States, 1986–2000. Arch Intern Med 2003;163(18):2147; with permission.)

Table 2	
Obesity-associated comorbidities	
Obesity-Related Disease Categories	**Selected Conditions**
Metabolic	Diabetes mellitus, gallstones, thromboembolic disease, NAFLD
Structural	Gastroesophageal reflux disease, arthritis in weight-bearing joints, obstructive sleep apnea, pseudotumor cerebri, compartment syndromes
Inflammatory	Asthma, hypothyroidism, psoriasis, arthritis in non–weight-bearing joints
Degenerative	Atherosclerotic vascular disease, pulmonary hypertension, cirrhosis
Neoplastic	Breast, ovarian, uterine, cervical, prostate, renal cell carcinomas; colorectal, pancreatic, gallbladder, esophageal adenocarcinomas; hepatocellular carcinoma
Psychological	Depression, anxiety and panic disorders, eating disorders

include obesity-related neurodegenerative and cognitive disorders. Obesity is a strong risk factor for the development of several malignancies, including all of the common reproductive tumors (breast, ovarian, uterine, cervical, and prostate), renal cell carcinoma, selected non-Hodgkin lymphomas, and several gastrointestinal (GI) cancers, including colorectal, pancreatic, and esophageal adenocarcinomas; cholangiocarcinoma; and hepatocellular carcinoma.[12] Finally, obesity has been shown to have a substantial detrimental impact on mental health and often leads to depression, anxiety disorders, and various forms of eating disorders.[13–15] As a result of these many comorbidities, obesity is associated with increased mortality. A recent systematic review found that, relative to normal-weight individuals, those with obesity had increased all-cause mortality; mortality was even higher in the subset with more severe (class 2–3) obesity.[16] Whitlock and colleagues[17] estimated that each 5 kg/m^2 increase in body mass index (BMI) is associated with a 30% increase in overall mortality over an 8-year follow-up period, suggesting a strong inverse relationship between BMI and lifespan.

PATHOPHYSIOLOGY OF OBESITY

Body energy content is stored almost exclusively within white adipose tissue, which is composed largely of triglycerides and comprises the body's fat mass (FM). An individual's total FM level is typically defended (defended adiposity level) to maintain available body energy content in a physiologically appropriate range. A stable FM is maintained through energy homeostasis (EH), a biologic process whereby energy intake (EI) and energy expenditure (EE) are matched over time to ensure FM stability. When an intervention or event (eg, acute illness, overeating, or restrictive dieting) alters the existing FM, a counter-regulatory process is activated to defend the original adiposity set point. On resolution of the acute illness or release of the imposed change in food intake, EI and EE are regulated to restore FM to its previous level. The physiologic regulation of FM is influenced by environmental, developmental, and genetic factors. Obesity appears to result from the disruption of these mechanisms such that the defended FM set point is abnormally high.

Role of the GI Tract in Energy Homeostasis

The GI tract plays a central role in normal EH and defense of the FM level. GI regulatory peptides, nerves innervating the GI tract (vagal afferents, sympathetic and enteric neurons), bile acids (BA), and the intestinal microbiota all contribute to the cellular and molecular mechanisms of energy regulation. Hunger and satiety play important roles in regulating energy balance. Postprandial satiety is generally stimulated by 2 mechanisms, gastric distention and signals produced by luminal nutrients transmitted to the central nervous system (CNS) through the release of gut-derived peptides and stimulation of vagal afferent nerves. GI regulatory peptides, including insulin, cholecystokinin, peptide YY, glucagonlike peptide-1 (GLP-1), leptin, glucose-sensitive insulinotropic peptide (GIP), and ghrelin play important roles in EH. Ghrelin promotes food intake and energy storage, GIP promotes lipogenesis, and the others generally promote *decreased* energy storage by regulating hunger, satiety, and lipolysis. Food consumption alters the secretion of these peptides, which act peripherally and centrally, and lead to coordinated regulation of perceptual cues (hunger, satiety, and reward-based eating), food intake behaviors, and energy expenditure that together regulate energy balance and adiposity.[18,19]

Gastric vagal afferents play a role in FM defense by responding to gastric distention, luminal nutrients, and secreted GI peptides. Following food intake, gastric distention activates gastric vagal mechanoreceptor-regulated afferents, which signal satiety to the CNS. After the placement of an adjustable gastric band (AGB), creation of a small gastric pouch as part of a Roux-en-Y gastric bypass (RYGB), or a narrow, tubelike stomach as part of a vertical sleeve gastrectomy (VSG), satiety signaling is altered and likely triggered by smaller meals, contributing to a decreased FM set point and consequent weight loss. Mucosal vagal afferents present in the small intestine also play a role in satiety. These nerves respond to chemical signals, including nutrient metabolites, and endogenous products, such as BA and endocannabinoids, to alter hunger, satiety and reward signals, energy balance, and body fat stores. In addition to responding to GI regulatory peptides, vagal afferent fibers innervate glucose sensors in the portal vein and play a role in the regulation of metabolic function, including glucose and lipid metabolism.

The suppression of food intake seen with vagal afferent stimulation is attenuated in obesity. In diet-induced obese rats, intestinal nutrients do not suppress food intake to the same degree as in control rats. GI regulatory peptide release is altered, with a decrease the sensitivity of vagal afferents to stimuli, thus, decreasing satiety, increasing defended FM, and increasing food intake.

Bile Acids

BA play an essential role in promoting lipid absorption from the GI tract. In addition, increasing evidence suggests that BA play an important role in regulating energy balance more broadly, both by modulating EE and diet-induced thermogenesis and by influencing hunger and satiety. Mice fed high-fat diets supplemented with cholic acid were resistant to the weight gain and increased adipocyte mass experienced by animals receiving a high-fat diet alone.[20] In addition, supplementation with cholic acid reversed diet-induced weight gain and improved glucose tolerance in mice receiving only the high-fat diet. Indirect calorimetry revealed increased energy expenditure in animals receiving BA supplementation, suggesting a role for BA in diet-induced thermogenesis. Circulating BA concentrations are increased after RYGB in humans and animal models, although the mechanisms by which they influence postoperative weight loss remain unknown.[21,22]

Microbiota

The gut microbiota also seems to play an important role in the development of obesity, suggesting that manipulation of the enteric microbial ecology may contribute to the effective treatment of obesity. Distinct bacterial species have been identified in the GI tracts of lean and obese individuals. Individuals with obesity have high numbers of hydrogen-producing bacterial groups that can increase fermentation of indigestible substances and increase short-chain fatty acid availability.[23] The altered microbiota observed in people with obesity may influence energy balance at multiple levels, including by enhancing energy harvest or by downregulating host energy expenditure.[24]

RYGB is associated with alterations in the microbiota that may contribute to the weight loss experienced following surgery. Transfer of gut microbiota from mice that had undergone RYGB to germ-free control mice resulted in significant weight loss.[25] RYGB is known to increase EE in these models, and recipients of microbiota from RYGB-treated mice seem to increase EE. These findings suggest that post-RYGB microbiota may induce signals that regulate EE.[26] However, the precise mechanisms by which alterations in the microbiota regulate energy balance and body weight are currently unknown.

The Liver and Weight Regulation

The liver plays an important role in glucose and lipid metabolism as well as in the control of energy balance and body weight. Hepatic carbohydrate and lipid metabolism influence satiety signaling. After food intake, hepatic portal venous glucose concentrations increase. It is hypothesized that glucose itself, increased glucose utilization, or a secondary regulatory peptide activated by glucose influences the fat mass set point to promote increased food intake, decreased energy expenditure, and increased fat storage.[27,28] Hepatic fatty acid oxidation may also be involved in weight regulation. Studies in both animals and humans have shown that medium-chain triglycerides (MCT) increase satiety to a greater extent than equivalent concentrations of long-chain triglycerides.[29] Medium-chain fatty acids, derived from MCT, can be directly absorbed in the hepatic portal vein and undergo rapid hepatic β-oxidation. This rapid oxidation may increase EE and slow weight gain.[30,31] Hepatic fatty acid oxidation can, thus, play a role in weight regulation, influenced by the type of fatty acid being oxidized, which itself is influenced by diet, intestinal metabolism, and lipid transport.

OBESITY AND LIVER DISEASE

Obesity affects multiple metabolic functions of the liver. It is associated with the development of NAFLD-associated steatosis and inflammation and promotes the progression of several other liver diseases, including hepatitis C and alcoholic liver disease.

NAFLD

NAFLD is the most common liver disease in the United States with an increasing prevalence worldwide. NAFLD can be considered in 2 forms, simple steatosis and NASH. Although long-term follow-up in people with NAFLD is limited, it is widely accepted that those with steatosis only are at a very low risk of progression, whereas those with significant inflammation (NASH) have a substantial risk of developing advanced disease.[32] NASH commonly leads to cirrhosis and/or hepatocellular carcinoma, and it is predicted that NASH-associated progressive liver disease will be the leading indication for liver transplantation in the United States within the next decade.[33,34]

The epidemiology of NAFLD and NASH has been frequently described in community-based cohorts. A study of 2287 individuals from the Dallas Heart Study evaluated the prevalence of NAFLD using magnetic resonance spectroscopy.[35] NAFLD, defined as more than 5% of hepatocytes with steatosis, was found in 31% of individuals. NASH is less prevalent but still affects a significant portion of the population.[32] A cohort of 328 individuals from Brooke Army Medical Center underwent ultrasonography (US) to assess for the presence of NAFLD.[36] Forty-six percent of the cohort was found to have NAFLD by US and underwent a liver biopsy. Of the total cohort, 12.2% were found to have NASH; among those who underwent liver biopsy, 29.9% had NASH. Thus, although less common than NAFLD overall, the prevalence of NASH in community-based cohorts is substantial.

Although NAFLD affects a third of the overall population, the prevalence of both NAFLD and NASH increases with increasing BMI and does so dramatically among those with obesity.[37,38] NAFLD is strongly associated with diabetes mellitus, obesity, and the metabolic syndrome.[39] The proportion of individuals with NAFLD directly parallels the increase in blood glucose seen in the development of diabetes. Jimba and colleagues[40] found that among Japanese adults, 27% with normal fasting glucose had NAFLD, 43% of those with impaired fasting glucose had NAFLD, and 62% of adults with newly diagnosed diabetes mellitus had NAFLD. Both increased BMI and diabetes mellitus are associated with advanced fibrosis in people with NASH.[41] Nonetheless, many individuals with NAFLD do not have obesity or diabetes mellitus. Despite not having obesity, however, these individuals often have central adiposity, which predisposes to the metabolic syndrome and is associated with insulin resistance.[42,43] Obesity and concurrent metabolic syndrome play a key role in the pathogenesis of NAFLD and the development of steatosis. Steatosis represents excess hepatic triglyceride storage. In the setting of obesity, diabetes mellitus, and/or the metabolic syndrome, there is increased delivery of free fatty acids to the liver. These free fatty acids are derived from both dietary sources and lipolysis within the excess adipose tissue that is characteristic of obesity. Steatosis is also exacerbated by increased de novo lipogenesis resulting from the combination of insulin resistance and hyperinsulinemia.[44] Thus, the milieu of obesity and its associated metabolic dysfunction create an environment ripe for the development of NAFLD.

Hepatitis C

Although the impact of obesity in the liver is most commonly manifest in NAFLD, obesity and hepatic steatosis also influence the development and progression of other forms of liver disease. Steatosis is frequently seen in individuals with concurrent hepatitis C infection. The steatosis observed may be metabolic in origin or a direct effect of viral infection as in the case of genotype 3 hepatitis C virus (HCV) infection. Steatosis also plays an important role in the progression of fibrosis in hepatitis C. The severity of steatosis is directly associated with the development of fibrosis.[45] In addition, weight gain and insulin resistance are both associated with progressive fibrosis in chronic HCV infection. In individuals with chronic hepatitis C, weight gain itself is associated with progressive liver disease. The Hepatitis C Antiviral Long-term Treatment Against Cirrhosis trial followed individuals with cirrhosis or advanced fibrosis with chronic hepatitis C for a median of 3.8 years.[46] Patients who had 5% or more weight gain over the first year of the study had a 35% increased risk of the composite outcome of death, hepatic decompensation, and increased fibrosis when compared with those with a stable weight.

Hepatocellular Carcinoma

Hepatocellular carcinoma (HCC) is the fifth most common cause of cancer in men and the seventh most common in women, with a steadily increasing incidence worldwide.[47] Obesity and diabetes mellitus are risk factors for the development of HCC in people with both alcoholic and nonalcoholic liver disease.[48–51] NASH cirrhosis is also associated with the development of HCC, and increasing reports cite HCC development in noncirrhotic NASH.[52–54]

Cirrhosis and Decompensated Liver Disease

Increased BMI is associated with development of fibrosis and progression to cirrhosis in individuals with chronic alcohol use.[46,55] BMI is an independent risk factor for the development of decompensation among individuals with cirrhosis of all causes.[56] In one study, 161 patients with cirrhosis followed for a median of 59 months were monitored for clinical decompensation (CD). CD occurred in 15% of people with a BMI less than 25 kg/m^2, in 31% of individuals with a BMI between 25 and 29, and in 43% of people with a BMI of 30 or more. Individuals with obesity were also noted to have a poor response to nonselective beta blockers administered for portal pressure reduction. The investigators hypothesized that the proinflammatory and profibrogenic phenotype associated with obesity may worsen portal hypertension and increase rates of CD. This finding suggests that obesity predisposes to liver disease progression independent of NAFLD. The effect of subsequent weight loss on that progress, however, has not yet been determined.

TREATMENT OF OBESITY

Because obesity is the root cause or at least a major contributor to many other metabolic disorders, there is good reason to consider weight loss as a primary therapy for the sequelae themselves. This point is particularly true for the comorbidities of obesity for which direct therapies are limited, such as OSA, musculoskeletal and venous disorders, and NAFLD. Because of the limited available options for treating NAFLD in particular, reducing the underlying obesity should be a prominent therapeutic strategy.

Treatment of obesity has been and remains a challenging endeavor. Although initial weight loss is relatively easy to achieve, long-term maintenance of weight loss is far less common, owing to the counter-regulatory effects of acute weight loss and the defense of the initial energy storage (body fat) set point. The goal of therapy, therefore, is to alter that set point so that the defended FM (and consequent body weight) is reduced. Reduction of the set point drives weight loss to that new equilibrium. Indeed, weight loss under these conditions is a natural consequence of the intervention rather than the result of acute manipulation of the quantity of food ingested or energy expended through voluntary action. By causing the body to defend a lower FM set point, successful therapy induces the mobilization of any excess, existing fat, a process that is achieved by a combination of reduced appetite and caloric intake and enhanced energy expenditure and fat oxidation.

Treatment of obesity is complicated by the wide patient-to-patient variation in response to each individual therapy for obesity, whether lifestyle intervention, medication, medical device, or bariatric surgery. For each of the available therapies, some patients exhibit substantial and durable weight loss; but many others experience only modest or transient effects on weight. A systematic trial-and-error approach is generally required to find the treatments that are most effective for an individual patient.

Lifestyle-Based Therapy

As with many other chronic diseases, optimal therapy for obesity consists of graded interventions, starting with the least invasive and progressing to more invasive (and generally more effective) approaches as required. Lifestyle-based therapies are the first step and should be the basis of all obesity treatment strategies because of their noninvasive nature and their associated weight-independent benefits. If lifestyle-based therapies are inadequate, pharmacologic therapy should then be considered to provide an additional benefit. As described below, there are several different lifestyle and pharmacologic treatments. Their effectiveness seems to vary in different patients. If these approaches fail, consideration should be given to bariatric surgery. Although invasive, surgical procedures are generally the most effective therapy, providing the greatest weight loss and improvement in obesity comorbidities. This benefit comes at a cost, however, both economically and in the potential for adverse events; so surgical therapy is generally reserved for patients who fail other interventions.

Table 3 depicts a scheme for the staged treatment of obesity. The first stage consists of self-directed modification of various components of lifestyle that may affect fat storage and body weight. Self-directed lifestyle modification is generally the most accessible and economical treatment of obesity. The overall goal of lifestyle-based treatment is to reduce the environmental drivers to obesity. It consists of one or more components, including (1) pursuing a more natural diet; (2) reducing caloric density, glycemic index, and overall calorie intake; (3) increasing aerobic and resistance exercise; (4) pursuing stress-reduction techniques; and (5) increasing the quantity and quality of nightly sleep. If self-directed lifestyle modification proves inadequate, its efficacy may be enhanced when administered by a medical professional (eg, physician, dietitian, psychologist, physical therapist, nurse, or other counselor) who provides guidance, ongoing assessment, and exhortation to optimize and maintain changes in behavior and lifestyle. Professional guidance can be particularly helpful in designing diet and exercise protocols most appropriate for patients, providing ongoing assessment and feedback about progress, and identifying and helping to mitigate the most prominent stressors that are likely to contribute to obesity.

The response to lifestyle modifications is highly variable; some patients exhibit substantial and durable weight loss, but many others experience only modest or transient effects on weight. It is important to note that mere dietary restriction or calorie reduction, without a change in diet composition, is unlikely to cause physiologic change in the defended set point for fat storage and is generally met with counter-regulatory changes in energy balance physiology that enhance appetite, decrease nonexercise energy expenditure, limit the degree of initial weight loss, and promote later regain of the lost weight.[57,58] These physiologic responses seem to account for the limited efficacy of the most common weight-loss diets. Hence, it is important to pursue lifestyle changes that can be maintained and tend to promote long-term physiologic change, including consumption of more complex and less processed foods, modest but regular exercise, normalization of eating and sleeping patterns, and means of chronically reducing life stressors. It is worth noting that many components of lifestyle treatment have substantial health and quality-of life benefits independent of weight

Table 3 Stages of obesity treatment	
Stage	**Intervention**
1	Self-directed lifestyle modification
2	Professionally directed lifestyle modification
3	Weight-loss medications
4	Bariatric surgery
5	Postsurgical combination therapies

loss itself, including weight-independent metabolic benefits that could aid in the treatment of diabetes, NAFLD, and other comorbidities. They should, therefore, be maintained regardless of weight outcomes. When lifestyle-based treatments do not adequately control the obesity, however, other treatment modalities should be considered, including medications and surgery.

Pharmacotherapy

Pharmacologic treatment of obesity can best be considered in 2 parts: (1) optimization of patients' current medical regimen to minimize its weight gain–promoting effects and (2) the addition of specific agents that promote long-term weight loss. There are many medications in common use that promote weight gain, including many used to treat complications of the obesity itself. Among the most common offenders are insulin, sulfonylureas, and thiazolidinediones for the treatment of type 2 diabetes; mood stabilizers, antidepressants, and other psychotropic drugs for the treatment of depression and anxiety; and corticosteroids for the treatment of several inflammatory and autoimmune disorders that are often associated with obesity.[59–63] As with other environmental factors that promote obesity, these medications have variable effects in different patients. Nonetheless, significant and durable weight loss can often be achieved by substituting weight-neutral or weight loss–promoting alternatives in each therapeutic category. For type 2 diabetes (and possibly NAFLD), such alternatives include metformin, GLP-1 agonists, and sodium-glucose linked transporter-2 inhibitors and, in some cases, may extend to dipeptidyl peptidase-4 inhibitors. Mood stabilizers that often promote weight loss include topiramate and zonisamide; others, including ziprasidone, seem to be far more weight neutral than other medications in this category.[64,65] Similarly, bupropion is more likely to promote weight loss than other antidepressants; among the commonly used selective serotonin reuptake inhibitors, fluoxetine and sertraline seem less weight-gain promoting than citalopram, escitalopram, or paroxetine.[66] Attention to the weight regulatory effects of all medications and adjustment of the patient's regimen to favor weight loss or at least minimize weight gain can often provide substantial amelioration of obesity.

There are several medications that have been shown to promote significant weight loss. They include 4 medications in common use that are specifically approved in the United States for the treatment of obesity (**Table 4**) and several others, approved for other purposes, that have been shown to promote weight loss in many patients (**Table 5**). The first category includes phentermine, an adrenergic agent approved in 1959 for the treatment of obesity and overweight. Among the many adrenergic agents approved by the Food and Drug Administration (FDA) in that era and since, phentermine has proven to have the best efficacy-safety profile and has, thus, supplanted agents with greater addictive potential and cardiovascular and other safety risks, such as diethylpropion and benzphetamine, which are still approved but rarely used to promote weight loss. Because many insurance plans specifically exclude coverage for medications to treat obesity, the full cost of these drugs must often be borne by the patients themselves. Phentermine has been the most widely used because of its low cost and long track record of safety and efficacy. There are few controlled studies of this agent, but the average 1-year weight loss seems to be about 5% to 7%.[66,67] As with all medications that affect weight and body fat stores, however, there is a wide patient-to-patient variation, with some patients experiencing little effect and others exhibiting profound appetite suppression and weight loss. The major side effects of phentermine include dry mouth, tachycardia, and increased blood pressure, so it should be avoided in patients at an increased risk of tachyarrhythmias, uncontrolled hypertension, or ischemic heart disease.

Table 4
Medications approved for the treatment of obesity

Medication	Average Weight Loss (a Placebo) (%)	Mechanism of Action	Potential Side Effects
Phentermine (Adipex, Ionamin, others)	6	Adrenergic (decreased appetite, increased energy expenditure)	Tachycardia, hypertension
Phentermine/topiramate ER (Qsymia)	10	Adrenergic, central nervous system effects	Tachycardia, hypertension, neuropathy, cognitive dysfunction, kidney stones
Lorcaserin (Belviq)	3.5	Serotonergic (5HT2c receptor activation)	Nausea
Orlistat (Xenical)	3	Lipase inhibition (reduced lipid absorption)	Steatorrhea, flatulence
Diethylpropion[a] (Tenuate)	NA[b]	Adrenergic	Tachycardia, hypertension, anxiety
Benzphetamine[a] (Didrex)	NA	Adrenergic	Tachycardia, hypertension, anxiety, addiction
Phendimetrazine[a] (Bontril, Prelu-2, others)	NA	Adrenergic	Tachycardia, hypertension, anxiety, addiction

Abbreviation: NA, not available.
[a] Approved by the Food and Drug Administration but rarely used.
[b] For several older medications, there are no published studies that precisely define average weight loss.

The FDA recently approved fixed-dose combinations of phentermine and extended-release topiramate for the treatment of obesity. This combination has demonstrated the greatest overall efficacy, with an average weight loss of approximately 10%. In the approved combinations,[68,69] the doses of phentermine are lower than typically

Table 5
Other medications that promote weight loss

Medication	Indicated Uses	Comments
Bupropion	Depression	—
Topiramate	Seizures Migraines Mood disorders	May produce neurologic side effects
Zonisamide	Seizures Mood disorders	Few published studies
Metformin	Type 2 diabetes PCOS	Rare liver toxicity
Liraglutide, exenatide	Type 2 diabetes	Injectable
Pramlintide	Type 2 diabetes	Injectable
Canagliflozin	Type 2 diabetes	Weight loss modest

Abbreviation: PCOS, polycystic ovary syndrome.

used for phentermine monotherapy, and the doses of topiramate are lower than typical for topiramate monotherapy for seizures, migraines, and mood disorders. The efficacy of the doses used suggests additive or synergistic effects of the 2 agents for weight loss and likely reduces the risk associated with the combination. Nonetheless, the same cautions should be used as with phentermine alone. In addition, the small but significant risk of peripheral neuropathy, cognitive dysfunction, and kidney stones with topiramate therapy must be considered in its use. Experience with higher-dose topiramate for other indications, however, has demonstrated that any neurologic sequelae are generally reversed on dose reduction or discontinuing the drug. Because of the potential for musculoskeletal birth defects (primarily cleft palate) from topiramate use during pregnancy, this agent should be used cautiously in women of childbearing age and stopped if pregnancy occurs or is anticipated.

Lorcaserin, a serotonin (5-hydroxytryptamine) 2c receptor agonist, is the newest agent approved for the treatment of obesity in the United States. It acts by selectively stimulating the serotonin receptor most responsible for regulating energy balance and body weight. As a result, it avoids the cardiac valvulopathic effects of earlier, nonspecific serotonergic agents for obesity, such as fenfluramine and dexfenfluramine. Weight loss from this agent averages approximately 4%; but, as with other weight loss medications, there is a wide variation in effect among patients, with a subset of patients exhibiting far more substantial weight loss (and others experiencing little benefit from this medication).[70,71] Side effects include mild GI distress, but there are no major contraindications to its use.

Orlistat, the other agent specifically approved for the treatment of obesity, works by inhibiting pancreatic and intestinal lipases, thereby reducing the absorption of ingested fats. Long-term weight loss from orlistat averages 3% to 4%, with the expected wide interpatient variability.[72] The potential side effects include mild steatorrhea, often experienced as urgency, malodorous stools, or oily rectal discharge. There is a modestly increased risk of malabsorption of fat-soluble vitamins in patients on orlistat, so daily supplementation with preparations of vitamins A, D, E, and K is recommended.

As noted earlier, weight loss with each of these agents varies widely from patient to patient. Because there are currently no clinically useful predictors of outcome in individual patients for any of them, their appropriate use is best determined by empiric testing. Many practitioners limit long-term use of these agents to those patients who experience a weight loss of at least 5% from baseline, an amount that has been frequently demonstrated to induce significant improvement in comorbid metabolic disorders, including type II diabetes mellitus. Patients themselves may use a higher threshold, being unwilling to continue medications that fail to provide a substantially greater weight loss. It must be emphasized, however, that as with all other therapies for obesity, medications seem to work by lowering the defended set point for body FM. A given patient is, thus, likely to exhibit a discrete amount of weight loss followed by a plateau. This effect is similar to the effects of other metabolically active medications, including those used to treat hypertension, dyslipidemia, or type 2 diabetes mellitus. Maintenance of the lower weight reflects continued effectiveness of the drug, and discontinuing it is almost always associated with the return to the pretreatment weight.

There are several additional medications approved for other indications that have been shown to have potent antiobesity effects. Some, including liraglutide, bupropion, zonisamide, and naltrexone, are currently being studied and developed specifically for this indication, either alone or as a component of fixed-dose combinations.[73,74] These medications, as well as others with demonstrated weight loss–promoting effects, including metformin, exenatide, pramlintide, and canagliflozin, have been used to good effect by obesity medicine specialists and other physicians.[75–78] As with the medications that have been FDA approved for treating obesity, there is a wide variation in response, and long-term use must be guided by their effect in individual patients. Most of the medications that promote weight loss seem to act through specific and largely independent mechanisms, so there are potential benefits to combining them to achieve greater benefit. Doing so follows the sequential and often combinatorial approach used in the treatment of most other chronic disorders. With the exception of the combination of phentermine and extended-release topiramate, however, the overall efficacy and safety profile of such combination therapy for obesity has not been well studied. Specific drug combinations need to be used carefully and their effects in individual patients followed closely. Moreover, there is likely to be little benefit to combining agents in the same class (eg, GLP-1 agonists, adrenergic agents, and so forth) or those with similar postulated mechanisms of action (eg, topiramate and zonisamide). For patients with NAFLD in particular, the insulin-sensitizing effect of metformin makes it a particularly attractive weight-loss agent, although substantial weight loss by any mechanism is likely to lead to decreased steatosis and its sequelae.

Bariatric Surgery

Among the available therapies for obesity, bariatric surgery is the most effective by far, with substantial weight loss, more than 75% of which is maintained for a decade or more.[79] (Recent data for RYGB demonstrate continued efficacy for at least 20 years.) The most widely used surgical procedures include RYGB, VSG, and AGB. All of these procedures are routinely performed laparoscopically, substantially decreasing the postoperative pain and risk of dehiscence, wound infection, and hernia. The average weight loss is approximately 40% for RYGB, 35% for VSG, and 20% for AGB; although as with all obesity therapies, there is broad variability in individual responses.[80] The magnitude and durability of weight loss after these operations is associated with profound improvements in many obesity comorbidities, including diabetes, dyslipidemia, hypertension, sleep apnea, and others. Recent studies demonstrate a 30% to 40% decrease in all-cause mortality within the 7 to 10 years after these procedures, with the greatest reductions in death from diabetes, cardiovascular disease, and obesity-associated cancers.[81]

Of course, surgery is the most invasive therapy for obesity, with a significant risk of acute complications, such as bleeding, intestinal leaks, and thromboembolic disease, and a perioperative mortality of 0.1% to 0.3%.[80] Long-term risks include the potential for micronutrient deficiencies and metabolic bone disease (most common after RYGB and BPD), esophageal motility disorders (most common after AGB), internal hernias, and adhesions. The most common micronutrient abnormalities are deficiencies in iron, vitamin B12, calcium, and vitamin D, with thiamine deficiency occurring most commonly in the setting of chronic vomiting after overinflation of the AGB.[82] Regular monitoring of iron status, vitamin B12, vitamin D, and thiamine levels, as well as plasma parathyroid hormone, with micronutrient supplementation as needed, can prevent these deficiencies and their complications.

Importantly, RYGB and VSG seem to induce improvement in type 2 diabetes that is greater than would be expected for the associated weight loss.[83] Indeed, dramatic improvement in diabetes occurs within days after these procedures, before significant weight loss has occurred. These observations have led to the designation of metabolic surgery for these procedures and the closely related biliopancreatic diversion (BPD). The situation is somewhat different for AGB whereby the improvement in diabetes seems to depend entirely on the associated weight loss.[84] Because of the profound weight loss induced by these procedures, they are associated with a substantial decrease in hepatic steatosis, with full remission in many cases. They have also been shown to decrease the inflammation and fibrosis of NASH. Because of the additional metabolic effects of RYGB and VSG, these operations are particularly attractive options for the treatment of NAFLD. Given the adverse impact of steatosis on other metabolic and liver diseases, the long-term risks associated with NASH itself, the beneficial effect of weight loss, and the limited benefit of other options, bariatric surgery is now recognized as a valuable treatment of severe fatty liver disease. In some cases, progressive NASH has been the primary indication for its use.

Endoscopic treatment of weight loss is currently undergoing rigorous evaluation. The duodenal-jejunal bypass barrier is a sleeve placed within the duodenum to decrease nutrient absorption in the proximal small bowel and increase delivery to the distal small bowel, mimicking the effect of RYGB. Barrier placement results in significant weight loss and improvement in diabetes parameters.[81,82] The impact on NAFLD is not yet known.

SUMMARY

Obesity is a highly prevalent condition worldwide with dramatic effects on health outcomes generally and liver disease in particular. Understanding the pathogenesis of obesity and its role in the development of NAFLD as well as the progression of other forms of liver disease will aid in the management of these complex and important disorders. Given its important role in the development of NAFLD and the limited available options for treating NAFLD directly, addressing the obesity epidemic is a critical component of addressing the problem of hepatic steatosis, NASH, and their sequelae. This effort is best done through a combination of more aggressive strategies for obesity prevention and more effective use of all of the available and emerging treatment options, including lifestyle-, medication-, surgery- and endoscopy-based interventions.

REFERENCES

1. Flegal KM, Carroll MD, Kit BK, et al. Prevalence of obesity and trends in the distribution of body mass index among US adults, 1999–2010. JAMA 2010;307(5): 491–7.
2. Finucane MM, Stevens GA, Cowan MJ, et al. National, regional, and global trends in body-mass index since 1980: systematic analysis of health examination surveys and epidemiological studies with 960 country-years and 9.1 million participants. Lancet 2011;377(9765):557–67.
3. Wang YC, McPherson K, Marsh T, et al. Health and economic burden of the projected obesity trends in the USA and the UK. Lancet 2011;378(9793):815–25.
4. Nguyen NT, Magno CP, Lane KT, et al. Association of hypertension, diabetes, dyslipidemia, and metabolic syndrome with obesity: findings from the National Health and Nutrition Examination Survey, 1999 to 2004. J Am Coll Surg 2008; 207(6):928–34.
5. Wang Y, Beydoun MA, Liang L, et al. Will all Americans become overweight or obese? Estimating the progression and cost of the US obesity epidemic. Obesity (Silver Spring) 2008;16(10):2323–30.
6. Egger G, Swinburn B. An "ecological" approach to the obesity pandemic. BMJ 1997;315(7106):477–80.
7. Sturm R. Increases in clinically severe obesity in the United States, 1986–2000. Arch Intern Med 2003;163(18):2146–8.
8. Daniels AB, Liu GT, Volpe NJ, et al. Profiles of obesity, weight gain, and quality of life in idiopathic intracranial hypertension (pseudotumor cerebri). Am J Ophthalmol 2007;143(4):635–41.

9. Setty AR, Curhan G, Choi HK. Obesity, waist circumference, weight change, and the risk of psoriasis in women: Nurses' Health Study II. Arch Intern Med 2007;167(15):1670–5.
10. Wilson PW, D'Agostino RB, Sullivan L, et al. Overweight and obesity as determinants of cardiovascular risk: the Framingham experience. Arch Intern Med 2002;162(16):1867–72.
11. Kenchaiah S, Evans JC, Levy D, et al. Obesity and the risk of heart failure. N Engl J Med 2002;347(5):305–13.
12. Calle EE, Rodriguez C, Walker-Thurmond K, et al. Overweight, obesity, and mortality from cancer in a prospectively studied cohort of U.S. adults. N Engl J Med 2003;348(17):1625–38.
13. Onyike CU, Crum RM, Lee HB, et al. Is obesity associated with major depression? Results from the Third National Health and Nutrition Examination Survey. Am J Epidemiol 2003;158(12):1139–47.
14. Luppino FS, de Wit LM, Bouvy PF, et al. Overweight, obesity, and depression: a systematic review and meta-analysis of longitudinal studies. Arch Gen Psychiatry 2010;67(3):220–9.
15. Gariepy G, Nitka D, Schmitz N. The association between obesity and anxiety disorders in the population: a systematic review and meta-analysis. Int J Obes (Lond) 2009;34(3):407–19.
16. Flegal KM, Kit BK, Orpana H, et al. Association of all-cause mortality with overweight and obesity using standard body mass index categories: a systematic review and meta-analysis. JAMA 2013;309(1):71–82.
17. Whitlock G, Lewington S, Sherliker P, et al. Body-mass index and cause-specific mortality in 900,000 adults: collaborative analyses of 57 prospective studies. Lancet 2009;373(9669):1083–96.
18. Morton GJ, Cummings DE, Baskin DG, et al. Central nervous system control of food intake and body weight. Nature 2006;443(7109):289–95.
19. Kaiyala KJ, Morton GJ, Leroux BG, et al. Identification of body fat mass as a major determinant of metabolic rate in mice. Diabetes 2010;59(7):1657–66.
20. Watanabe M, Houten SM, Mataki C, et al. Bile acids induce energy expenditure by promoting intracellular thyroid hormone activation. Nature 2006;439(7075):484–9.
21. Kohli R, Bradley D, Setchell KD, et al. Weight loss induced by Roux-en-Y gastric bypass but not laparoscopic adjustable gastric banding increases circulating bile acids. J Clin Endocrinol Metab 2013;98(4):E708–12.
22. Steinert RE, Peterli R, Keller S, et al. Bile acids and gut peptide secretion after bariatric surgery - a 1-year prospective randomized pilot trial. Obesity (Silver Spring) 2013. [Epub ahead of print].
23. Zhang H, DiBaise JK, Zuccolo A, et al. Human gut microbiota in obesity and after gastric bypass. Proc Natl Acad Sci U S A 2009;106(7):2365–70.
24. Turnbaugh PJ, Ley RE, Mahowald MA, et al. An obesity-associated gut microbiome with increased capacity for energy harvest. Nature 2006;444(7122):1027–31.
25. Liou AP, Paziuk M, Luevano JM Jr, et al. Conserved shifts in the gut microbiota due to gastric bypass reduce host weight and adiposity. Sci Transl Med 2013;5(178):178ra41.
26. Stylopoulos N, Hoppin AG, Kaplan LM. Roux-en-Y gastric bypass enhances energy expenditure and extends lifespan in diet-induced obese rats. Obesity (Silver Spring) 2009;17(10):1839–47.
27. Langhans W, Grossmann F, Geary N. Intrameal hepatic-portal infusion of glucose reduces spontaneous meal size in rats. Physiol Behav 2001;73(4):499–507.

28. Mithieux G, Misery P, Magnan C, et al. Portal sensing of intestinal gluconeogenesis is a mechanistic link in the diminution of food intake induced by diet protein. Cell Metab 2005;2(5):321–9.
29. Langhans W. Role of the liver in the control of glucose-lipid utilization and body weight. Curr Opin Clin Nutr Metab Care 2003;6(4):449–55.
30. Rolland V, Roseau S, Fromentin G, et al. Body weight, body composition, and energy metabolism in lean and obese Zucker rats fed soybean oil or butter. Am J Clin Nutr 2002;75(1):21–30.
31. Newbold RR. Impact of environmental endocrine disrupting chemicals on the development of obesity. Hormones (Athens) 2010;9(3):206–17.
32. Vernon G, Baranova A, Younossi ZM. Systematic review: the epidemiology and natural history of non-alcoholic fatty liver disease and non-alcoholic steatohepatitis in adults. Aliment Pharmacol Ther 2011;34(3):274–85.
33. Charlton M. Cirrhosis and liver failure in nonalcoholic fatty liver disease' Molehill or Mountain? Hepatology 2008;47(5):1431–3.
34. Yatsuji S, Hashimoto E, Tobari M, et al. Clinical features and outcomes of cirrhosis due to non-alcoholic steatohepatitis compared with cirrhosis caused by chronic hepatitis C. J Gastroenterol Hepatol 2009;24(2):248–54.
35. Browning JD, Szczepaniak LS, Dobbins R, et al. Prevalence of hepatic steatosis in an urban population in the United States: impact of ethnicity. Hepatology 2004;40(6):1387–95.
36. Williams CD, Stengel J, Asike MI, et al. Prevalence of nonalcoholic fatty liver disease and nonalcoholic steatohepatitis among a largely middle-aged population utilizing ultrasound and liver biopsy: a prospective study. Gastroenterology 2011;140(1):124–31.
37. Dixon JB, Bhathal PS, O'Brien PE. Nonalcoholic fatty liver disease: predictors of nonalcoholic steatohepatitis and liver fibrosis in the severely obese. Gastroenterology 2001;121(1):91–100.
38. Patt CH, Yoo HY, Dibadj K, et al. Prevalence of transaminase abnormalities in asymptomatic, healthy subjects participating in an executive health-screening program. Dig Dis Sci 2003;48(4):797–801.
39. Farrell GC, Larter CZ. Nonalcoholic fatty liver disease: from steatosis to cirrhosis. Hepatology 2006;43(2 Suppl 1):S99–112.
40. Jimba S, Nakagami T, Takahashi M, et al. Prevalence of non-alcoholic fatty liver disease and its association with impaired glucose metabolism in Japanese adults. Diabet Med 2005;22(9):1141–5.
41. Angulo P, Keach JC, Batts KP, et al. Independent predictors of liver fibrosis in patients with nonalcoholic steatohepatitis. Hepatology 1999;30(6):1356–62.
42. Thomas EL, Hamilton G, Patel N, et al. Hepatic triglyceride content and its relation to body adiposity: a magnetic resonance imaging and proton magnetic resonance spectroscopy study. Gut 2005;54(1):122–7.
43. Kral JG, Schaffner F, Pierson RN Jr, et al. Body fat topography as an independent predictor of fatty liver. Metabolism 1993;42(5):548–51.
44. Ferre P, Foufelle F. Hepatic steatosis: a role for de novo lipogenesis and the transcription factor SREBP-1c. Diabetes Obes Metab 2010;12(Suppl 2):83–92.
45. Hu KQ, Kyulo NL, Esrailian E, et al. Overweight and obesity, hepatic steatosis, and progression of chronic hepatitis C: a retrospective study on a large cohort of patients in the United States. J Hepatol 2004;40(1):147–54.
46. Everhart JE, Lok AS, Kim HY, et al. Weight-related effects on disease progression in the hepatitis C antiviral long-term treatment against cirrhosis trial. Gastroenterology 2009;137(2):549–57.

47. El-Serag HB. Hepatocellular carcinoma. N Engl J Med 2011;365(12):1118–27.
48. Marrero JA, Fontana RJ, Fu S, et al. Alcohol, tobacco and obesity are synergistic risk factors for hepatocellular carcinoma. J Hepatol 2005;42(2):218–24.
49. Nair S, Mason A, Eason J, et al. Is obesity an independent risk factor for hepatocellular carcinoma in cirrhosis? Hepatology 2002;36(1):150–5.
50. Turati F, Talamini R, Pelucchi C, et al. Metabolic syndrome and hepatocellular carcinoma risk. Br J Cancer 2012;108(1):222–8.
51. Bosetti C, Rosato V, Polesel J, et al. Diabetes mellitus and cancer risk in a network of case-control studies. Nutr Cancer 2012;64(5):643–51.
52. Ascha MS, Hanouneh IA, Lopez R, et al. The incidence and risk factors of hepatocellular carcinoma in patients with nonalcoholic steatohepatitis. Hepatology 2010;51(6):1972–8.
53. Baffy G, Brunt EM, Caldwell SH. Hepatocellular carcinoma in non-alcoholic fatty liver disease: an emerging menace. J Hepatol 2012;56(6):1384–91.
54. Liu B, Balkwill A, Reeves G, et al. Body mass index and risk of liver cirrhosis in middle aged UK women: prospective study. BMJ 2010;340:c912.
55. Raynard B, Balian A, Fallik D, et al. Risk factors of fibrosis in alcohol-induced liver disease. Hepatology 2002;35(3):635–8.
56. Berzigotti A, Garcia-Tsao G, Bosch J, et al. Obesity is an independent risk factor for clinical decompensation in patients with cirrhosis. Hepatology 2010;54(2):555–61.
57. Leibel RL, Rosenbaum M, Hirsch J. Changes in energy expenditure resulting from altered body weight. N Engl J Med 1995;332(10):621–8.
58. Sumithran P, Proietto J. The defence of body weight: a physiological basis for weight regain after weight loss. Clin Sci (Lond) 2013;124(4):231–41.
59. Schwartz TL, Nihalani N, Jindal S, et al. Psychiatric medication-induced obesity: a review. Obes Rev 2004;5(2):115–21.
60. Inzucchi SE. Oral antihyperglycemic therapy for type 2 diabetes: scientific review. JAMA 2002;287(3):360–72.
61. Nair S, Wilding JP. Sodium glucose cotransporter 2 inhibitors as a new treatment for diabetes mellitus. J Clin Endocrinol Metab 2010;95(1):34–42.
62. Vilsboll T, Christensen M, Junker AE, et al. Effects of glucagon-like peptide-1 receptor agonists on weight loss: systematic review and meta-analyses of randomised controlled trials. BMJ 2012;344. d7771.
63. Karagiannis T, Paschos P, Paletas K, et al. Dipeptidyl peptidase-4 inhibitors for treatment of type 2 diabetes mellitus in the clinical setting: systematic review and meta-analysis. BMJ 2012;344. e1369.
64. Wang PW, Hill SJ, Childers ME, et al. Open adjunctive ziprasidone associated with weight loss in obese and overweight bipolar disorder patients. J Psychiatr Res 2011;45(8):1128–32.
65. Gadde KM, Kopping MF, Wagner HR 2nd, et al. Zonisamide for weight reduction in obese adults: a 1-year randomized controlled trial. Arch Intern Med 2012;172(20):1557–64.
66. Hendricks EJ, Greenway FL, Westman EC, et al. Blood pressure and heart rate effects, weight loss and maintenance during long-term phentermine pharmacotherapy for obesity. Obesity (Silver Spring) 2011;19(12):2351–60.
67. Valle-Jones JC, Brodie NH, O'Hara H, et al. A comparative study of phentermine and diethylpropion in the treatment of obese patients in general practice. Pharmatherapeutica 1983;3(5):300–4.
68. Gadde KM, Allison DB, Ryan DH, et al. Effects of low-dose, controlled-release, phentermine plus topiramate combination on weight and associated

comorbidities in overweight and obese adults (CONQUER): a randomised, placebo-controlled, phase 3 trial. Lancet 2011;377(9774):1341–52.

69. Garvey WT, Ryan DH, Look M, et al. Two-year sustained weight loss and metabolic benefits with controlled-release phentermine/topiramate in obese and overweight adults (SEQUEL): a randomized, placebo-controlled, phase 3 extension study. Am J Clin Nutr 2012;95(2):297–308.

70. Smith SR, Weissman NJ, Anderson CM, et al. Multicenter, placebo-controlled trial of lorcaserin for weight management. N Engl J Med 2010;363(3):245–56.

71. Fidler MC, Sanchez M, Raether B, et al. A one-year randomized trial of lorcaserin for weight loss in obese and overweight adults: the BLOSSOM trial. J Clin Endocrinol Metab 2011;96(10):3067–77.

72. Davidson MH, Hauptman J, DiGirolamo M, et al. Weight control and risk factor reduction in obese subjects treated for 2 years with orlistat: a randomized controlled trial. JAMA 1999;281(3):235–42.

73. Greenway FL, Fujioka K, Plodkowski RA, et al. Effect of naltrexone plus bupropion on weight loss in overweight and obese adults (COR-I): a multicentre, randomised, double-blind, placebo-controlled, phase 3 trial. Lancet 2010;376(9741):595–605.

74. Astrup A, Rossner S, Van Gaal L, et al. Effects of liraglutide in the treatment of obesity: a randomised, double-blind, placebo-controlled study. Lancet 2009; 374(9701):1606–16.

75. Knowler WC, Fowler SE, Hamman RF, et al. 10-year follow-up of diabetes incidence and weight loss in the Diabetes Prevention Program Outcomes Study. Lancet 2009;374(9702):1677–86.

76. Rosenstock J, Aggarwal N, Polidori D, et al. Dose-ranging effects of canagliflozin, a sodium-glucose cotransporter 2 inhibitor, as add-on to metformin in subjects with type 2 diabetes. Diabetes Care 2012;35(6):1232–8.

77. Hollander P, Maggs DG, Ruggles JA, et al. Effect of pramlintide on weight in overweight and obese insulin-treated type 2 diabetes patients. Obes Res 2004;12(4):661–8.

78. Buse JB, Drucker DJ, Taylor KL, et al. DURATION-1: exenatide once weekly produces sustained glycemic control and weight loss over 52 weeks. Diabetes Care 2010;33(6):1255–61.

79. Sjostrom L, Peltonen M, Jacobson P, et al. Bariatric surgery and long-term cardiovascular events. JAMA 2012;307(1):56–65.

80. Hutter MM, Schirmer BD, Jones DB, et al. First report from the American College of Surgeons Bariatric Surgery Center Network: laparoscopic sleeve gastrectomy has morbidity and effectiveness positioned between the band and the bypass. Ann Surg 2011;254(3):410–20; discussion 20–2.

81. Sjostrom L, Narbro K, Sjostrom CD, et al. Effects of bariatric surgery on mortality in Swedish obese subjects. N Engl J Med 2007;357(8):741–52.

82. Bloomberg RD, Fleishman A, Nalle JE, et al. Nutritional deficiencies following bariatric surgery: what have we learned? Obes Surg 2005;15(2):145–54.

83. Schauer PR, Kashyap SR, Wolski K, et al. Bariatric surgery versus intensive medical therapy in obese patients with diabetes. N Engl J Med 2012;366(17): 1567–76.

84. Dixon JB, O'Brien PE, Playfair J, et al. Adjustable gastric banding and conventional therapy for type 2 diabetes: a randomized controlled trial. JAMA 2008; 299(3):316–23.

Obesity-Associated Nonalcoholic Fatty Liver Disease

Yusuf Yilmaz, MD[a,b], Zobair M. Younossi, MD, MPH, AGAF[c,*]

KEYWORDS

• Obesity • Nonalcoholic fatty liver disease • Epidemiology • Pathophysiology

KEY POINTS

• Obesity is strongly associated with the prevalence of nonalcoholic fatty liver disease (NAFLD) in both adult and pediatric populations.
• NAFLD is not invariably associated with obesity; in particular, there is evidence suggesting that NAFLD associated with the carriage of the high-risk rs738409 C>G single-nucleotide polymorphism in PNPLA3 is characterized by an increase in liver fat but no insulin resistance or adipose tissue inflammation.
• Nutrition, physical activity, and behavioral modifications are a critical component of the treatment regimen for all obese patients with NAFLD.
• Bariatric surgeries that affect or restrict the flow or absorption of food through the gastrointestinal tract may improve liver histology in morbidly obese patients with nonalcoholic steatohepatitis (NASH), although randomized clinical trials and quasi-randomized clinical studies are lacking.
• Although primary prevention is the long-term goal for diminishing obesity, early detection of both NASH and hepatic fibrosis using noninvasive biochemical and imaging markers that may replace liver biopsy is the current challenge.

INTRODUCTION

In past decades, the prevalence of obesity and overweight has been largely on the rise and this condition is on the brink of replacing smoking as the leading cause of preventable death.[1,2] Because of its association with an increased risk of suffering from multiple diseases, obesity takes enormous health and personal tolls on modern societies

Conflicts of Interest: The authors have nothing to disclose.
[a] Department of Gastroenterology, School of Medicine, Marmara University, Fevzi Cakmak Mah, Mimar Sinan Cad. No. 41 Ust Kaynarca, Pendik, Istanbul 34899, Turkey; [b] Institute of Gastroenterology, Marmara University, Karaciger Arastirmalari Birimi, Basibuyuk, Maltepe, Istanbul 34840, Turkey; [c] Department of Medicine, Betty and Guy Beatty Center for Integrated Research, Center for Liver Diseases, Inova Health System, Inova Fairfax Hospital, Claude Moore Health Education and Research Building, 3rd Floor, 3300 Gallows Road, Falls Church, VA 22042, USA
* Corresponding author. Betty and Guy Beatty Center for Integrated Research, Claude Moore Health Education and Research Building, 3rd Floor, 3300 Gallows Road, Falls Church, VA.
E-mail address: zobair.younossi@inova.org

(Box 1).[3–17] In fact, recently, the American Medical Association classified obesity as a disease. The obesity pandemic is likely the result of dramatic changes in the health, financial, and cultural environment over the past century.[18,19] Historically, in the years before the development of medical advancements that prevented debilitating diseases that caused their victims to become dreadfully feeble as they slowly died, being heavy was considered a sign of strength.[20] Indeed, at times when food was scarce, having a rotund physique was regarded as a status symbol and an indicator of prosperity and good health. But as times changed, the detrimental effects that overweight and obesity had on health were discovered and the conditions became so prevalent that they are currently recognized as leading risk factors for morbidity and mortality worldwide.[20] Although the fundamental cause of obesity is a positive imbalance between energy intake and energy expenditure, the etiology of obesity is multifactorial and involves a complex interaction among genetic, environmental, psychosocial, and behavioral factors.[21,22] From a pathophysiological standpoint, the development of obesity is associated with adipose tissue remodeling,[23] which leads to adipocyte dysfunction, abnormal cytokine secretion, and chronic low-grade inflammation.[24] Obesity also contributes to fat deposition in nonadipose tissues as ectopic fat, and it is a major risk factor for nonalcoholic fatty liver disease (NAFLD).[8]

NAFLD is a clinicopathological condition characterized by lipid accumulation in the liver causing liver damage similar to alcohol, but occurring in individuals without a history of chronic alcohol consumption.[25–30] NAFLD represents a wide spectrum of liver diseases ranging from simple steatosis to nonalcoholic steatohepatitis (NASH) and fibrosis to irreversible cirrhosis. Simple steatosis is defined histologically as greater than 5% hepatic lipid accumulation that rarely progresses to advanced liver diseases, whereas NASH constitutes an inflammation and hepatocellular damage having a strong potential to progress into cirrhosis, end-stage liver failure, and hepatocellular

---

Box 1
Main obesity-associated diseases

Disease

Type 2 diabetes

Malignancies

Ischemic heart disease and heart failure

Venous thrombosis

Gastroesophageal reflux disease

Nonalcoholic fatty liver disease

Erectile dysfunction

Stroke

Hypertension

Osteoarthritis

Gout

Gallbladder disease

Obstructive sleep apnea

Asthma

Depression

carcinoma (HCC).[31,32] Although NAFLD is an independent risk for cardiovascular disease and mortality, only NASH is associated with advanced liver disease. Therefore, treatment strategies to address NAFLD will be important, primarily, from a cardiovascular disease standpoint. On the other hand, clinical trials focused on liver disease must focus on patients with established diagnosis of NASH.

Concomitant with obesity, NAFLD is an increasingly recognized condition; up to 30% of adults in Western countries have NAFLD.[33] Insulin resistance is the key pathogenic abnormality associated with obesity-associated NAFLD.[34] A fatty liver is insulin resistant and overproduces glucose and very low density lipoprotein, and also other proinflammatory molecules, such as C-reactive protein and interleukin-6, which lead to hyperglycemia, hyperinsulinemia, and lipid disorders.[34] Due to those metabolic consequences, NAFLD is closely linked to the metabolic syndrome and is considered its hepatic expression.[25,35] However, not all obese persons deposit fat in the liver[35] and liver fat content is recognized to be independent of age, sex, and body mass index.[36] The deviation in liver fat accumulation between individuals is thought to explain, at least in part, why some obese and even lean individuals develop metabolic syndrome and insulin resistance, whereas others equally obese do not.[37] Similarly, not all patients with NAFLD have a diagnosis of metabolic syndrome.[38]

Over the past several years, epidemiologic studies have informed the public health impact of obesity-associated NAFLD. The aim of the present review is to give an overview of the epidemiology and the possible mechanisms underlying the observed association between obesity and NAFLD.

PREVALENCE AND INCIDENCE OF OBESITY-ASSOCIATED NAFLD

The prevalence of obesity has increased dramatically worldwide (**Fig. 1**), and the rate of obesity has more than doubled since 1980.[39] At least 1.46 billion adults were overweight or obese and 170 million of the world's children were overweight or obese in 2008.[40] In future prospects this number will only increase further.[41] In Europe, obesity

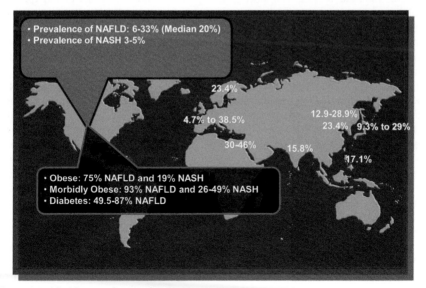

Fig. 1. Worldwide prevalence of NAFLD.

has increased 10% to 40% in the past 10 years, and 10% to 25% of men and 10% to 30% of women are obese depending on the European country.[42] In the United States, 64% and 50% of the population are currently estimated to be overweight or obese, respectively.[43] The trend of the obesity epidemics is not only true for adults, but has also trickled down to affect children of all ages.[44] For children between the ages of 2 and 5, the prevalence of overweight and obesity increased from 5.0% to almost 14.0%, from 6.5% to almost 19.0% for children aged 6 to 11 years, and from 5.0% to 17.5% for adolescents between the ages of 12 and 19.[45]

Owing largely to the obesity epidemic, NAFLD is now the most common chronic liver condition worldwide. Based on the available data, NAFLD is estimated to occur in one-third of the general population in the United States.[46] In adults, women are most frequently diagnosed with NAFLD,[47] but this likely to represent a bias because men traditionally drink more alcohol than women and therefore may get excluded from a diagnosis based on alcohol intake. Concerning ethnicity, the lowest rates of NAFLD are seen in African American individuals and the highest in Asian and Hispanic individuals, with White in between.[48,49] Differently from NAFLD that can be screened by ultrasound and liver enzymes, determining the true prevalence of NASH is complicated.[28,29] Liver biopsy provides the only definitive diagnosis of NASH,[32] but its invasiveness and cost complicate its use as a diagnostic tool in the general population.[33] However, NASH seems to occur in approximately 3% of the lean population, 19% of the obese population, and the almost half of morbidly obese persons.[50,51] Importantly, the increasing burden of obesity-associated NAFLD will be transposed in the future to an increased need for hepatic transplantation for NASH. In fact, currently, NASH ranks as the third most common indication for liver transplantation (2001: 1.2%; 2009: 9.7%).[52] Another important future consequence of the epidemic of obesity-associated NAFLD will likely be a higher incidence of HCC. In a recent study conducted in 6 European countries, a total of 160 cases of HCC were detected during a 22-month follow-up; of note, 43% of the cases occurred in the absence of any other risk factor, such as alcohol abuse, cirrhosis, or infection with hepatitis B or C.[53] Therefore, the high prevalence of obesity-associated NAFLD will lead to a higher incidence of HCC in the general population with a concomitant burden on treatment availability, including liver transplantation.

Data on the incidence, predictive factors, and remission rates of NAFLD remain scanty. In particular, it is still difficult to draw firm conclusions regarding people from the general population who do not drink alcohol. A recent study conducted in a sample of the 147 patients who did not have NAFLD at baseline showed that 28 (19%) developed NAFLD at a 7-year follow-up.[54] Baseline body mass index, homeostasis model assessment of insulin resistance (HOMA-IR) score, blood cholesterol, triglycerides, leptin levels, and weight gain were significantly higher and adiponectin was lower among those who developed NAFLD at 7-year follow-up, compared with those who remained NAFLD-free. However, only weight gain and baseline HOMA-IR were independent predictors for the development of NAFLD.[54] Collectively, these longitudinal results suggest that obesity (and associated insulin resistance) is an important driving force behind the development of NAFLD. Conversely, one-third of patients with NAFLD showed improvement of their disease within the 7-year follow-up; such cases were chiefly dependent on modest weight reduction. Taken together, these data indicate that weight gain is an independent predictor of incident NAFLD in initially healthy subjects. Therefore, weight loss interventions represent the optimal (and probably the only effective) population-based strategy to reduce the future burden of NAFLD.

WORLDWIDE DIFFERENCES IN OBESITY-ASSOCIATED NAFLD

Although obesity and NAFLD are major health concerns worldwide, there are significant geographic differences in the prevalence of these conditions. In the United States, obesity is particularly associated with a heavy reliance on high-fat, high-calorie meals ("junk food"), which is more common among people of low socioeconomic position.[55] However, the opposite phenomenon can be found in developing countries, where it is the better-educated population that has the highest prevalence of obesity.[56] In general, robust comparisons of obesity prevalence between countries are difficult because of different methodological approaches in data collection.[57] The most important of these differences is probably that between measured and self-reported measures, with self-reported data more likely to underestimate the presence of obesity compared with actual measurements.[58–60] The worldwide prevalence of obesity is monitored by the World Health Organization through the Global Database on body mass index.[61,62] Although methodological caveats limit the reliability of comparisons between countries, Asia has the lowest and the Pacific Islands have the highest estimates of obesity prevalence.[62] Overall, most countries have rising trends of obesity. However, decreasing trends in the prevalence of obesity have been noted in men from Denmark and Saudi Arabia, as well as among women living in Denmark, Ireland, Saudi Arabia, Finland, and Spain.[62]

In parallel with the obesity epidemics, NAFLD has become the most common form of liver disease in the United States and most countries worldwide. Importantly, estimates in the US general population suggest that approximately 6 million individuals have progressed to NASH and about 600,000 to NASH-related cirrhosis.[63] NAFLD is also considered a major health issue in Japan, Australia, Europe, and the Middle East.[64–68] Studies conducted in the United States have suggested the presence of racial and ethnic variations in NAFLD, which result in a nonuniform distribution, with the disorder being most common among Latino individuals and least prevalent among African American individuals.[48,69–72] In general, Hispanic individuals have the highest prevalence of NAFLD, followed by non-Hispanic white individuals, whereas African American individuals have the lowest rates.[73] Such differences do not seem to be entirely explained by variations in the prevalence of the stereotypical metabolic risk factors and the effect of HOMA-IR on the risk of NASH is modified by ethnicity.[74] In particular, HOMA-IR does not seem to be a significant risk factor for NASH among Latinos, but it is significant among non-Latino whites.[75] Therefore, ethnicity may act as an important modifier of the association between obesity and NAFLD. It is also possible that these ethnic variations may reflect differences in genetic susceptibility to visceral adiposity, including hepatic involvement.[70] In general, the ongoing search for relevant genetic variants should result in a better understanding of energy metabolism and hopefully clarify the molecular mechanisms underlying the association between obesity and NAFLD. For example, Lallukka and colleagues[75] recently showed that NAFLD associated with the carriage of the high-risk rs738409 C>G single-nucleotide polymorphism in PNPLA3 is characterized by an increase in liver fat but no insulin resistance or adipose tissue inflammation, whereas obesity-associated NAFLD has all 3 of these features. Moreover, the Genetics of Obesity-Related Liver Disease (GOLD) Consortium has shown that NAFLD is about 26% to 27% heritable with 5 single-nucleotide polymorphisms in the PNPLA3, NCAN, GCKR, LYPLAL1, and PPP1R3B genes found to be associated with hepatic steatosis as measured using computed tomography in individuals of European ancestry.[76] In the future, it will be necessary to understand how specific combinations of environmental and genetic factors can give rise to ethnic differences in obesity-associated NAFLD. In this context, eliminating ethnic disparities in health should be an international priority, and obesity and NAFLD are prime targets.

CLINICAL CORRELATIONS

As discussed previously, NAFLD is a complex phenotype that arises from numerous genetic, environmental, behavioral, and even social origins.[34,63] The lifestyle factors contributing to the rising epidemic of obesity, and hence obesity-related NAFLD, are embedded in changes in society worldwide, mainly increased sedentary or inactive lifestyles[77] and consumption of calorie-rich foods in the form of soft drinks,[78] fast foods,[79] and sugar-enriched products.[80] Importantly, the clustering of unhealthy behaviors in obese children, such as poor nutritional habits, low levels of physical activity, and "junk-food" consumption dictate the need for multifaceted global programs to tackle global NAFLD risk at an early stage.[81,82] However, further research is needed to identify culturally sensitive strategies for obesity prevention and their impact not only on body weight, but also on NAFLD morbidity and mortality.

The importance of lifestyle management in the treatment of patients with obesity-related NAFLD cannot be overemphasized.[82] Adoption of a healthy lifestyle facilitates weight loss and decreases insulin resistance, and produces independent beneficial effects on the liver.[83–86] It is noteworthy that obesity-related metabolic abnormalities and fatty infiltration of the liver may be present even at a young age, and progress asymptomatically for decades before clinical manifestations set in.[87,88] In this scenario, nutrition, physical activity, and behavioral modifications aimed at weight loss are a critical component of the treatment regimen for all obese patients with NAFLD, even at a young age. Besides exercise and dieting, many therapeutic targets have been recently identified, on both the intake and the expenditure side of the energy balance equation, thereby providing hope that new agents may become available in the future.[89] For obese patients with NAFLD who do not respond to a trial of diet, exercise, and behavioral therapy, pharmacotherapy can be tried.[90] The use of drugs should be individualized, taking into account the severity of liver disease, comorbidities, and practical considerations related to cost, side effects, and frequency of dosing. Randomized trials and carefully constructed observational studies are needed to optimize effectiveness of nonsurgical weight loss interventions in obese patients and determine if the small weight losses they produce can have an impact on NAFLD incidence and clinical course. Moreover, intensive counseling and behavioral treatments need to be implemented to support long-term weight loss maintenance.

Among weight loss interventions, bariatric surgery results in the most dramatic weight loss, and, thus, studies of obese patients are the most likely to show reduced risk of NAFLD. Restrictive surgical procedures are indeed capable of inducing earlier satiety by decreasing the volume of the stomach (laparoscopic-adjustable gastric banding) or restricting the stomach and bypassing the small bowel (Roux-en-Y gastric bypass). Bariatric surgeries that affect or restrict the flow of food through the gastrointestinal tract have been shown to be an important therapeutic option that may result in a histologic improvement of NASH in morbidly obese patients (body mass index ≥ 35 kg/m^2).[91] Although long-term weight loss and resolution of obesity-associated NAFLD have been reported in most patients,[92] the lack of randomized clinical trials and quasi-randomized clinical studies still does not allow assessment of the benefits and harms of bariatric surgery as a therapeutic approach for patients with NASH.[93] Taken together, these data indicate that preventing and managing obesity-related NAFLD requires multiple, parallel efforts.

Table 1
Example of therapeutic interventions for NASH

Therapy	Histologic Improvement	Liver Enzymes	Impact on Hepatic Fibrosis	Use Recommended
Metformin	Not consistently	Not consistently improved	Unknown	Not recommended
Rosiglitazone	Not consistently	Improvement noted	Unknown	Not recommended
Pioglitazone	Not consistently	Not consistently	No	Considered to treat diabetes but not solely for NASH
Vitamin E	Improvement	Improvement	No	Recommended for nondiabetic individuals with biopsy-proven NASH
Statins	Unknown	Unknown	Unknown	Not recommended for treatment of NASH but can be used to treat hyperlipidemia in patients with NAFLD
Orlistat	No	Possible improvement with weight loss	Unknown	Not recommended solely for NASH
Ursodeoxycholic acid	No improvement	Not consistently	No	Not recommended

In addition to weight reduction strategies to address obesity-related NAFLD, there have been a number of medical therapies designed to treat histologic NASH. These include antioxidants, such as vitamin E, insulin sensitizers, such as pioglitazone and metformin, lipid-lowering agents, such as statins, and cytoprotective agents, such as ursodeoxycholic acid (**Table 1**).[94,95] Despite decades of clinical trials, current evidence suggests that only vitamin E may be beneficial for treatment of nondiabetic patients with NASH, but no single treatment can be recommended to all patients with NASH.[94,95]

SUMMARY

The main conclusions from this review are the following: (1) obesity is strongly associated with the prevalence of NAFLD in both adult and pediatric populations[95,96]; (2) obesity is an independent predictor of incident NAFLD in initially healthy subjects; (3) NAFLD is not invariably associated with obesity, in particular there is evidence suggesting that NAFLD associated with high-risk rs738409 C>G single-nucleotide polymorphism in PNPLA3 is characterized by an increase in liver fat but no insulin resistance or adipose tissue inflammation; (4) there are significant ethnic variations in the prevalence of obesity-related NAFLD, which may be explained by both environmental and genetic factors; (5) nutrition, physical activity, and behavior modifications aimed at weight loss are a critical component of the treatment regimen for all obese patients with NAFLD; (6) bariatric surgeries that affect or restrict the flow of food through the gastrointestinal tract may improve liver histology in morbidly obese patients with NASH, although randomized clinical trials and quasi-randomized clinical studies are lacking; (7) because only patients with histologically proven NASH are shown to have progressive liver disease, clinical trials must focus on this subtype of NAFLD; and (8) although vitamin E is recommended for nondiabetic individuals with NASH, no single treatment could be recommended to all patients with NASH.

In general, obesity-associated NAFLD should be considered an important and often underrecognized public health problem. As the prevalence of obesity increases, the prevalence of NAFLD with its associated morbidity and mortality will increase as well. Although primary prevention is the long-term goal for diminishing the prevalence of obesity, early detection of both NASH and hepatic fibrosis using noninvasive biochemical and imaging markers that may replace liver biopsy is the overriding current challenge.[97–102] From a clinical standpoint, treating NAFLD in the obese requires addressing obesity as part of the therapeutic plan. Lifestyle management is required in every case, with a focus on weight loss and risk reduction. In most patients, additional therapies, including medications, aggressive diet counseling, behavioral techniques, and sometimes bariatric surgery in morbidly obese subjects, will be required. Data showing improved liver histology among individuals who lose weight and maintain the loss strengthen confidence in the obesity-NAFLD link, and also provide a note of hope that weight loss in obese individuals may help them prevent end-stage liver disease. Research on the biologic mechanisms underlying the obesity-NAFLD link is still in early stages, but may lead to potential treatments and preventive agents.

REFERENCES

1. Flegal KM, Williamson DF, Pamuk ER, et al. Estimating deaths attributable to obesity in the United States. Am J Public Health 2004;94:1486–9.
2. Hurt RT, Frazier TH, McClave SA, et al. Obesity epidemic: overview, pathophysiology, and the intensive care unit conundrum. JPEN J Parenter Enteral Nutr 2011;35:4S–13S.
3. Kautzky-Willer A, Lemmens-Gruber R. Obesity and diabetes. Handb Exp Pharmacol 2012;214:307–40.
4. Vucenik I, Stains JP. Obesity and cancer risk: evidence, mechanisms, and recommendations. Ann N Y Acad Sci 2012;1271:37–43.
5. Nikolopoulou A, Kadoglou NP. Obesity and metabolic syndrome as related to cardiovascular disease. Expert Rev Cardiovasc Ther 2012;10:933–9.
6. Braekkan SK, Siegerink B, Lijfering WM, et al. Role of obesity in the etiology of deep vein thrombosis and pulmonary embolism: current epidemiological insights. Semin Thromb Hemost 2013;39:533–40.
7. Nocon M, Labenz J, Jaspersen D, et al. Association of body mass index with heartburn, regurgitation and esophagitis: results of the progression of gastroesophageal reflux disease study. J Gastroenterol Hepatol 2007;22:1728–31.
8. Fabbrini E, Sullivan S, Klein S. Obesity and nonalcoholic fatty liver disease: biochemical, metabolic, and clinical implications. Hepatology 2010;51:679–89.
9. Diaz-Arjonilla M, Schwarcz M, Swerdloff RS, et al. Obesity, low testosterone levels and erectile dysfunction. Int J Impot Res 2009;21:89–98.
10. Kernan WN, Inzucchi SE, Sawan C, et al. Obesity: a stubbornly obvious target for stroke prevention. Stroke 2013;44:278–86.
11. Aghamohammadzadeh R, Heagerty AM. Obesity-related hypertension: epidemiology, pathophysiology, treatments, and the contribution of perivascular adipose tissue. Ann Med 2012;44(Suppl 1):S74–84.

12. Berenbaum F, Eymard F, Houard X. Osteoarthritis, inflammation and obesity. Curr Opin Rheumatol 2013;25:114–8.
13. Juraschek SP, Miller ER 3rd, Gelber AC. Body mass index, obesity, and prevalent gout in the United States in 1988–1994 and 2007–2010. Arthritis Care Res (Hoboken) 2013;65:127–32.
14. Dittrick GW, Thompson JS, Campos D, et al. Gallbladder pathology in morbid obesity. Obes Surg 2005;15:238–42.
15. Drager LF, Togeiro SM, Polotsky VY, et al. Obstructive sleep apnea: a cardiometabolic risk in obesity and metabolic syndrome. J Am Coll Cardiol 2013. http://dx.doi.org/10.1016/j.jacc.2013.05.045.
16. Boulet LP. Asthma and obesity. Clin Exp Allergy 2013;43:8–21.
17. Luppino FS, de Wit LM, Bouvy PF, et al. Overweight, obesity, and depression: a systematic review and meta-analysis of longitudinal studies. Arch Gen Psychiatry 2010;67:220–9.
18. Novak NL, Brownell KD. Role of policy and government in the obesity epidemic. Circulation 2012;126:2345–52.
19. Matthews CM. Exploring the obesity epidemic. Proc (Bayl Univ Med Cent) 2012; 25:276–7.
20. Eknoyan G. A history of obesity, or how what was good became ugly and then bad. Adv Chronic Kidney Dis 2006;13:421–7.
21. Nammi S, Koka S, Chinnala KM, et al. Obesity: an overview on its current perspectives and treatment options. Nutr J 2004;3:3.
22. Lee YS. The role of genes in the current obesity epidemic. Ann Acad Med Singapore 2009;38:45–53.
23. Sun K, Kusminski CM, Scherer PE. Adipose tissue remodeling and obesity. J Clin Invest 2011;121:2094–101.
24. Lee MJ, Wu Y, Fried SK. Adipose tissue remodeling in pathophysiology of obesity. Curr Opin Clin Nutr Metab Care 2010;13:371–6.
25. Kim CH, Younossi ZM. Nonalcoholic fatty liver disease: a manifestation of the metabolic syndrome. Cleve Clin J Med 2008;75:721–8.
26. Younossi ZM. Review article: current management of non-alcoholic fatty liver disease and non-alcoholic steatohepatitis. Aliment Pharmacol Ther 2008;28: 2–12.
27. Nugent C, Younossi ZM. Evaluation and management of obesity-related nonalcoholic fatty liver disease. Nat Clin Pract Gastroenterol Hepatol 2007;4:432–41.
28. Ong JP, Younossi ZM. Epidemiology and natural history of NAFLD and NASH. Clin Liver Dis 2007;11:1–16.
29. Milić S, Stimac D. Nonalcoholic fatty liver disease/steatohepatitis: epidemiology, pathogenesis, clinical presentation and treatment. Dig Dis 2012;30:158–62.
30. Paredes AH, Torres DM, Harrison SA. Nonalcoholic fatty liver disease. Clin Liver Dis 2012;16:397–419.
31. Kleiner DE, Brunt EM. Nonalcoholic fatty liver disease: pathologic patterns and biopsy evaluation in clinical research. Semin Liver Dis 2012;32:3–13.
32. Brunt EM, Tiniakos DG. Histopathology of nonalcoholic fatty liver disease. World J Gastroenterol 2010;16:5286–96.
33. Bellentani S, Scaglioni F, Marino M, et al. Epidemiology of non-alcoholic fatty liver disease. Dig Dis 2010;28:155–61.
34. Tuyama AC, Chang CY. Non-alcoholic fatty liver disease. J Diabetes 2012;4: 266–80.
35. Liu CJ. Prevalence and risk factors for non-alcoholic fatty liver disease in Asian people who are not obese. J Gastroenterol Hepatol 2012;27:1555–60.

36. Jakobsen MU, Berentzen T, Sørensen TI, et al. Abdominal obesity and fatty liver. Epidemiol Rev 2007;29:77–87.
37. Kotronen A, Yki-Järvinen H. Fatty liver: a novel component of the metabolic syndrome. Arterioscler Thromb Vasc Biol 2008;28:27–38.
38. Yilmaz Y. NAFLD in the absence of metabolic syndrome: different epidemiology, pathogenetic mechanisms, risk factors for disease progression? Semin Liver Dis 2012;32:14–21.
39. Flegal KM, Carroll MD, Ogden CL, et al. Prevalence and trends in obesity among US adults, 1999–2008. JAMA 2010;303:235–41.
40. Swinburn BA, Sacks G, Hall KD, et al. The global obesity pandemic: shaped by global drivers and local environments. Lancet 2011;378:804–14.
41. Shamseddeen H, Getty JZ, Hamdallah IN, et al. Epidemiology and economic impact of obesity and type 2 diabetes. Surg Clin North Am 2011;91: 1163–72.
42. Tsigos C, Hainer V, Basdevant A, et al. Management of obesity in adults: European clinical practice guidelines. Obes Facts 2008;1:106–16.
43. Ogden CL, Carroll MD. Prevalence of overweight, obesity, and extreme obesity among adults: United States, trends 1960–1962 through 2007–2008. Hyattsville, MD: National Center for Health Statistics; 2010.
44. Skelton JA, Irby MB, Grzywacz JG, et al. Etiologies of obesity in children: nature and nurture. Pediatr Clin North Am 2011;58:1333–54.
45. Ben-Sefer E, Ben-Natan M, Ehrenfeld M. Childhood obesity: current literature, policy and implications for practice. Int Nurs Rev 2009;56:166–73.
46. Sanyal AJ. NASH: a global health problem. Hepatol Res 2011;41:670–4.
47. Sheth SG, Gordan FD, Chopra S. Nonalcoholic steatohepatitis. Ann Intern Med 1997;126:137–45.
48. Browning JD, Szczepaniak LS, Dobbins R, et al. Prevalence of hepatic steatosis in an urban population in the United States: impact of ethnicity. Hepatology 2004;40:1387–95.
49. Petersen KF, Dufour S, Feng J, et al. Increased prevalence of insulin resistance and nonalcoholic fatty liver disease in Asian-Indian men. Proc Natl Acad Sci U S A 2006;103:18273–7.
50. Silverman JF, O'Brien KF, Long S, et al. Liver pathology in morbidly obese patients with and without diabetes. Am J Gastroenterol 1990;85:1349–55.
51. Wanless IR, Lentz JS. Fatty liver hepatitis (steatohepatitis) and obesity: an autopsy study with analysis of risk factors. Hepatology 1990;12:1106–10.
52. Charlton MR, Burns JM, Pedersen RA, et al. Frequency and outcomes of liver transplantation for nonalcoholic steatohepatitis in the United States. Gastroenterology 2011;141:1249–53.
53. Reeves H, Villa E, Bellentani S, et al. The emerging impact of hepatocellular carcinoma arising on a background of NAFLD. J Hepatol 2012;56(Suppl 2):S3.
54. Zelber-Sagi S, Lotan R, Shlomai A, et al. Predictors for incidence and remission of NAFLD in the general population during a seven-year prospective follow-up. J Hepatol 2012;56:1145–51.
55. Jeffery RW, French SA. Epidemic obesity in the United States: are fast foods and television viewing contributing? Am J Public Health 1998;88:277–80.
56. Drewnowski A, Specter SE. Poverty and obesity: the role of energy density and energy costs. Am J Clin Nutr 2004;79:6–16.
57. Ford ES, Mokdad AH, Giles WH, et al. Geographic variation in the prevalence of obesity, diabetes, and obesity-related behaviors. Obes Res 2005;13: 118–22.

58. Shields M, Connor Gorber S, Janssen I, et al. Bias in self-reported estimates of obesity in Canadian health surveys: an update on correction equations for adults. Health Rep 2011;22:35–45.
59. Dauphinot V, Wolff H, Naudin F, et al. New obesity body mass index threshold for self-reported data. J Epidemiol Community Health 2009;63:128–32.
60. Bolton-Smith C, Woodward M, Tunstall-Pedoe H, et al. Accuracy of the estimated prevalence of obesity from self reported height and weight in an adult Scottish population. J Epidemiol Community Health 2000;54:143–8.
61. Nguyen DM, El-Serag HB. The epidemiology of obesity. Gastroenterol Clin North Am 2010;39:1–7.
62. Nishida C, Mucavele P. Monitoring the rapidly emerging public health problem of overweight and obesity: the WHO global database on body mass index. SCN News 2005;29:5–12.
63. Erickson SK. Nonalcoholic fatty liver disease. J Lipid Res 2009;50(Suppl):S412–6.
64. Bacon BR, Farahvash MJ, Janney CG, et al. Nonalcoholic steatohepatitis: an expanded clinical entity. Gastroenterology 1994;107:1103–9.
65. Matteoni CA, Younossi ZM, Gramlich T, et al. Nonalcoholic fatty liver disease: a spectrum of clinical and pathological severity. Gastroenterology 1999;116:1413–9.
66. Powell EE, Cooksley WG, Hanson R, et al. The natural history of nonalcoholic steatohepatitis: a follow-up study of forty-two patients for up to 21 years. Hepatology 1990;11:74–80.
67. Nonomura A, Mizukami Y, Unoura M, et al. Clinicopathologic study of alcohol-like liver disease in non-alcoholics; non-alcoholic steatohepatitis and fibrosis. Gastroenterol Jpn 1992;27:521–8.
68. el Hassan AY, Ibrahim EM, al Mulhim FA, et al. Fatty infiltration of the liver: analysis of prevalence, radiological and clinical features and influence on patient management. Br J Radiol 1992;65:774–8.
69. Clark JM, Brancati FL, Diehl AM. The prevalence and etiology of elevated aminotransferase levels in the United States. Am J Gastroenterol 2003;98:960–7.
70. Weston SR, Leyden W, Murphy R, et al. Racial and ethnic distribution of nonalcoholic fatty liver in persons with newly diagnosed chronic liver disease. Hepatology 2005;41:372–9.
71. Caldwell SH, Harris DM, Patrie JT, et al. Is NASH underdiagnosed among African Americans? Am J Gastroenterol 2002;97:1496–500.
72. Mohanty SR, Troy TN, Huo D, et al. Influence of ethnicity on histological differences in non-alcoholic fatty liver disease. J Hepatol 2009;50:797–804.
73. Attar BM, Van Thiel DH. Current concepts and management approaches in nonalcoholic fatty liver disease. ScientificWorldJournal 2013;2013:481893.
74. Bambha K, Belt P, Abraham M, et al. Ethnicity and nonalcoholic fatty liver disease. Hepatology 2012;55:769–80.
75. Lallukka S, Sevastianova K, Perttilä J, et al. Adipose tissue is inflamed in NAFLD due to obesity but not in NAFLD due to genetic variation in PNPLA3. Diabetologia 2013;56:886–92.
76. Speliotes EK, Yerges-Armstrong LM, Wu J, et al. Genome-wide association analysis identifies variants associated with nonalcoholic fatty liver disease that have distinct effects on metabolic traits. PLoS Genet 2011;7:e1001324.
77. Rector RS, Thyfault JP. Does physical inactivity cause nonalcoholic fatty liver disease? J Appl Physiol 2011;111:1828–35.

78. Zelber-Sagi S, Nitzan-Kaluski D, Goldsmith R, et al. Long term nutritional intake and the risk for non-alcoholic fatty liver disease (NAFLD): a population based study. J Hepatol 2007;47:711–7.

79. Zelber-Sagi S, Ratziu V, Oren R. Nutrition and physical activity in NAFLD: an overview of the epidemiological evidence. World J Gastroenterol 2011;17:3377–89.

80. Yilmaz Y. Review article: fructose in non-alcoholic fatty liver disease. Aliment Pharmacol Ther 2012;35:1135–44.

81. Caporaso N, Morisco F, Camera S, et al. Dietary approach in the prevention and treatment of NAFLD. Front Biosci 2012;17:2259–68.

82. Centis E, Marzocchi R, Suppini A, et al. The role of lifestyle change in the prevention and treatment of NAFLD. Curr Pharm Des 2013;19(29):5270–9.

83. Rodriguez B, Torres DM, Harrison SA. Physical activity: an essential component of lifestyle modification in NAFLD. Nat Rev Gastroenterol Hepatol 2012;9:726–31.

84. Thoma C, Day CP, Trenell MI. Lifestyle interventions for the treatment of non-alcoholic fatty liver disease in adults: a systematic review. J Hepatol 2012;56:255–66.

85. Patel AA, Torres DM, Harrison SA. Effect of weight loss on nonalcoholic fatty liver disease. J Clin Gastroenterol 2009;43:970–4.

86. Harrison SA, Day CP. Benefits of lifestyle modification in NAFLD. Gut 2007;56:1760–9.

87. Pacifico L, Anania C, Martino F, et al. Management of metabolic syndrome in children and adolescents. Nutr Metab Cardiovasc Dis 2011;21:455–66.

88. Nobili V, Svegliati-Baroni G, Alisi A, et al. A 360-degree overview of paediatric NAFLD: recent insights. J Hepatol 2013;58:1218–29.

89. Malinowski SS, Byrd JS, Bell AM, et al. Pharmacologic therapy for nonalcoholic fatty liver disease in adults. Pharmacotherapy 2013;33:223–42.

90. Nakajima K. Multidisciplinary pharmacotherapeutic options for nonalcoholic fatty liver disease. Int J Hepatol 2012;2012:950693.

91. Rabl C, Campos GM. The impact of bariatric surgery on nonalcoholic steatohepatitis. Semin Liver Dis 2012;32:80–91.

92. Pillai AA, Rinella ME. Non-alcoholic fatty liver disease: is bariatric surgery the answer? Clin Liver Dis 2009;13:689–710.

93. Chavez-Tapia NC, Tellez-Avila FI, Barrientos-Gutierrez T, et al. Bariatric surgery for non-alcoholic steatohepatitis in obese patients. Cochrane Database Syst Rev 2010;(1):CD007340.

94. Sanyal AJ, Chalasani N, Kowdley KV, et al, NASH CRN. Pioglitazone, vitamin E, or placebo for nonalcoholic steatohepatitis. N Engl J Med 2010;362(18):1675–85.

95. Chalasani N, Younossi Z, Lavine JE, et al. The diagnosis and management of non-alcoholic fatty liver disease: practice guideline by the American Gastroenterological Association, American Association for the Study of Liver Diseases, and American College of Gastroenterology. Gastroenterology 2012;143(2):503.

96. Younossi ZM, Stepanova M, Afendy M, et al. Changes in the prevalence of the most common causes of chronic liver diseases in the United States from 1988 to 2008. Clin Gastroenterol Hepatol 2011;9(6):524–30.

97. Yilmaz Y, Ulukaya E. Toward a biochemical diagnosis of NASH: insights from pathophysiology for distinguishing simple steatosis from steatohepatitis. Curr Med Chem 2011;18:725–32.

98. Wieckowska A, Feldstein AE. Diagnosis of nonalcoholic fatty liver disease: invasive versus noninvasive. Semin Liver Dis 2008;28:386–95.

99. Wieckowska A, McCullough AJ, Feldstein AE. Noninvasive diagnosis and monitoring of nonalcoholic steatohepatitis: present and future. Hepatology 2007;46: 582–9.

100. Miele L, Forgione A, Gasbarrini G, et al. Noninvasive assessment of fibrosis in non-alcoholic fatty liver disease (NAFLD) and non-alcoholic steatohepatitis (NASH). Transl Res 2007;149:114–25.

101. Younossi ZM, Page S, Rafiq N, et al. A biomarker panel for non-alcoholic steatohepatitis (NASH) and NASH-related fibrosis. Obes Surg 2011;21:431–9.

102. Younossi ZM, Jarrar M, Nugent C, et al. A novel diagnostic biomarker panel for obesity-related nonalcoholic steatohepatitis (NASH). Obes Surg 2008;18: 1430–7.

The Impact of Obesity on Liver Histology

Zachary D. Goodman, MD, PhD

KEYWORDS

- Nonalcoholic fatty liver disease • Steatosis • Nonalcoholic steatohepatitis
- Cryptogenic cirrhosis • Hepatocellular adenoma • Hepatocellular carcinoma

KEY POINTS

- Obesity and metabolic syndrome produce changes in the liver's normal role in lipid and energy metabolism that cause a sequence of histopathologic changes.
- Steatosis is caused by an increase in hepatocellular fat vacuoles that parallels increased body mass index. Death of a small number of steatotic hepatocytes can produce liver enzyme elevation and focal nonspecific inflammation.
- Steatohepatitis occurs when there is cytoskeletal damage in genetically susceptible individuals resulting in loss of normal keratin filaments, ballooning degeneration of affected liver cells, and formation of Mallory-Denk bodies.
- In patients with steatohepatitis, activation of hepatic stellate cells produces intralobular fibrosis in the perisinusoidal spaces, whereas periportal ductular reaction causes activation of portal myofibroblasts and periportal fibrosis. With continuing fibrogenesis, there is progression to bridging fibrosis and cirrhosis.
- Hepatocellular carcinoma may develop in the cirrhotic liver, but both hepatocellular adenoma and hepatocellular carcinoma may occur in fatty liver disease before cirrhosis develops.

NORMAL LIVER AND NONSPECIFIC OR PHYSIOLOGIC STEATOSIS

The liver plays a central role in lipid metabolism, and consequently lipids (primarily triglycerides) may accumulate in the liver (primarily in hepatocytes) whenever there is an imbalance between the delivery of fat to the liver from the diet or from adipose tissue stores and the export of fat as a component of very-low-density lipoproteins. Small lipid droplets, identifiable only by electron microscopy or fat stains, are normally present in the cytoplasm of hepatocytes,[1] but under conditions of metabolic imbalance, stress, or cellular injury in many pathologic processes, lipid droplets become large enough to visualize by light microscopy as clear vacuoles in hepatocytes cytoplasm.

Disclosure Statement: The author has nothing to disclose.
Center for Liver Diseases, Inova Fairfax Hospital, 3300 Gallows Road, Falls Church, VA 22042, USA
E-mail address: zachary.goodman@inova.org

Fat stains performed on frozen sections of livers from autopsies of hospitalized adults[2] and children dying of trauma[3] have shown that some degree of microvesicular steatosis is nearly always present, even though it is often not appreciated with routine paraffin-embedded sections. Similar population-based histologic studies of liver biopsies have not been performed in normal living subjects, because liver biopsies are seldom performed without a clinical indication, but proton nuclear magnetic resonance spectroscopy detects some hepatic triglyceride in all normal individuals, with a minimum of 1.9% of tissue by weight.[4]

OBESITY-RELATED STEATOSIS AND NONALCOHOLIC FATTY LIVER DISEASE

The presence of hepatocyte fat vacuoles that can be detected in routine hematoxylin-eosin–stained sections can be considered steatosis. Any alteration of the lipid transport and lipoprotein secretion may cause sufficient enlargement of normal lipid droplets to qualify, and minor degrees of unexplained steatosis are common. Traditionally, steatosis has been graded histologically by the proportion of affected parenchyma as mild (<1/3), moderate (1/3 to 2/3), or marked (>2/3) (**Fig. 1**).[5] This grading has the disadvantage of including many cases with only a few affected hepatocytes in the same category as those that have 32% fat; so, in recent years, a lower limit of 5% fat, as estimated by a pathologist, has often been used as a defining feature of NAFLD.[6] This practice is supported by the nuclear magnetic resonance studies showing that 95% of individuals with normal body mass index (BMI) and no risk factors for fatty liver disease had less than 5.5% hepatic triglyceride by weight.[4] Even experienced pathologists, however, routinely overestimate the amount of fat when compared with quantitative measurements by digital image analysis and computer-assisted morphometry,[7] with estimates typically doubling the amount of fat that is actually present, so liver biopsies estimated to have 5% fat may actually have much less.

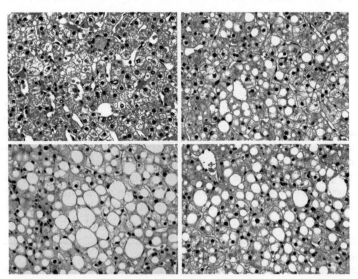

Fig. 1. Degrees of steatosis. None (*upper left*)—hepatocytes have no visible cytoplasmic fat vacuoles. Mild (*upper right*)—fat vacuoles occupy greater than 5% but less than 33% of hepatocyte cytoplasm. Moderate (*lower right*)—fat vacuoles occupy greater than 33% of hepatocyte cytoplasm. Marked (*lower left*)—fat vacuoles occupy greater than 66% of hepatocyte cytoplasm.

Although many genetic, environmental, and other factors seem to play a role in the pathogenesis of hepatocellular fat accumulation, and there is wide variation among individuals, the degree of histologic hepatic steatosis seems to correlate approximately with BMI. As previously noted, population-based data are impossible to obtain, and studies of obese patients are typically limited to those with an indication for liver biopsy, usually elevated liver-associated enzymes, or to morbidly obese patients undergoing bariatric surgery. There is evidence, however, of a correlation of steatosis with BMI in patients with chronic hepatitis C biopsied before therapeutic trials. In one study of more than 1400 patients, those with absolutely no steatosis on liver biopsy had a mean BMI of 26; those with microscopic steatosis up to 5% had a mean BMI of 28; those with 5% to 33% steatosis had average mean BMI of 30; and those with greater that 33% fat, as estimated by a pathologist, had a mean BMI of 31.[8] Similarly, another study of 400 hepatitis C patients found a mean BMI of 27; fewer than 5% had mean BMI of 29, and those with 5% or greater had mean BMI of 32.[9] In contrast, in patients with morbid obesity, the degree of steatosis does not correlate significantly with the BMI,[10] perhaps because both weight and steatosis are skewed toward the high end of the scale in this population. Liver biopsies performed during bariatric surgery routinely detect some degree of steatosis in approximate 90% of morbidly obese patients.

Metabolic syndrome, in particular insulin resistance, is much more important than obesity alone in the development of hepatic steatosis and steatohepatitis.[11,12] Many other genetically determined metabolic diseases are characterized by hepatocellular fat accumulation,[13] but these are generally rare compared with common metabolic syndrome–associated nonalcoholic fatty liver disease (NAFLD). Hyperinsulinemia promotes both triglyceride synthesis with hepatocellular fat accumulation and lipoprotein secretion leading to hyperlipidemia. The resulting steatosis is the first hit of the two-hit theory of the pathogenesis of steatohepatitis.[14] Oxidative stress or other poorly understood factors may cause minor degrees of hepatocellular injury in the fatty liver with focal hepatocyte dropout and minor degrees of inflammation characterized by focal clusters of inflammatory cells, mainly lymphocytes and hypertrophied Kupffer cells. Depending on the degree of inflammation, these changes may be regarded as simple steatosis or steatosis with nonspecific inflammation.

NONALCOHOLIC STEATOHEPATITIS

In 1979 and 1980 there were several reports of series of patients who did not consume alcohol but who had liver disease that histologically mimicked alcoholic hepatitis.[15–17] Most of these patients were obese, diabetic, or both. There had been earlier descriptions of the same phenomenon, but these received little attention, and the prevailing view up to that time had been that if the liver biopsy showed alcoholic hepatitis, then the patient must have been secretly drinking. Ludwig and colleagues[16] were especially instrumental in establishing this as a disease entity, and their name, nonalcoholic steatohepatitis (NASH), became the preferred term for what is now considered the severe form of NAFLD. Although obesity plays a role in NASH, metabolic syndrome and insulin resistance are considered more important in its pathogenesis in combination with oxidative stress and genetic predisposition.[14]

In addition to hepatocellular fat accumulation, livers with steatohepatitis contain variable numbers of liver cells with cytoskeletal damage that can be recognized by the presence of hepatocellular ballooning and Mallory-Denk bodies (**Fig. 2**). Epithelial cell cytoskeletons are composed of keratin proteins, which in hepatocytes are predominantly K8 and K18, that can be demonstrated by specific immunostaining.

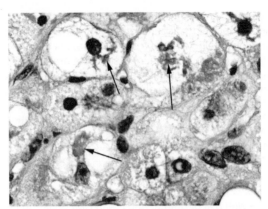

Fig. 2. NASH. Ballooned hepatocytes that contain Mallory-Denk bodies (*arrows*).

Oxidative stress–related cytoskeletal damage causes the normal keratin filaments to aggregate and form Mallory-Denk bodies associated with stress-related proteins, such as ubiquitin and p62. The cell that has lost its skeleton swells like an inflated balloon, losing the normal cytoplasmic staining for K8/18, which is now confined to the Mallory-Denk body.[18] The injury in steatohepatitis is most severe in zone 3 of the hepatic acinus (ie, centrilobular areas, where ballooned cells and Mallory-Denk bodies are most readily found). Because the ballooned hepatocytes are enlarged, up to 100 μm in diameter, the Mallory-Denk body may be out of the plane of a 4-μm–thick microscopic section, which is the most likely reason why every ballooned cell does not seem to contain one of these inclusions. Immunostaining for ubiquitin or p62 can be helpful in identification of Malory-Denk bodies and can establish a diagnosis of NASH in equivocal cases (**Fig. 3**). Apoptotic bodies may also be present, and there is typically an inflammatory response with a predominance of lymphocytes and Kupffer cells and occasionally some neutrophils in more severe cases. Most patients who undergo liver biopsy have some degree of fibrosis. Centrilobular pericellular/perisinusoidal fibrosis produced by activated stellate cells in association with inflammation and

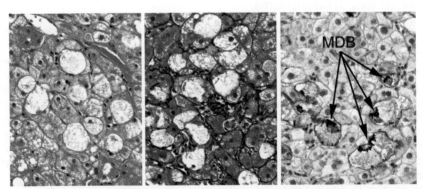

Fig. 3. NASH. Hepatocellular ballooning in NASH is characterized by swollen liver cells with thin strands of cytoplasm (*left*). The Masson trichrome stain shows deposition of delicate strands of blue-staining collagen in the perisinusoidal spaces surrounding ballooned liver cells (*center*), and an immunostain for ubiquitin demonstrates small Mallory-Denk bodies (MDB) (*arrows*) in some of the ballooned hepatocytes (*right*).

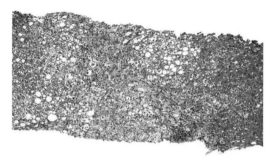

Fig. 4. Bridging fibrosis in NASH (Masson trichrome stain). Collagenous fibrous tissue, stained blue, extends from a centrilobular area at lower right, to a portal area at upper left. Trapped hepatocytes are incorporated into the scar.

ballooning is the earliest stage (see **Fig. 3**) and is characteristic of the steatohepatitis pattern of injury. Portal fibrosis associated with ductular reaction follows the centrilobular fibrosis,[19] and both processes seem to play a role in the development of bridging fibrosis (**Fig. 4**) and cirrhosis (**Fig. 5**), whereas chronic portal inflammation also increases and may play a role in advancing fibrosis.[20] Population-based data on the relative incidence of these lesions are not available, and some degree of selection bias is inevitable in published series based on liver biopsies. In a large series of adults with NAFLD accumulated by the Nonalcoholic Steatohepatitis Clinical Research Network, of 693 patients, 26% had no fibrosis, 49% had mild or moderate fibrosis, 17% had bridging fibrosis, and 8% had cirrhosis.[21]

CRYPTOGENIC CIRRHOSIS

Some obese or diabetic patients are found to have otherwise unexplained cirrhosis on liver biopsy or at autopsy. In one autopsy series, 14% of obese patients had cirrhosis,[22] and cirrhosis is 2 to 3 times more frequent in diabetics than in the general population. Although the cause is often uncertain, it is likely that most of these are the result of clinically silent NASH. Furthermore, more than 70% of patients with so-called cryptogenic cirrhosis are obese and/or diabetic, suggesting previous NASH that had

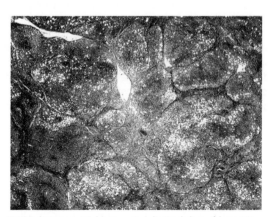

Fig. 5. Cirrhosis in NASH (Masson trichrome stain). Nodules of hepatic parenchyma are surrounded by bands of blue-staining fibrous scars with loss of normal architecture.

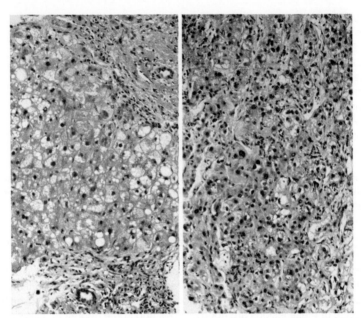

Fig. 6. Liver biopsy showing hepatocellular carcinoma (*right*) in a liver with NASH (*left*).

become histologically inapparent after the development of cirrhosis.[23,24] A recent investigation found that loss of fat correlated well with elevation of serum adiponectin levels in patients with cirrhosis, suggesting that this may be the mechanism leading to cryptogenic cirrhosis as a form of burned-out NASH.[25]

PRIMARY HEPATIC NEOPLASMS—HEPATOCELLULAR ADENOMA AND HEPATOCELLULAR CARCINOMA

Hepatocellular adenoma is an uncommon benign neoplasm that occurs most often in women with long-term exposure to contraceptive steroids. Three subtypes have been described, and all have been noted to be increasing in frequency in association with overweight and obesity.[26,27] Some of these have evolved into hepatocellular carcinoma.[28]

Hepatocellular carcinoma (**Fig. 6**) has an increased incidence in patients with obesity and diabetes.[29,30] A majority of these are in individuals with NASH-related cirrhosis or cryptogenic cirrhosis presumably due to NASH.[31] A recent review, however, documented 116 reported cases of hepatocellular carcinoma in precirrhotic NAFLD, including some patients with no fibrosis at all.[32] Such cases can be expected to become more common in future years with the growing epidemic of obesity.

REFERENCES

1. Phillips MJ, Poucell S, Patterson J, et al. The Liver: an atlas and text of ultrastructural pathology. New York: Raven Press; 1987.
2. Fraser JL, Antonioli DA, Chopra S, et al. Prevalence and nonspecificity of microvesicular fatty change in the liver. Mod Pathol 1995;8:65–70.
3. Bonnell HJ, Beckwith JB. Fatty liver in sudden childhood death. Am J Dis Child 1986;140:30–3.

4. Browning JD, Szczepaniak LS, Dobbins R, et al. Prevalence of hepatic steatosis in an urban population in the United States: impact of ethnicity. Hepatology 2004; 40:1387–95.
5. Burt AD, Mutton A, Day CP. Diagnosis and interpretation of steatosis and steatohepatitis. Semin Diagn Pathol 1998;15:246–58.
6. Kleiner DE, Brunt EM, Van Natta M, et al. Design and validation of a histological scoring system for nonalcoholic fatty liver disease. Hepatology 2005;41:1313–21.
7. Hall AR, Dhillon AP, Green AC, et al. Hepatic steatosis estimated microscopically versus digital image analysis. Liver Int 2013;33:926–35.
8. Poynard T, Ratziu V, McHutchison J, et al. Effect of treatment with peginterferon or interferon alfa-2b and ribavirin on steatosis in patients infected with hepatitis C. Hepatology 2003;38:75–85.
9. Conjeevaram HS, Kleiner DE, Everhart JE, et al. Race, insulin resistance and hepatic steatosis in chronic hepatitis C. Hepatology 2007;45:80–7.
10. Dixon JB, Bhathal PS, O'Brien PE. Nonalcoholic fatty liver disease: predictors of nonalcoholic steatohepatitis and liver fibrosis in the severely obese. Gastroenterology 2001;121:91–100.
11. Marceau P, Biron S, Hould FS, et al. Liver pathology and the metabolic syndrome X in severe obesity. J Clin Endocrinol Metab 1999;84:1513–7.
12. Bugianesi E, McCullough AJ, Marchesini G. Insulin resistance: a metabolic pathway to chronic liver disease. Hepatology 2005;42:987–1000.
13. Hooper AJ, Adams LA, Burnett JR. Genetic determinants of hepatic steatosis in man. J Lipid Res 2011;52:593–617.
14. Day CP. Pathogenesis of steatohepatitis. Best Pract Res Clin Gastroenterol 2002; 16:663–78.
15. Adler M, Schaffner F. Fatty liver hepatitis and cirrhosis in obese patients. Am J Med 1979;67:811–6.
16. Ludwig J, Viggiano TR, McGill DB, et al. Nonalcoholic steatohepatitis. Mayo Clinic experiences with a hitherto unnamed disease. Mayo Clin Proc 1980;55: 434–8.
17. Falchuk KR, Fiske SC, Haggitt RC, et al. Pericentral hepatic fibrosis and intracellular hyalin in diabetes mellitus. Gastroenterology 1980;78:535–41.
18. Lackner C, Gogg-Kamerer M, Zatloukal K, et al. Ballooned hepatocytes in steatohepatitis: the value of keratin immunohistochemistry for diagnosis. J Hepatol 2008;48:821–8.
19. Skoien R, Richardson MM, Jonsson JR, et al. Heterogeneity of fibrosis patterns in non-alcoholic fatty liver disease supports the presence of multiple fibrogenic pathways. Liver Int 2013;33:624–32.
20. Brunt EM, Kleiner DE, Wilson LA, et al. Portal chronic inflammation in nonalcoholic fatty liver disease (NAFLD): a histologic marker of advanced NAFLD-Clinicopathologic correlations from the nonalcoholic steatohepatitis clinical research network. Hepatology 2009;49:809–20.
21. Neuschwander-Tetri BA, Clark JM, Bass NM, et al. Clinical, laboratory and histological associations in adults with nonalcoholic fatty liver disease. Hepatology 2010;52:913–24.
22. Wanless IR, Lentz JS. Fatty liver hepatitis (steatohepatitis) and obesity: an autopsy study with analysis of risk factors. Hepatology 1990;12:1106–10.
23. Caldwell SH, Oelsner DH, Iezzoni JC, et al. Cryptogenic cirrhosis: clinical characterization and risk factors for underlying disease. Hepatology 1999;29:664–9.
24. Caldwell SH, Crespo DM. The spectrum expanded: cryptogenic cirrhosis and the natural history of nonalcoholic fatty liver disease. J Hepatol 2004;40:578–84.

25. van der Poorten D, Samer CF, Ramezani-Moghadam M, et al. Hepatic fat loss in advanced nonalcoholic steatohepatitis: are alterations in serum adiponectin the cause? Hepatology 2013;57:2180–8.

26. Paradis V, Champault A, Ronot M, et al. Telangiectatic adenoma: an entity associated with increased body mass index and inflammation. Hepatology 2007;46: 140–6.

27. Biolulac-Sage P, Taouji S, Possenti L, et al. Hepatocellular adenoma subtypes: the impact of overweight and obesity. Liver Int 2012;32:1217–21.

28. Paradis V, Zalinski S, Chelbi E, et al. Hepatocellular carcinomas in patients with metabolic syndrome often develop without significant liver fibrosis: a pathological analysis. Hepatology 2009;49:851–9.

29. Larsson SC, Wolk A. Overweight, obesity and risk of liver cancer: a meta-analysis of cohort studies. Br J Cancer 2007;97:1005–8.

30. El-Serag HB, Hampel H, Javadi F. The association between diabetes and hepatocellular carcinoma: a systematic review of epidemiologic evidence. Clin Gastroenterol Hepatol 2006;4:369–80.

31. White DL, Kanwal F, El-Serag HB. Association between nonalcoholic fatty liver disease and risk for hepatocellular cancer, based on systematic review. Clin Gastroenterol Hepatol 2012;10:1342–59.

32. Baffy G, Brunt EM, Caldwell SH. Hepatocellular carcinoma in non-alcoholic fatty liver disease: an emerging menace. J Hepatol 2012;56:1384–91.

Adipose Tissue as an Endocrine Organ

Christine McGown, MS[a], Aybike Birerdinc, PhD[a,b],
Zobair M. Younossi, MD, MPH, AGAF[a,b,c],*

KEYWORDS

- Obesity • Adipose tissue • Endocrine • Hypoxia • Inflammation • Insulin resistance

KEY POINTS

- Obesity is a strong risk factor for developing numerous chronic diseases, primarily insulin resistance, type 2 diabetes, heart disease, and nonalcoholic fatty liver disease.
- Visceral fat is a functional endocrine organ with important influences on numerous metabolic and hormonal responses.
- Visceral adipose tissue is known to produce inflammatory adipokines, regulatory adiponectin, as well as other regulatory molecules such as leptin, cocaine and amphetamine–regulated transcript and nuclear factor κB that play important roles in the cause of these chronic diseases.
- The endocrine effects of adipose tissue during obesity and the systemic impact of this signaling need to be investigated in greater detail to understand the progression of chronic metabolic diseases.

INTRODUCTION

Obesity is one of the most important health issues in developed countries. Statistics taken between 1999 and 2004 indicate that in the United States the obesity rate for men increased from 27.5% to 31.3% and the rate for women remained steady at 33%, indicating that a significant proportion of American adults are obese as defined by a body mass index (BMI) more than 30.[1] In the past decade a growing number of children have also become obese, with 16% of girls and 18% of boys fitting the definition of obese for their age groups in 2004.[1] The root causes of obesity are diverse and can differ from simply a high-calorie diet and lack of exercise to an underlying

[a] College of Science, Center for the Study of Chronic Metabolic Diseases, George Mason University, 4400 University Drive, Fairfax, VA 22030, USA; [b] Betty and Guy Beatty Center for Integrated Research, Inova Health System, 3300 Gallows Road, Falls Church, VA 22042, USA; [c] Department of Medicine, Center for Liver Diseases, Inova Fairfax Hospital, VCU-Inova Campus, Falls Church, VA, USA
* Corresponding author. Beatty Center for Integrated Research, 3300 Gallows Road, Falls Church, VA 22042.
E-mail address: zobair.younossi@inova.org

Clin Liver Dis 18 (2014) 41–58
http://dx.doi.org/10.1016/j.cld.2013.09.012
1089-3261/14/$ – see front matter © 2014 Elsevier Inc. All rights reserved.
liver.theclinics.com

medical condition such as diabetes.[2,3] Although obesity may seem simple, on a functional and metabolic level it is highly complex. Obesity has an important influence on numerous metabolic and hormonal responses including changes in sex hormones,[4] inflammation,[5,6] and insulin resistance.[2,7] Fat, visceral fat in particular, is increasingly considered to be a functional endocrine organ. Recent studies have found that, in addition to fat storage, adipose tissue is known to store lipid-based hormones[4] and to produce inflammatory adipokines,[5,6] regulatory adiponectin,[8] and other regulatory molecules such as leptin,[9] cocaine and amphetamine–regulated transcript[2] and nuclear factor κB (NFκB).[6] The organism-wide impact of this signaling cannot be underestimated, and strongly supports the theory that obesity is essentially a systemic medical condition with adipose tissue deregulation the underlying force driving the change.

Obesity is also a considerable risk factor for developing numerous other chronic diseases, such as insulin resistance, type 2 diabetes (T2D), heart disease, and nonalcoholic fatty liver disease (NAFLD). In the United States, NAFLD is currently estimated to exist in about 60% to 90% of the adult obese population,[10] compared with 15% to 30% of the general population.[11] NAFLD is not just a concern for adults but a growing number of adolescents as well.[12] Current estimates for the years 2007 to 2010 indicate that 10.7% of children in the United States are at risk for NAFLD, compared with estimates of 3.9% in 1994 to 1998.[12] Just as with adults, obesity is a major risk factor for the development of NAFLD, with estimates in obese children increasing from 20.7% in 1994 to 1998 to 38.2% in 2007 to 2010 (ie, nearly doubling).[12]

Some patients with NAFLD are at risk to progress to more severe forms of liver disease, including steatohepatosis, hepatic steatosis, nonalcoholic steatohepatosis (NASH), and ultimately cirrhosis.[11,13] About 20% of all patients with NASH are projected to develop cirrhosis of the liver within 20 years of initial diagnosis.[14]

Although the risk factors contributing to progression from NAFLD to NASH are largely unknown, adipose tissue signaling is thought to be an important driver via its promotion of both insulin resistance and proinflammatory signaling (**Fig. 1**).[15] Numerous lines of research have implicated adipose tissue via hypoxia,[6,16] inflammation[3,5,6,17] and overall endocrine disruption[18,19] in the impairment of many different organ systems, including the liver. This article discusses the endocrine effects of adipose tissue during obesity and the systemic impact of this signaling.

VISCERAL FAT COMPOSITION

In order to properly understand adipose tissue on a whole-organism level it is important to understand the components of adipose tissue and the functions of these various components. Two main types of adipose tissue are found in the human body: white adipose tissue (WAT) and brown adipose tissue (BAT).[20,21,22] Both are unique in structure, function, and when and where they occur in the body.[20] Both types of adipocytes store lipids to some extent in the form of triglycerides, but other functions of these cells are unique.[3] BAT in humans is typically associated with fetuses and infants and is defined by its main characteristic of being able to use fat to create heat in a unique process known as nonshivering thermogenesis via the expression of uncoupling protein 1 (UCP1) in the mitochondria.[20] It was widely thought that BAT represented at most 1% of adipose tissue in adult humans[23] until recent studies found areas of tissue resembling the metabolic profile of BAT in adult humans,[24] localized to areas such as the upper thoracic cavity and neck.[24,25]

In contrast, WAT is the more common type of adipose tissue in human adults and is designed for quick storage and release of lipids in response to metabolic conditions,

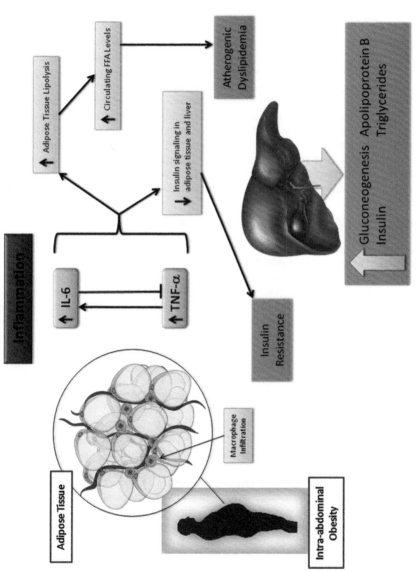

Fig. 1. Systemic impact of increased visceral adipose tissue and subsequent downstream signaling.

and lacks the energy-burning ability of BAT.[20,23] WAT cells contain 1 large lipid droplet (LD) that takes up most of the space in the cell to hold as much as possible, whereas BAT cells contain multiple smaller LDs that provide easy access to lipases to speed up the thermogenesis process.[26] In addition to storing fats, adipocytes produce several signaling molecules,[2,5,6,9] and can also store lipid-based hormones.[4] Energy homeostasis is linked directly to the proper endocrine functions of adipose tissue[2,3,9] and dysregulation can cause insulin resistance[3] as well as other serious health issues included under the umbrella term of metabolic syndrome.[4,27]

In addition to traditional BAT there is a third type of adipose tissue with the metabolic functions of BAT and the developmental origins of WAT (Myf5 positive).[20,28] This type of adipose tissue is called brite or beige and is localized inside regions of WAT tissue.[20] Beige tissue produces small amounts of UCP1, which allows it to create heat similarly to BAT.[20] Beige cells develop through a process known as browning in which WAT cells differentiate into beige cells because of chemical signaling or cold exposure.[20,21] A recent study by Sharp and colleagues[28] found that adult BAT cells share the molecular profile of beige cells rather than traditional BAT, suggesting that most human adult BAT may be beige cells. Thiazolidinediones, which are insulin-sensitizing agents used in the treatment of T2D, have strongly been associated with BAT activity and may also be involved in the browning of WAT.[29]

ADIPOKINES AND CYTOKINES DERIVED FROM VISCERAL FAT

Adipose tissue also contains several other cell types, including macrophages and monocytes,[30] which makes it difficult to determine the source of the endocrine signals sent from visceral adipose tissue. Some endocrine factors released from visceral adipose tissue (including the important and highly investigated adiponectin; leptin; resistin; and the cytokines tumor necrosis factor alpha [TNF-α] and interleukin [IL]-6) are discussed later.[31,32] However, there are other adipokines and chemokines that are gaining increasing interest, particularly in the context of insulin signaling, such as visfatin, vaspin, apelin, nesfatin, omentin, chemerin, and chemokines such as monocyte chemoattractant protein 1 (MCP-1), which require further study in obese patients with NAFLD and NASH. These are summarized in **Table 1**.

Some lines of research indicate that human adipose tissue, particularly in situations of obesity, releases substantial amounts of the proinflammatory cytokines IL-6 and IL-8,[53] most likely via the obesity-related increase in the TNF-α production involving the p38 MAPK and NF-κB pathways.[54] In addition, MCP-1 serum levels are increased in patients with NAFLD and these levels positively correlate with both BMI and the levels of fasting glucose.[55]

Visfatin, the extracellular secreted form of nicotinamide phosphoribosyltransferase, has been shown to be upregulated in obesity and to be involved in the regulation of glucose homeostasis via its impact on insulin secretion, insulin receptor phosphorylation, as well as the expression of several beta-cell function–associated genes in the pancreas.[56] However, vaspin (a visceral adipose tissue–derived member of the serine protease inhibitor [serpin] family)[57] has a less clear role in humans, because serum vaspin concentrations have been shown to have a circadian rhythm, with a preprandial increase and postprandial decrease.[58] A study of diabetic patients suggests that serum vaspin levels correlate with Homeostatic Model Assessment (HOMA) scores for insulin resistance rather than with BMI and that the strongest indicator of vaspin mRNA expression in human subcutaneous adipose tissue (SAT) was insulin sensitivity, all of which highlights the importance of the continued study of this adipokine as a potential insulin sensitizer.[59]

Another adipokine found to be increased in obese patients is apelin, which is thought to inhibit glucose-stimulated insulin secretion by acting on its receptor, expressed in beta cells of pancreatic islands. Apelin levels in patients with NAFLD correlated positively with BMI and the HOMA indexes.[60] Chemerin, encoded by the retinoic acid receptor responder 2 gene RARRES2, which has been largely studied in obese/diabetic but not normoglycemic mice, exacerbated glucose intolerance, lowered serum insulin levels, and decreased tissue glucose uptake.[61] In humans, receptors for chemerin were detected in primary hepatocytes, Kupffer cells, bile-duct cells, and hepatic stellate cells and its production was strongly induced by treatment with exogenous adiponectin, suggesting this adipokine as an additional target of study within the context of insulin signaling.[62]

Nesfatin, encoded by *NUCB2*, seems also to be involved in glucose homeostasis regulation. In patients with newly diagnosed T2D and glucose intolerant subjects the levels of nesfatin were increased,[63] whereas in patients with insulin resistance–associated polycystic ovary syndrome (PCOS) these levels were shown to be decreased.[64] Nesfatin is thought to act on beta cells by exerting a direct, glucose-dependent insulinotropic action.[65,66] In contrast, omentin is expressed in the stromal vascular cells of the visceral adipose and has been shown to enhance insulin-stimulated glucose uptake without affecting the basal influx of glucose.[67] Levels of omentin in the serum of fasting patients have been shown to negatively correlate with Homeostasis Model of Assessment - Insulin Resistance (HOMA-IR) scores and positively correlate with serum levels of adiponectin.[68]

All of these newly identified players involved in adipose tissue signaling have substantive roles in insulin regulation and glucose homeostasis, and additional roles in the endocrine function of adipose tissue are being elucidated.

HYPOXIA

Hypoxia is the deprivation of adequate oxygen from tissues in the body and is a common issue found in obese patients, particularly in adipose tissue, and is thought to be one of the mechanisms by which proinflammatory adipose signaling is initiated and maintained.[16] Hypoxia is associated with obesity because of hypertrophy increasing the size of adipose cell to 140 to 180 μm, which is more than the 100 μm diffusion distance of oxygen.[69] One of the key symptoms of obesity-related hypoxia on adipose tissue is the release of adipokines (adipose-originated cytokines) that cause widespread systemic inflammation.[6] On a molecular level the hypoxic response is complex with an alternative mRNA expression profile unique to hypoxic adipose tissue[16] that in recent years has been investigated in terms of adipose endocrine signaling.

Hepcidin

In 2011, Hintze and colleagues[70] studied the effect of hypoxic adipose tissue on hepatocyte expression of hepcidin, a signaling molecule activated by inflammation and that impairs both macrophages and enterocytes from releasing iron into the bloodstream. In a healthy body, hepcidin expression causes an important host-defense response that blocks pathogen access to the limited resource of free iron in the bloodstream.[70] Sites of pathogen infection are often also sites of inflammation, so the signaling of hepcidin works to the body's benefit under most circumstances.[70] However, obesity causes widespread inflammation, so this signal is always present, especially in regions of hypoxic adipose tissue, resulting in iron deficiency.[70] One study found that hepatocytes exposed to hypoxic adipose cell serum produced a significantly greater amount of hepcidin mRNA than the controls and the hypoxic

Table 1
Summary of the role of important adipokines in inflammation, insulin resistance and fibrosis

Adipokine	Inflammation	Insulin Resistance	Fibrosis
Adiponectin	Antiinflammatory	Suppresses	Suppresses
Leptin	Proinflammatory	Suppression effects are low because of leptin resistance	Fibrogenic action
Resistin	Proinflammatory	Possibly involved in insulin resistance; difficult to study in humans	Possibly fibrogenic
TNF-α	Proinflammatory	Impairs insulin signaling	Fibrogenic action
IL-6	Proinflammatory	No apparent effect on insulin resistance, but insulin suppresses the expression of many proinflammatory cytokines (including IL-6)	No apparent fibrogenic action, serum levels are increased in NAFLD but not significantly in more advanced stages of fibrosis
Visfatin	Proinflammatory	Regulates insulin secretion, insulin receptor phosphorylation	At least some fibrogenic effects
Vaspin	Possibly Antiinflammatory, serum levels are negatively correlated with IL-6	Insulin sensitizer	Unknown
Apelin	Possibly proinflammatory or inflammatory biomarker, serum concentrations correlate with increased inflammation	Inhibits glucose-stimulated insulin secretion	Profibrotic in the liver; antifibrogenic in cardiac tissue
Chemerin	Chemoattractant of immune cells including macrophages, regulates activity of macrophages, proinflammatory or antiinflammatory depending on tissue type	Exacerbates glucose intolerance, lowers serum insulin levels, and decreases tissue glucose uptake	Unknown

Nesfatin	Possibly antiinflammatory; antiinflammatory activity shown in rat brain model but no clear correlation in human adipose tissues	Exerts both central and peripheral insulin-sensitizing effects	Unknown
Omentin	Antiinflammatory, suppresses a key TNF-α inflammation pathway in both smooth muscle and endothelial cells	Enhances insulin-stimulated glucose uptake	Unknown
LCN2	Possibly proinflammatory, subcutaneous adipose tissue concentration is correlated with IL-6	Possibly has a role, suppresses TNF-α signaling in mouse model, but no clear link in humans	Stabilizes MMP-9 in MMP-9/LCN complex to enhance MMP-mediated matrix degradation during liver fibrosis, potential fibrosis biomarker
TSP1	Possibly proinflammatory, TSP1 expression correlates with key inflammatory factors CD68 and MCP-1, TSP1 downregulated with antiinflammatory pioglitazone treatment	Possible role, correlated with insulin resistance in both human and mouse models	Activates TGF-β to enhance progression of cardiac fibrosis during diabetes, evidence in rat models
B-cell activation factor	Proinflammatory, treatment of human adipocytes with BAFF upregulates other proinflammatory adipokines	Glucose uptake impaired in BAFF-treated adipocytes, insulin pathways possibly regulated through interaction between BAFF and BAFF receptor	Possibly profibrogenic in skin, treatment of mice with antagonist of BAFF significantly reduces fibrogenic symptoms

Abbreviations: LCN, lipocalin; MMP, matrix metallopeptidase; TGF, transforming growth factor; TSP1, thrombospondin-1.
Data from Refs.[30,33–52]

cultured adipocytes also produced significantly more IL-6 and leptin than adipocytes cultured in normal oxygen conditions.[70] The STAT3 promoter, upregulated in the hypoxic group, was the source of this expression because the mutation of the STAT3 promoter highly inhibited the activity of the hypoxic adipocyte group, reducing expression to that of the controls.[70]

H1F1

Many different cellular processes are altered in adipose tissue during hypoxia conditions. H1F1 is a key controlling element in many hypoxic responses and in adipose tissue, inducing the buildup of the Extracellular Matrix (ECM) that brings inflammatory cells and overall dysregulation to adipose tissue.[71] The H1F1 response is unique to adipose tissue because in most tissues it produces a beneficial effect.[71] H1F1 (Histone Cluster 1, H1a) is part of the hypoxia-inducible factor (HIF) family and is a heterodimer composed of H1F1α and H1F1β (also known as Aryl Hydrocarbon Receptor Nuclear [ARNT]), which are each transcribed under different circumstances.[72] H1F1β or ARNT is constitutively expressed at low levels, whereas H1F1α is both expressed and induced constitutively.[71,72] H1F1α is unstable under oxygenated conditions and so is only functionally present at high levels during hypoxia, allowing it to sense and produce a response in hypoxic conditions.[71,72] In 2011, Jiang and colleagues[72] studied both H1F1α knockout mice and ARNT knockout mice to see the effect of HIF1 signaling inhibition on insulin resistance in the adipose tissue of mice fed a high-fat diet (HFD) and found that inhibition of HIF1 in adipose tissue improves obesity and insulin resistance. Furthermore, this improvement is associated with decreased expression of SOC3 and the induction of adiponectin. Adiponectin has far-reaching consequences, and increased secretion has been consistently linked to higher insulin sensitivity in muscle and liver tissues, further showing how adipose tissue carries an important endocrine affect.[72] The study also found that the inflammatory and insulin resistance–linked molecules TNF-α and PAI-1had decreased expression in the transgene mice, further exhibiting the importance of HIF1 signaling.[72] In addition, although several adipogenesis genes were upregulated by HFD in the transgene mice, the size and amount of adipoctyes did not increase.[72] This indicates that adipogenesis depends on HIF1, not just diet, and in some way alterations in that signaling contribute to obesity.[72]

Sun and colleagues[71] studied the effects of inhibiting H1F1α on the WAT pads of obese mice fed an HFD, and mice treated with the H1F1α inhibitor PX-478 experienced a wide range of metabolic benefits including increased glucose tolerance and lower glucose and triacylglycerides in the bloodstream. The important adipokine, leptin, reached normal levels of circulation in HFD PX-478 mice with higher overall metabolism levels and increased energy expenditure than the HFD control.[71] The HFD PX-478 mice also showed browning of white adipose cells, suggesting further metabolic improvement compared with the HFD control group.[71] Fibrosis through the ECM and inflammation were also lower in PX-478 mice than in the HFD control.[71]

Mitochondrial Dysfunction

Mitochondrial dysfunction is one of the key issues that contribute to insulin resistance in obese individuals.[69] In adipocytes, failure of mitochondria decreases the release of adiponectin, contributing to insulin resistance and low glucose utilization.[69] Two pathways control mitochondrial disruption: an HIF-1α and a non–HIF-1α route.[69] A 2013 study by Jang and colleagues[69] found that ATF3 could be the factor involved in the non–HIF-1α route. The same team discovered that ATF3 has higher expression in obese mouse WAT, and that ATF3 lowered the expression of adiponectin and inhibits the expression of adiponectin receptors in 3T3-L1 preadipose tissue cells.[69] Cell cultures with ATF3 overexpression or that were hypoxic had considerable mitochondrial impairment as measured by lower ATP production; lower mitochondrial membrane potential; lower nicotinamide adenine dinucleotide dehydrogenase, reduced form, dehydrogenase activity; and lower expression of mitochondrial genes compared with the control.[69] Of particular importance was the lowered expression of NRF-1, a key controlling gene of mitochondrial function.[69] ATF3 lowered NRF-1 promoter activity and is a good candidate for the pathway being disrupted in adipose tissue by ATF3.[69] Further evidence pointing to ATF3 is that the knockdown or deletion of ATF3 recovered some mitochondrial function, also possibly presenting ATF3 as a potential drug target in treating obesity.[69]

INFLAMMATION

Along with the hypoxic response, the accumulation of adipose tissue causes the release of inflammatory cytokines (referred to as adipokines when associated with adipose tissue), which typically result in low-grade inflammation throughout adipose tissue.[73] Adipose tissue inflammation is not always direct and involves several different molecular pathways from the direct release of inflammatory signals, to the lowering of antiinflammatory signals, to the release of signals that lead to the recruitment of macrophages.[74] Macrophage recruitment is a key component of inflammation in human adipose tissue because macrophages also secrete signals that influence the inflammatory response.[75] Many proinflammatory cytokines, such as TNF-α and IL-6 are secreted by macrophages once imbedded in adipose tissue.[30] Macrophage recruitment is so central to inflammation that CD68, expressed on macrophages, is considered to be an indicator of adipose inflammation, even though its direct role is macrophage recruitment (**Fig. 2**).[74]

Resistin, a cysteine-rich adipose-derived peptide hormone encoded by the RETN gene, is probably the best-characterized adipokine with a primary inflammatory role in adipose tissue during obesity.[5] Resistin also plays a role in insulin resistance, which occurs alongside the inflammation of adipose tissue during obesity and is thought to be a mechanistic link between these two symptoms.[5] Resistin has also been shown to influence several metabolic disorders, including heart disease.[5,76] A 2012 study of Indian postmenopausal women found that, in SAT resistin mRNA expression was directly correlated with serum resistin and, controversially, increased BMI.[77]

Also important to inflammation during obesity is the 244-amino-acid polypeptide, adiponectin, an antiinflammatory adipokine produced by adipocytes with several therapeutic benefits.[73,74] Adiponectin has many different functions in the body and is able to boost the expression of antiinflammatory signals such as IL-10 and IL-1RA to lower inflammation.[73] Adiponectin also lowers the expression of C-reactive protein, a metabolic biomarker of inflammation in the body.[78] The expression of adiponectin is decreased during obesity[79] and is thought to lead to a widespread low-grade inflammation in adipose tissue,[73] whereas weight loss has a positive impact on adiponectin recovery, as shown in a 2012 study on patients who had had bariatric surgery and who showed significantly increased adiponectin as they lost weight.[73] Even without weight loss, aerobic exercise can have a positive effect on recovering adiponectin levels during obesity, but this effect may vary based on underlying genetics.[80] Much like resistin, adiponectin plays an important role in heart disease inflammation; decreasing levels of adiponectin have been correlated with vascular inflammation.[81]

Newly discovered adipokines are filling in a lot of the blanks in the pathways involved in obesity-related inflammation. One of these new adipokines is thrombospondin-1

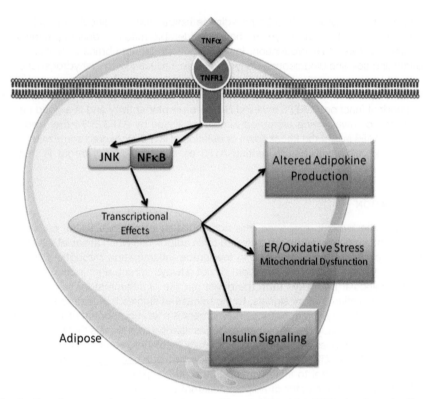

Fig. 2. Signaling cascades and downstream effects initiated by TNF-α in visceral adipose tissue. ER, endoplasmic reticulum; TNFR, tumor necrosis factor receptor.

(TSP1), which was first to be recognized as a proinflammatory adipokine in a 2010 study by Varma and colleagues[30] from human adipose biopsy tissue. In addition to TSP1 expression being correlated with increased BMI and insulin resistance, the concentration of TSP1 production also correlated with several macrophage-related inflammatory biomarkers.[30] The most intriguing component of TSP1 is that it is produced by both adipocytes and macrophages in adipose tissue during obesity, suggesting a strong crosstalk between the pathways of macrophage-induced and adipose-induced inflammation.[30]

Another new adipokine is B-cell activation factor (BAFF), which was recently discovered to be expressed with the BAFF receptor in adipose tissue by Kim and colleagues[47] in a 2009 study. Outside of adipose tissue, BAFF has an important role in the immune system and contributes to B-cell maturation and survival.[47] BAFF mRNA was detected in cultured 3T3-L1 cells and tested under inflammatory and antiinflammatory conditions.[47] BAFF increased during adipocyte differentiation and briefly under TNF-α stimulation.[47] BAFF decreased when exposed to the antiinflammatory drug rosiglitazone, suggesting a possible inflammatory role.[47]

INSULIN RESISTANCE

In addition to inflammation, perhaps the most common and well-recognized symptom of obesity is insulin resistance. Disruptions in insulin signaling, especially growing insensitivity to insulin, not only result in diabetes, but are strongly associated with all of the other comorbidities of metabolic syndrome.[82] Many adipokines have a potential role in insulin resistance, although not all of these are well understood. For instance, the role of resistin in insulin resistance has been heavily contested, with different studies showing different results.[77] Adiponectin is thought to play a crucial role in insulin sensitivity, via increased glucose use and fatty acid oxidation,[83] inhibition of serine kinases that antagonize insulin signaling,[84] and increased mitochondrial biogenesis,[84] and it is thought to involve the receptor-dependent activation of the 5'-AMP to activated protein kinase. Recent research has indicated that the insulin-sensitizing and antiapoptotic actions of adiponectin may in part be caused by its effects on sphingolipid metabolism.[85]

Leptin is also an important adipokine involved in insulin signaling, with high leptin expression correlating directly with insulin resistance.[86] A 2013 study on weight loss through calorie restriction on obese women found that leptin was correlated with insulin resistance during obesity and was also inversely correlated with increasing insulin sensitivity after weight loss.[86] However, these correlations with leptin were not as strong as the correlations observed in the same study with adiponectin.[86]

TNF-α is perhaps the best investigated of the various cytokines within this context.[87] TNF-α has a proinflammatory role and is produced at higher levels in the adipose tissues of obese individuals compared with lean individuals.[88] Two forms of TNF-α exist: soluble TNF-α, and membrane-bound TNF-α (mTNF-α).[87] Both types of TNF-α can end up in the bloodstream, with mTNF-α being released through a more complex route involving ectodomain shedding[87] and proteolytic cleavage.[89] TNF-α influences metabolic functions and insulin resistance in obesity through a variety of pathways that are not all well understood.[89] One proposed pathway through which TNF-α affects insulin resistance is through the phosphatidylinositol 3-kinase and the p80 TNF receptor, which is overexpressed in obesity.[89] Chronic exposure to TNF-α correlated with plasminogen activator inhibitor-1 (PAI-1) expression in 3T3-L1 adipocytes via the protein kinase C (PKC) pathway.[90] PAI-1 is another adipokine[86] that is correlated with cardiovascular dysfunction and metabolic insulin resistance.[90] One study found that the longer the cells were exposed to TNF-α, the more complex and alternative pathways were activated in the induction of PAI-1 expression, showing the large variety in potential signaling pathways involving TNF-α.[90] TNF-α has also been found to cause insulin resistance through the inhibitor of kappa light polypeptide (IKK)-NFκB and Janus N-terminal Kinase (JNK)-AP1 pathways.[91] Recent research indicates that chemokines expressed by adipocytes under obesity-associated chronic inflammation are reduced by NF-κB inactivation and increased by NF-κB activation, suggesting that their expression is heavily regulated by NF-κB.[92] Despite these promising advances, more research needs to be done to fully elucidate the role of TNF-α in insulin resistance (see **Fig. 2**).

HORMONE IMBALANCES

Hormone imbalances are also a side effect of obesity and tend to result in certain gender-specific symptoms.[4] A comprehensive 9-year study of the effect of reproductive hormones in women across different stages of menopause and with different BMIs found increased concentrations of serum free androgens and decreased serum concentrations of sex hormone–binding globulin (SHBG) in obese women.[93] Overexpression of androgens in women can result in metabolic disorders, most notably PCOS, which itself may contribute to the risk of developing NAFLD.[4,94] SHBG binds to androgens in the body, sequestering the molecules from the serum and effectively lowering the hormonal effect.[4] Therefore, decreased expression of SHBG multiplies the effect of high concentrations of androgens, and the production of SHBG is blocked by serum insulin.[4] A 2012 study of hyperexpression of testosterone in women with PCOS and women without PCOS found no correlation between testosterone and BMI in either group, whereas SHBG did have an inverse relationship with increasing BMI, suggesting a connection with the expression of insulin.[4]

SUMMARY

Obesity is currently one the largest epidemics in the industrialized world. It is also the nexus on which numerous costly chronic diseases, such as hypertension, hyperlipidemia, T2D, and many others cross. In light of both the health and health care impacts of these ranges of diseases, obesity must be studied as a progenitor condition rather than an incidental condition deriving from other disease states. Over the last decade, important contributions have been made to the understanding of adipose as an endocrine organ. However, the interplay between the signaling cascades connecting the major outcomes of obesity (namely, inflammation, insulin resistance, and hormone deregulation) have yet to be untangled. Adipose is a highly functional endocrine organ, and, in obese persons, one of the most prolific sources of proinflammatory signaling with organism-wide impact. Thus, the role of adipose tissue as an endocrine organ needs to be further studied from the isolated disease perspective as well as the systemic chronic disease perspective.

REFERENCES

1. Ogden CL, Carroll MD, Curtin LR. Prevalence of overweight and obesity in the United States, 1999-2004. JAMA 2006;295(13):1549–55. http://dx.doi.org/10.1001/jama.295.13.1549.
2. Banke E, Riva M, Shcherbina L, et al. Cocaine- and amphetamine-regulated transcript is expressed in adipocytes and regulate lipid-and glucose homeostasis. Regul Pept 2013;182:35–40. Available at: http://www.sciencedirect.com/science/article/pii/S0167011513000128. Accessed June 8, 2013.
3. Guo C-A, Kogan S, Amano SU, et al. CD40 deficiency in mice exacerbates obesity-induced adipose tissue inflammation, hepatic steatosis, and insulin resistance. Am J Physiol Endocrinol Metab 2013;304(9):E951–63. http://dx.doi.org/10.1152/ajpendo.00514.2012.
4. Yasmin E, Balen AH, Barth JH. The association of body mass index and biochemical hyperandrogenaemia in women with and without polycystic ovary syndrome. Eur J Obstet Gynecol Reprod Biol 2012. Available at: http://www.sciencedirect.com/science/article/pii/S0301211512004484. Accessed June 8, 2013.
5. Kang S-W, Kim MS, Kim H-S, et al. Celastrol attenuates adipokine resistin-associated matrix interaction and migration of vascular smooth muscle cells. J Cell Biochem 2013;114(2):398–408. Available at: http://onlinelibrary.wiley.com/doi/10.1002/jcb.24374/full. Accessed June 8, 2013.
6. Tkacova R, Ukropec J, Skyba P, et al. Effects of hypoxia on adipose tissue expression of NFκB, IκBα, IKKγ and IKAP in patients with chronic obstructive pulmonary disease. Cell Biochem Biophys 2012;1–6. Available at: http://link.springer.com/article/10.1007/s12013-012-9391-9. Accessed June 8, 2013.
7. Suzuki K, Harada N, Yamane S, et al. Transcriptional regulatory factor X6 (Rfx6) increases gastric inhibitory polypeptide (GIP) expression in enteroendocrine K-cells and is involved in GIP hypersecretion in high fat diet-induced obesity. J Biol Chem 2013;288(3):1929–38. Available at: http://www.jbc.org/content/288/3/1929.short. Accessed June 8, 2013.

8. Kiezun M, Maleszka A, Smolinska N, et al. Expression of adiponectin receptors 1 (AdipoR1) and 2 (AdipoR2) in the porcine pituitary during the oestrous cycle. Reprod Biol Endocrinol 2013;11:18. http://dx.doi.org/10.1186/1477-7827-11-18.
9. Hsuchou H, Jayaram B, Kastin AJ, et al. Endothelial cell leptin receptor mutant mice have hyperleptinemia and reduced tissue uptake. J Cell Physiol 2013; 228(7):1610–6. http://dx.doi.org/10.1002/jcp.24325.
10. Coulon S, Francque S, Colle I, et al. Evaluation of inflammatory and angiogenic factors in patients with non-alcoholic fatty liver disease. Cytokine 2012;59(2): 442–9. http://dx.doi.org/10.1016/j.cyto.2012.05.001.
11. Younossi ZM, Stepanova M, Rafiq N, et al. Pathologic criteria for nonalcoholic steatohepatitis: interprotocol agreement and ability to predict liver-related mortality. Hepatology 2011;53(6):1874–82. http://dx.doi.org/10.1002/hep.24268.
12. Welsh JA, Karpen S, Vos MB. Increasing Prevalence of nonalcoholic fatty liver disease among United States adolescents, 1988-1994 to 2007-2010. J Pediatr 2013;162(3):496–500.e1. http://dx.doi.org/10.1016/j.jpeds.2012.08.043.
13. Fuchs CD, Claudel T, Kumari P, et al. Absence of adipose triglyceride lipase protects from hepatic endoplasmic reticulum stress in mice. Hepatology 2012; 56(1):270–80. http://dx.doi.org/10.1002/hep.25601.
14. Gentile CL, Nivala AM, Gonzales JC, et al. Experimental evidence for therapeutic potential of taurine in the treatment of nonalcoholic fatty liver disease. Am J Physiol Regul Integr Comp Physiol 2011;301(6):R1710–22. http://dx.doi.org/10.1152/ajpregu.00677.2010.
15. Valenti L, Rametta R, Ruscica M, et al. The i148m Pnpla3 polymorphism influences serum adiponectin in patients with fatty liver and healthy controls. BMC Gastroenterol 2012;12. http://dx.doi.org/10.1186/1471-230X-12-111.
16. Hodson L, Humphreys SM, Karpe F, et al. Metabolic signatures of human adipose tissue hypoxia in obesity. Diabetes 2013;62(5):1417–25. http://dx.doi.org/10.2337/db12-1032.
17. Gonzalez-Rodriguez A, Mas-Gutierrez JA, Mirasierra M, et al. Essential role of protein tyrosine phosphatase 1B in obesity-induced inflammation and peripheral insulin resistance during aging. Aging Cell 2012;11(2):284–96. http://dx.doi.org/10.1111/j.1474-9726.2011.00786.x.
18. Ho GY, Wang T, Gunter MJ, et al. Adipokines linking obesity with colorectal cancer risk in postmenopausal women. Cancer Res 2012;72(12):3029–37. http://dx.doi.org/10.1158/0008-5472.CAN-11-2771.
19. Al Awadhi SA, Al Khaldi RM, Al Rammah T, et al. Associations of adipokines & insulin resistance with sex steroids in patients with breast cancer. Indian J Med Res 2012;135(4):500–5.
20. Lasar D, Julius A, Fromme T, et al. Browning attenuates murine white adipose tissue expansion during postnatal development. Biochim Biophys Acta 2013; 1831(5):960–8. http://dx.doi.org/10.1016/j.bbalip.2013.01.016.
21. Frontini A, Vitali A, Perugini J, et al. White-to-brown transdifferentiation of omental adipocytes in patients affected by pheochromocytoma. Biochim Biophys Acta 2013;1831(5):950–9. http://dx.doi.org/10.1016/j.bbalip.2013.02.005.
22. Shan T, Liang X, Bi P, et al. Myostatin knockout drives browning of white adipose tissue through activating the AMPK-PGC1 alpha-Fndc5 pathway in muscle. FASEB J 2013;27(5):1981–9. http://dx.doi.org/10.1096/fj.12-225755.
23. Gaffney EF, Hargreaves HK, Semple E, et al. Hibernoma: distinctive light and electron microscopic features and relationship to brown adipose tissue. Hum Pathol 1983;14(8):677–87.

24. Cypess AM, Lehman S, Williams G, et al. Identification and importance of brown adipose tissue in adult humans. N Engl J Med 2009;360(15):1509–17. http://dx.doi.org/10.1056/NEJMoa0810780.

25. Cypess AM, White AP, Vernochet C, et al. Anatomical localization, gene expression profiling and functional characterization of adult human neck brown fat. Nat Med 2013;19(5):635–9. http://dx.doi.org/10.1038/nm.3112.

26. Barneda D, Frontini A, Cinti S, et al. Dynamic changes in lipid droplet-associated proteins in the "browning" of white adipose tissues. Biochim Biophys Acta 2013;1831(5):924–33. http://dx.doi.org/10.1016/j.bbalip.2013.01.015.

27. Diaz ES, Karlan BY, Li AJ. Obesity-associated adipokines correlate with survival in epithelial ovarian cancer. Gynecol Oncol 2013;129(2):353–7. http://dx.doi.org/10.1016/j.ygyno.2013.02.006.

28. Sharp LZ, Shinoda K, Ohno H, et al. Human BAT possesses molecular signatures that resemble beige/brite cells. PLoS One 2012;7(11). http://dx.doi.org/10.1371/journal.pone.0049452.

29. Colca JR, McDonald WG, Cavey GS, et al. Identification of a mitochondrial target of thiazolidinedione insulin sensitizers (mTOT)—Relationship to newly identified mitochondrial pyruvate carrier proteins. PLoS One 2013;8(5):e61551. http://dx.doi.org/10.1371/journal.pone.0061551.

30. Varma V, Yao-Borengasser A, Bodles AM, et al. Thrombospondin-1 is an adipokine associated with obesity, adipose inflammation, and insulin resistance. Diabetes 2008;57(2):432–9. http://dx.doi.org/10.2337/db07-0840.

31. Auguet T, Terra X, Porras JA, et al. Plasma visfatin levels and gene expression in morbidly obese women with associated fatty liver disease. Clin Biochem 2013; 46(3):202–8. http://dx.doi.org/10.1016/j.clinbiochem.2012.11.006.

32. Terra X, Auguet T, Quesada I, et al. Increased levels and adipose tissue expression of visfatin in morbidly obese women: the relationship with pro-inflammatory cytokines. Clin Endocrinol (Oxf) 2012;77(5):691–8. http://dx.doi.org/10.1111/j.1365-2265.2011.04327.x.

33. Kazama K, Usui T, Okada M, et al. Omentin plays an anti-inflammatory role through inhibition of TNF-α-induced superoxide production in vascular smooth muscle cells. Eur J Pharmacol 2012;686(1–3):116–23. http://dx.doi.org/10.1016/j.ejphar.2012.04.033.

34. Saldanha JF, Carrero JJ, Lobo JC, et al. The newly identified anorexigenic adipokine nesfatin-1 in hemodialysis patients: are there associations with food intake, body composition and inflammation? Regul Pept 2012;173(1–3):82–5. http://dx.doi.org/10.1016/j.regpep.2011.09.010.

35. Tang C-H, Fu X-J, Xu X-L, et al. The anti-inflammatory and anti-apoptotic effects of nesfatin-1 in the traumatic rat brain. Peptides 2012;36(1):39–45. http://dx.doi.org/10.1016/j.peptides.2012.04.014.

36. Chakaroun R, Raschpichler M, Klöting N, et al. Effects of weight loss and exercise on chemerin serum concentrations and adipose tissue expression in human obesity. Metabolism 2012;61(5):706–14. http://dx.doi.org/10.1016/j.metabol.2011.10.008.

37. Yamawaki H, Kameshima S, Usui T, et al. A novel adipocytokine, chemerin exerts anti-inflammatory roles in human vascular endothelial cells. Biochem Biophys Res Commun 2012;423(1):152–7. http://dx.doi.org/10.1016/j.bbrc.2012.05.103.

38. Herenius MM, Oliveira AS, Wijbrandts CA, et al. Anti-TNF therapy reduces serum levels of chemerin in rheumatoid arthritis: a new mechanism by which

anti-TNF might reduce inflammation. PLoS One 2013;8(2):e57802. http://dx.doi. org/10.1371/journal.pone.0057802.

39. Leite NC, Salles GF, Cardoso CR, et al. Serum biomarkers in type 2 diabetic patients with non-alcoholic steatohepatitis and advanced fibrosis. Hepatol Res 2013;43(5):508–15. http://dx.doi.org/10.1111/j.1872-034X.2012.01106.x.

40. Manning PJ, Sutherland WH, Williams SM, et al. Oral but not intravenous glucose acutely decreases circulating interleukin-6 concentrations in overweight individuals. PLoS One 2013;8(6):e66395. http://dx.doi.org/10.1371/journal.pone. 0066395.

41. Yamawaki H, Kuramoto J, Kameshima S, et al. Omentin, a novel adipocytokine inhibits TNF-induced vascular inflammation in human endothelial cells. Biochem Biophys Res Commun 2011;408(2):339–43. http://dx.doi.org/10.1016/j.bbrc. 2011.04.039.

42. Ordoñez FJ, Fornieles-Gonzalez G, Rosety MA, et al. Anti-inflammatory effect of exercise, via reduced leptin levels, in obese women with Down syndrome. Int J Sports Physiol Perform 2012. [Epub ahead of print].

43. Das S, Kumar A, Seth RK, et al. Proinflammatory adipokine leptin mediates disinfection byproduct bromodichloromethane-induced early steatohepatitic injury in obesity. Toxicol Appl Pharmacol 2013;269(3):297–306. http://dx.doi. org/10.1016/j.taap.2013.02.003.

44. Matsushita T, Fujimoto M, Hasegawa M, et al. BAFF antagonist attenuates the development of skin fibrosis in tight-skin mice. J Invest Dermatol 2007; 127(12):2772–80. http://dx.doi.org/10.1038/sj.jid.5700919.

45. Li Y, Tong X, Rumala C, et al. Thrombospondin1 deficiency reduces obesity-associated inflammation and improves insulin sensitivity in a diet-induced obese mouse model. PLoS One 2011;6(10):e26656. http://dx.doi.org/10.1371/journal. pone.0026656.

46. Law IK, Xu A, Lam KS, et al. Lipocalin-2 deficiency attenuates insulin resistance associated with aging and obesity. Diabetes 2010;59(4):872–82. http://dx.doi. org/10.2337/db09-1541.

47. Kim YH, Choi BH, Cheon HG, et al. B cell activation factor (BAFF) is a novel adipokine that links obesity and inflammation. Exp Mol Med 2009;41(3):208–16. http://dx.doi.org/10.3858/emm.2009.41.3.024.

48. Kim J-W, Lee SH, Jeong S-H, et al. Increased urinary lipocalin-2 reflects matrix metalloproteinase-9 activity in chronic hepatitis C with hepatic fibrosis. Tohoku J Exp Med 2010;222(4):319–27.

49. Hamada M, Abe M, Miyake T, et al. B cell-activating factor controls the production of adipokines and induces insulin resistance. Obesity (Silver Spring) 2011; 19(10):1915–22. http://dx.doi.org/10.1038/oby.2011.165.

50. Belmadani S, Bernal J, Wei C-C, et al. A thrombospondin-1 antagonist of transforming growth factor-beta activation blocks cardiomyopathy in rats with diabetes and elevated angiotensin II. Am J Pathol 2007;171(3):777–89. http://dx. doi.org/10.2353/ajpath.2007.070056.

51. Avouac J, Clemessy M, Distler JH, et al. Enhanced expression of ephrins and thrombospondins in the dermis of patients with early diffuse systemic sclerosis: potential contribution to perturbed angiogenesis and fibrosis. Rheumatology (Oxford) 2011;50(8):1494–504. http://dx.doi.org/10.1093/rheumatology/ keq448.

52. Auguet T, Quintero Y, Terra X, et al. Upregulation of lipocalin 2 in adipose tissues of severely obese women: positive relationship with proinflammatory cytokines.

Obesity (Silver Spring) 2011;19(12):2295–300. http://dx.doi.org/10.1038/oby.2011.61.

53. Fain JN, Madan AK, Hiler ML, et al. Comparison of the release of adipokines by adipose tissue, adipose tissue matrix, and adipocytes from visceral and subcutaneous abdominal adipose tissues of obese humans. Endocrinology 2004; 145(5):2273–82. http://dx.doi.org/10.1210/en.2003-1336.

54. Fain JN, Bahouth SW, Madan AK. Involvement of multiple signaling pathways in the post-bariatric induction of IL-6 and IL-8 mRNA and release in human visceral adipose tissue. Biochem Pharmacol 2005;69(9):1315–24. http://dx.doi.org/10.1016/j.bcp.2005.02.009.

55. Kirovski G, Dorn C, Huber H, et al. Elevated systemic monocyte chemoattractant protein-1 in hepatic steatosis without significant hepatic inflammation. Exp Mol Pathol 2011;91(3):780–3. http://dx.doi.org/10.1016/j.yexmp.2011.08.001.

56. Brown JE, Onyango DJ, Ramanjaneya M, et al. Visfatin regulates insulin secretion, insulin receptor signalling and mRNA expression of diabetes-related genes in mouse pancreatic beta-cells. J Mol Endocrinol 2010;44(3):171–8. http://dx.doi.org/10.1677/JME-09-0071.

57. Hida K, Wada J, Eguchi J, et al. Visceral adipose tissue-derived serine protease inhibitor: a unique insulin-sensitizing adipocytokine in obesity. Proc Natl Acad Sci U S A 2005;102(30):10610–5. http://dx.doi.org/10.1073/pnas.0504703102.

58. Jeong E, Youn B-S, Kim DW, et al. Circadian rhythm of serum vaspin in healthy male volunteers: relation to meals. J Clin Endocrinol Metab 2010;95(4):1869–75. http://dx.doi.org/10.1210/jc.2009-1088.

59. Klöting N, Berndt J, Kralisch S, et al. Vaspin gene expression in human adipose tissue: association with obesity and type 2 diabetes. Biochem Biophys Res Commun 2006;339(1):430–6. http://dx.doi.org/10.1016/j.bbrc.2005.11.039.

60. Ercin CN, Dogru T, Tapan S, et al. Plasma apelin levels in subjects with nonalcoholic fatty liver disease. Metabolism 2010;59(7):977–81. http://dx.doi.org/10.1016/j.metabol.2009.10.019.

61. Ernst MC, Issa M, Goralski KB, et al. Chemerin exacerbates glucose intolerance in mouse models of obesity and diabetes. Endocrinology 2010;151(5):1998–2007. http://dx.doi.org/10.1210/en.2009-1098.

62. Wanninger J, Bauer S, Eisinger K, et al. Adiponectin upregulates hepatocyte CMKLR1 which is reduced in human fatty liver. Mol Cell Endocrinol 2012; 349(2):248–54. http://dx.doi.org/10.1016/j.mce.2011.10.032.

63. Zhang Z, Li L, Yang M, et al. Increased plasma levels of nesfatin-1 in patients with newly diagnosed type 2 diabetes mellitus. Exp Clin Endocrinol Diabetes 2012;120(2):91–5. http://dx.doi.org/10.1055/s-0031-1286339.

64. Deniz R, Gurates B, Aydin S, et al. Nesfatin-1 and other hormone alterations in polycystic ovary syndrome. Endocrine 2012;42(3):694–9. http://dx.doi.org/10.1007/s12020-012-9638-7.

65. Gonzalez R, Reingold BK, Gao X, et al. Nesfatin-1 exerts a direct, glucose-dependent insulinotropic action on mouse islet β- and MIN6 cells. J Endocrinol 2011;208(3):R9–16. http://dx.doi.org/10.1530/JOE-10-0492.

66. Nakata M, Manaka K, Yamamoto S, et al. Nesfatin-1 enhances glucose-induced insulin secretion by promoting Ca(2+) influx through L-type channels in mouse islet β-cells. Endocr J 2011;58(4):305–13.

67. Yang R-Z, Lee M-J, Hu H, et al. Identification of omentin as a novel depot-specific adipokine in human adipose tissue: possible role in modulating insulin

action. Am J Physiol Endocrinol Metab 2006;290(6):E1253–61. http://dx.doi.org/10.1152/ajpendo.00572.2004.

68. Yan P, Liu D, Long M, et al. Changes of serum omentin levels and relationship between omentin and adiponectin concentrations in type 2 diabetes mellitus. Exp Clin Endocrinol Diabetes 2011;119(4):257–63. http://dx.doi.org/10.1055/s-0030-1269912.

69. Jang M-K, Son Y, Jung MH. ATF3 plays a role in adipocyte hypoxia-mediated mitochondria dysfunction in obesity. Biochem Biophys Res Commun 2013; 431(3):421–7. http://dx.doi.org/10.1016/j.bbrc.2012.12.154.

70. Hintze KJ, Snow D, Nabor D, et al. Adipocyte hypoxia increases hepatocyte hepcidin expression. Biol Trace Elem Res 2011;143(2):764–71. http://dx.doi.org/10.1007/s12011-010-8932-6.

71. Sun K, Halberg N, Khan M, et al. Selective inhibition of hypoxia-inducible factor 1α ameliorates adipose tissue dysfunction. Mol Cell Biol 2013;33(5):904–17. http://dx.doi.org/10.1128/MCB.00951-12.

72. Jiang C, Qu A, Matsubara T, et al. Disruption of hypoxia-inducible factor 1 in adipocytes improves insulin sensitivity and decreases adiposity in high-fat diet-fed mice. Diabetes 2011;60(10):2484–95. http://dx.doi.org/10.2337/db11-0174.

73. Illán-Gómez F, Gonzálvez-Ortega M, Orea-Soler I, et al. Obesity and inflammation: change in adiponectin, C-reactive protein, tumour necrosis factor-alpha and interleukin-6 after bariatric surgery. Obes Surg 2012;22(6):950–5. http://dx.doi.org/10.1007/s11695-012-0643-y.

74. Lallukka S, Sevastianova K, Perttila J, et al. Adipose tissue is inflamed in NAFLD due to obesity but not in NAFLD due to genetic variation in PNPLA3. Diabetologia 2013;56(4):886–92. http://dx.doi.org/10.1007/s00125-013-2829-9.

75. Johnston A, Arnadottir S, Gudjonsson JE, et al. Obesity in psoriasis: leptin and resistin as mediators of cutaneous inflammation. Br J Dermatol 2008;159(2): 342–50. http://dx.doi.org/10.1111/j.1365-2133.2008.08655.x.

76. Bobbert P, Jenke A, Bobbert T, et al. High leptin and resistin expression in chronic heart failure: adverse outcome in patients with dilated and inflammatory cardiomyopathy. Eur J Heart Fail 2012;14(11):1265–75. http://dx.doi.org/10.1093/eurjhf/hfs111.

77. Sadashiv SK, Tiwari S, Paul BN, et al. Over expression of resistin in adipose tissue of the obese induces insulin resistance. World J Diabetes 2012;3(7): 135–41. http://dx.doi.org/10.4239/wjd.v3.i7.135.

78. Ahonen TM, Saltevo JT, Kautiainen HJ, et al. The association of adiponectin and low-grade inflammation with the course of metabolic syndrome. Nutr Metab Cardiovasc Dis 2012;22(3):285–91. http://dx.doi.org/10.1016/j.numecd.2010.07.001.

79. Arita Y, Kihara S, Ouchi N, et al. Paradoxical decrease of an adipose-specific protein, adiponectin, in obesity. Biochem Biophys Res Commun 1999;257(1): 79–83. http://dx.doi.org/10.1006/bbrc.1999.0255.

80. Lee K-Y, Kang H-S, Shin Y-A. Exercise improves adiponectin concentrations irrespective of the adiponectin gene polymorphisms SNP45 and the SNP276 in obese Korean women. Gene 2013;516(2):271–6. http://dx.doi.org/10.1016/j.gene.2012.12.028.

81. Choi HY, Kim S, Yang SJ, et al. Association of adiponectin, resistin, and vascular inflammation: analysis with 18F-fluorodeoxyglucose positron emission tomography. Arterioscler Thromb Vasc Biol 2011;31(4):944–9. http://dx.doi.org/10.1161/ATVBAHA.110.220673.

82. Brännmark C, Nyman E, Fagerholm S, et al. Insulin signaling in type 2 diabetes: experimental and modeling analyses reveal mechanisms of insulin resistance in human adipocytes. J Biol Chem 2013;288(14):9867–80. http://dx.doi.org/10.1074/jbc.M112.432062.

83. Yamauchi T, Kamon J, Minokoshi Y, et al. Adiponectin stimulates glucose utilization and fatty-acid oxidation by activating AMP-activated protein kinase. Nat Med 2002;8(11):1288–95. http://dx.doi.org/10.1038/nm788.

84. Shibata R, Sato K, Pimentel DR, et al. Adiponectin protects against myocardial ischemia-reperfusion injury through AMPK- and COX-2-dependent mechanisms. Nat Med 2005;11(10):1096–103. http://dx.doi.org/10.1038/nm1295.

85. Holland WL, Miller RA, Wang ZV, et al. Receptor-mediated activation of ceramidase activity initiates the pleiotropic actions of adiponectin. Nat Med 2011; 17(1):55–63. http://dx.doi.org/10.1038/nm.2277.

86. Golubović MV, Dimić D, Antić S, et al. Relationship of adipokine to insulin sensitivity and glycemic regulation in obese women–the effect of body weight reduction by caloric restriction. Vojnosanit Pregl 2013;70(3):284–91.

87. Xu H, Uysal KT, Becherer JD, et al. Altered tumor necrosis factor-alpha (TNF-alpha) processing in adipocytes and increased expression of transmembrane TNF-alpha in obesity. Diabetes 2002;51(6):1876–83.

88. Hotamisligil GS, Arner P, Caro JF, et al. Increased adipose tissue expression of tumor necrosis factor-alpha in human obesity and insulin resistance. J Clin Invest 1995;95(5):2409–15. Available at: http://www.ncbi.nlm.nih.gov/pmc/articles/PMC295872/. Accessed July 12, 2013.

89. Hauner H, Bender M, Haastert B, et al. Plasma concentrations of soluble TNF-alpha receptors in obese subjects. Int J Obes Relat Metab Disord 1998;22(12):1239–43.

90. Pandey M, Loskutoff DJ, Samad F. Molecular mechanisms of tumor necrosis factor-α-mediated plasminogen activator inhibitor-1 expression in adipocytes. FASEB J 2005. http://dx.doi.org/10.1096/fj.04-3459fje.

91. Matsubara T, Mita A, Minami K, et al. PGRN is a key adipokine mediating high fat diet-induced insulin resistance and obesity through IL-6 in adipose tissue. Cell Metab 2012;15(1):38–50. http://dx.doi.org/10.1016/j.cmet.2011.12.002.

92. Tourniaire F, Romier-Crouzet B, Lee JH, et al. Chemokine expression in inflamed adipose tissue is mainly mediated by NF-κB. PLoS One 2013;8(6):e66515. http://dx.doi.org/10.1371/journal.pone.0066515.

93. Sutton-Tyrrell K, Zhao X, Santoro N, et al. Reproductive hormones and obesity: 9 years of observation from the Study of Women's Health Across the Nation. Am J Epidemiol 2010;171(11):1203–13. http://dx.doi.org/10.1093/aje/kwq049.

94. Baranova A, Tran TP, Afendy A, et al. Molecular signature of adipose tissue in patients with both non-alcoholic fatty liver disease (NAFLD) and polycystic ovarian syndrome (PCOS). J Transl Med 2013;11(1):133. http://dx.doi.org/10.1186/1479-5876-11-133.

Obesity and NAFLD
The Role of Bacteria and Microbiota

Ajay Duseja, MBBS, MD, DM, Yogesh Kumar Chawla, MBBS, MD, DM*

KEYWORDS

- Nonalcoholic fatty liver disease • Nonalcoholic steatohepatitis
- Small intestinal bacterial overgrowth • Intestinal permeability • Endotoxemia
- Toll-like receptors • Probiotics

KEY POINTS

- The term "gut microbiota" incorporates not just bacteria but also viruses and other microorganisms, such as protozoa, archaeal spp, yeasts, and parasites.
- Gut–liver axis plays a central role in the pathogenesis of obesity and NAFLD, mainly through the crosstalk of the intestinal microbiota with the host immune system modulating inflammation, insulin resistance, and intestinal permeability.
- Gut microbiota are linked to obesity through increased energy harvesting and storage and to NAFLD though the systemic inflammation, cytokines, and insulin resistance secondary to endotoxemia resulting from SIBO and increased gut permeability.

INTRODUCTION

The liver is a unique organ that receives blood supply from the portal vein and the hepatic artery. The blood in the portal vein, which drains from the mesenteric veins, contains not only products of digestion but also microbial products derived from microbes that colonize the gut. Therefore, the liver, which acts as the first site of filtration for such products, also becomes the first site of exposure to microbial products from the gut. Microbial products have been recognized to be responsible pathogenically for several disease situations of the liver and were earlier shown to be associated with hepatic encephalopathy and spontaneous bacterial peritonitis. What initially was termed as "gut flora" is now termed as "gut microbiota," which is a preferred terminology because it incorporates not just bacteria but also viruses and other microorganisms, such as protozoa, archaeal spp, yeasts, and parasites. The human gut contains more than 1000 different bacterial species with 99% belonging to about 40 species.[1] The bacterial number increases from 10^4 in the jejunum to 10^7 colony-forming units per gram of luminal content in the ileum

Disclosure and Conflict of Interest: The authors have nothing to disclose.
Department of Hepatology, Post Graduate Institute of Medical Education and Research, Sector 12, Chandigarh 160012, India
* Corresponding author.
E-mail addresses: ykchawla@hotmail.com; ykchawla@gmail.com

http://dx.doi.org/10.1016/j.cld.2013.09.002
1089-3261/14/$ – see front matter

and are mainly gram-negative aerobes and nonobligate anaerobes, whereas in the colon the number increases to 10^{12} colony-forming units per gram and are predominantly anaerobes. Genome of microbiota (microbiome) contains 100 times more genes than the human genome.[2] The human gut is sterile in utero and the acquired microbiota at the time of birth depends on the mode of delivery (ie, vaginal or caesarean section). Establishment of further bacterial flora depends on whether the infant is on breast or bottle feed. Introduction of solid food in the diet establishes the adult-type of bacterial flora.[3] The adult human gut bacterial flora consists predominantly of gram-positive Firmicutes (60%–80%) and gram-negative Bacteroidetes (20%–40%) that usually remains stable over time and is only subject to minor changes caused by age, diet, medication, infection, and intestinal surgery.[4,5] Other bacteria in the human gut include, Bifidobacteria, Proteobacteria, Fusobacteria, Cyanobacteria, Verrcomicrobia, and Spirochaetes spp. Even though most of the adult gut flora consists of Firmicutes and Bacteroidetes there are differences at the species and strain level with less than 1% similarity in the bacterial species among individuals. The gut microbiota in addition to the energy harvesting by way of digestion of complex indigestible polysaccharides, synthesis of vitamins, and fat storage (discussed later) are an important source of energy to the colonocytes. Microorganisms also secrete several bioactive metabolites with diverse functions. Thus, the gut microbiota may be regarded as a microbial organ within the gut that contributes to multiple host processes including defense against pathogens by maintaining immunity at the level of gut, synthesis of several vitamins, and development of intestinal microvilli.[1,6]

This article reviews the literature on the association of gut microbiota with obesity and nonalcoholic fatty liver disease (NAFLD).

GUT MICROBIOTA AND OBESITY

Estimated prevalence of overweight and obesity in US adults is close to 65% and 30%, respectively.[7] The figures are likely to worsen in future because of the rising problem of overweight and obesity in children.[8] Obesity is a lifestyle disease resulting from increased food intake and decreased physical activity especially in genetically predisposed individuals and has always been considered to be a state of "nutritional disequilibrium." The gut microbiota are involved in energy harvesting and its storage in the adipose tissue. Microbiota help in extracting calories from otherwise indigestible polysaccharides in the diet with the help of glycoside hydrolases and polysaccharide lysases, enzymes that are absent in humans. Microbes convert these polysaccharides to monosaccharides and short-chain fatty acids in the colon, which after absorption cause the triglyceride synthesis in the liver.[9] Microbes also suppress the intestinal epithelial expression of fasting-induced adipocyte protein (Fiaf), an inhibitor of lipoprotein lipase. Inhibition of the activity of Fiaf increases the lipoprotein lipase activity in the adipose tissue with increased storage of liver-synthesized triacyglycerols in the adipose tissue.[1] Recent literature suggests the emerging role of gut microbiota in the development of obesity and its consequence including NAFLD. Most of the data are based on animal experiments but there is emerging human data that establishes the link between the gut microbiota, obesity, and NAFLD.

One of the earlier animal studies evaluating the role of gut microbiota in obesity used germ-free (GF) mice and found that these animals despite consuming more food had 42% less body fat compared with normal animals.[2] After transplantation of cecal microbiota from normal to GF mice there was 57% increase in the total body fat without any change in the energy expenditure and food intake. The results of the study suggested the role of gut microbiota in energy harvesting and fat storage.[2] Similar results were shown in another study from the same group where despite high-calorie diet there was no gain in body weight in the mice in the absence of gut microbiota.[10] Turnbaugh and colleagues[11] transplanted the gut microbiota from obese ob/ob and lean (ob/+ or +/+) mice into lean wild-type (WT) GF mice and found that animals that received the obese-type microbiota had higher fat gain (47% ± 8.3%) than the animals that received the lean-type microbiota (27% ± 3.6%) with no difference in energy expenditure and food intake between the two groups, thereby again suggesting the role of gut microbiota in the genesis of obesity.

Studies have shown not only the quantitative difference in the gut microbiota between the obese and lean animals but also the differences in the bacterial species. A study comparing genetically obese leptin deficient (ob/ob) mice with lean (ob/+, +/+) siblings and mothers, found that obese mice had less of Bacteroidetes (50% less) and more of Firmicutes in their gut compared with lean mice.[12] Moreover the differences in the bacterial species between the two groups were not related to the difference in the food intake or total body mass. The same group also studied the microbial profiles in 12 obese human subjects and found that compared with lean subjects, obese subjects had lesser Bacteroidetes and more of Firmicutes.[13] On assigning these subjects a fat-restricted or carbohydrate-restricted low-calorie diet for 1 year and sequencing 16 S rRNA genes from their stool samples, these subjects had an increase in Bacteroidetes spp and decrease in Firmicutes spp. The change in gut microbiota correlated with the weight loss of 6% in the fat-restricted group and 2% on carbohydrate-restricted diet.[13] In another study, children were followed up until 7 years of age after baseline stool sample collection for gut microbiota at the age of 6 and 12 months. The study found that compared with lean, children who were overweight or obese at age 7 had less of Bacteroidetes spp and more of *Staphylococcus aureus* at the age 6 and 12 months.[14] These studies support the concept that gut microbiota has a relationship with body weight and different gut microbiota composition has a bearing on determining the overweight and obesity in an individual.

Pathogenesis of Microbiota-associated Obesity

Pathogenesis of microbiota-associated obesity is still unclear. Possible mechanism include increased energy harvest and fat storage, as described previously; induction of systemic inflammation; and its consequences and central effects on satiety (**Box 1**). The gut microbiota help in extracting calories from otherwise indigestible polysaccharides in the diet, converting these polysaccharides to monosaccharides and short-chain fatty acids in the colon, which after absorption cause triglyceride synthesis in the liver.[11] Microbial inhibition of the activity of Fiaf increases the lipoprotein lipase

---

Box 1
Pathogenesis of microbiota-associated obesity

- Increased energy harvest and fat storage
  - Conversion of polysaccharides to monosaccharides and short-chain fatty acids
  - Inhibition of the activity of Fiaf
- Induction of systemic inflammation
  - Altering gut permeability and endotoxemia
  - Increased eCB system tone
- Central effects on satiety

activity in the adipose tissue with increased storage of triacyglycerols in the adipose tissue. This concept has been supported by animal studies showing the increased energy harvest and increase in body fat after transplantation of obese-type microbiota in GF mice.[1] Stool examination of these animals showed more end products of fermentation and fewer calories suggesting increased energy extraction and storage by the obese-type microbiota.[11] The decreased Bacteroidetes spp and increased Firmicutes spp in obese animals and humans could also suggest that Firmicutes spp possess more diverse enzymes capable of digesting and extracting calories from complex polysaccharides.

By altering the gut permeability, the gut microbiota are also responsible for causing the endotoxemia and the systemic inflammation secondary to the downward signaling following the Toll-like receptor (TLR) stimulation (discussed later). Low-grade inflammation secondary to endotoxemia may be linked to obesity through increased endocannabinoid (eCB) system tone. Muccioli and colleagues[15] showed in an animal model that gut microbiota modulate the intestinal eCB system tone, which in turn regulates gut permeability and plasma lipopolysaccharide (LPS) levels. By using CB(1) agonist and antagonist in lean and obese mouse models, they found that the eCB system controls gut permeability and adipose tissue physiology through LPS-eCB system regulatory loops and plays an important role in adipogenesis and obesity.[15]

GUT MICROBIOTA AND NAFLD

NAFLD is a constellation of conditions histologically characterized by mainly macrovesicular hepatic steatosis in individuals who do not consume alcohol in amounts generally considered to be harmful to the liver. It is a broad term consisting of patients with simple steatosis at one end of the spectrum, nonalcoholic steatohepatitis (NASH), NASH-related cirrhosis, and hepatocellular carcinoma at the other end. For some differences, NAFLD/NASH is an important cause of unexplained rise in hepatic transaminases, cryptogenic cirrhosis, and hepatocellular carcinoma worldwide.[16,17] NAFLD is an extremely common liver disease with a prevalence as high as 46% in the general population.[18] The figures increase with presence of risk factors, such as obesity and diabetes mellitus. In a systematic review including 1620 patients with severe obesity, prevalence of steatosis and NASH was 91% (range, 85%–98%) and 37% (range, 24%–98%), respectively, with cirrhosis in 1.7% (range, 1%–7%) of patients.[19]

Pathophysiologic Basis of NAFLD

In most of the subjects, NAFLD starts with an imbalance between energy intake and expenditure that leads to adipose tissue expansion. In addition, development of NAFLD is affected by genetic predisposition and environmental factors, such as diet and physical activity.

Insulin resistance plays a major role in the pathogenesis of NAFLD. Originally, the pathogenesis of NAFLD was considered as two-hit process.[20] Liver fat accumulation was the suggested first hit or the first step because of excessive triglyceride accumulation caused by a discrepancy between influx (from diet, increased hepatic uptake from subcutaneous and visceral adipose tissue, and de novo synthesis of hepatic fat) and decreased β-oxidation, decreased apolipoprotein B100 synthesis, and decreased very-low-density lipoprotein export from the liver. After the first hit (steatosis) a second hit, such as oxidative stress with accompanying inflammation, may cause progression to NASH in some patients.[20] Recently, a modified two-hit, three-hit, and multiple-hit theories have been proposed as the possible pathophysiologic mechanisms in patients with NAFLD.[21] According to the modified two-hit hypothesis, the accumulation of free fatty acids alone has been suggested to be sufficient to induce liver damage (concept of lipotoxicity), without recourse for a second hit, and triglyceride accumulation in the form of steatosis is considered protective by preventing free fatty acid–induced injury. According to the three-hit hypothesis, a third hit has been proposed as the inadequate hepatocyte regeneration and apoptosis. The multiple-hit hypotheses suggests that multiple events acting in parallel including lipotoxicity, increased oxidative stress, mitochondrial dysfunction, iron overload, and proinflammatory cytokines lead to NASH.[21]

Risk factors for NAFLD include increasing age, overweight or obesity, diabetes mellitus, hypertension, dyslipidemia, or metabolic syndrome usually associated with insulin resistance. The interethnic difference in the prevalence of NAFLD is believed to be related not only to different lifestyles but also to a strong genetic predisposition. Several genetic polymorphisms including hemochromatosis gene, apolipoprotein C3, MC4R, and Patatin-like phospholipase domain-containing protein 3 and TLR gene polymorphisms are associated with NAFLD.[22,23] With respect to environmental factors influencing the risk of NAFLD and NASH, diet, exercise, and possibly gut microbiota are some of the candidates. The gut microbiota are involved in the pathogenesis of NAFLD by increasing gut permeability, causing low-grade inflammation, affecting dietary choline and bile acid metabolism, and by producing endogenous ethanol, ammonia, and acetaldehyde that are generally metabolized by the liver and are able to control Kupffer cell activity and cytokine production (**Box 2**).

Small intestinal bacterial overgrowth and intestinal permeability
Tight junctions link the intestinal cells and play an important role in maintaining the integrity of the intestinal barrier. Occurrence of small intestinal bacterial overgrowth (SIBO) and increased intestinal permeability because of leaky tight junctions has been reported in patients with NAFLD. In an experimental study, Gäbele and colleagues[24] induced NASH by feeding C57BL/6 mice a high-fat diet and then studied the effects of exposing the mice to 1% dextran sulfate sodium. By causing intestinal injury, combined administration of high-fat diet and dextran sulfate sodium not only worsened steatohepatitis, but also induced a profibrogenic response in the liver. The study suggested that the induction of intestinal inflammation by dextran sulfate sodium led to damage to intestinal barrier, LPS translocation, hepatic inflammation, and fibrogenesis in mice model of NASH.[24] In one of the earlier human studies that assessed SIBO by a combined C-D-xylose and lactulose breath test and intestinal permeability by a dual lactulose rhamnose sugar test, it was found that 50% of patients with NASH had SIBO compared with 22% of SIBO in control subjects.[25] In another study 18 patients with NASH were compared with age- and gender-matched control subjects and SIBO was assessed by the lactulose

---

Box 2
Pathogenesis of microbiota-associated NAFLD

- Small intestinal overgrowth, increased gut permeability
- Endotoxemia causing low-grade inflammation
  - Role of TLRs and inflammasomes
- Altered dietary choline metabolism
- Altered bile acid metabolism
  - Role of FXR receptors
- Production of endogenous ethanol

hydrogen breath test. SIBO was found to be more common in patients with NASH (77.78% vs 31.25%; *P*<.0001) compared with control subjects. Patients with NASH also had enhanced expression of TLR-4/myeloid differentiation factor 2 suggesting the interaction between SIBO and TLR-4 expression in patients with NAFLD.[26] In a study by Miele and colleagues,[27] 35 biopsy-proved patients with NAFLD were compared with patients with untreated celiac disease and healthy subjects for the presence of SIBO and gut permeability. Increased gut permeability and SIBO correlated with the severity of steatosis but not with the presence of NASH.[27] These studies suggest that SIBO by altering the intestinal integrity can promote bacterial translocation from the gut into the portal circulation, and through interaction with TLRs in the liver can induce the inflammatory and fibrogenic response. There is now evidence that high-fat diet can lead to the translocation of not only bacterial products but also of complete living bacteria from intestinal lumen toward tissues, such as adipose tissue. Accumulation of translocated bacteria in metabolically active tissues can also participate in exacerbating hepatic inflammation and fibrosis.[28,29]

Innate immunity, TLRs, and inflammasomes

The liver is a major component of the immune system, consisting of a large number of tissue macrophages, dendritic cells, and specialized lymphocytes, such as natural killer T cells acting as first-line defense against invading micro-organisms and endotoxins. TLRs present on the innate immune cells are the major sensors for the microorganisms. Although there is lot of literature on TLR signaling in patients with liver disease and NAFLD, there is sparse literature on the functional status of the cells of innate immunity in patients with NAFLD.[30] We recently showed that dendritic cells in patients with NAFLD exhibit immature yet functionally activated phenotype in response to LPS stimulation because they secrete inflammatory cytokines, which further contribute in exacerbating the symptoms.[31] Inefficient antigen presentation and continuous presence of endotoxin in these patients might be responsible for inducing activation of the innate immune system resulting in chronic subclinical inflammation.[31]

TLRs present on the cells of the innate immunity recognize highly conserved motifs in pathogens termed pathogen-associated molecular patterns (PAMPs) and damage-associated molecular patterns (DAMPs) present on endogenous ligands. TLRs, acting as immune sensors of PAMPs and DAMPs, initiate an adaptive immune response and a signaling cascade leading to activation of proinflammatory genes, such as tumor necrosis factor (TNF)-α and interleukins-6, -8, and -12.[32] The most studied PAMP is the LPS, a component of the gram-negative bacterial cell membrane, the active component of endotoxin. The latter binds to LPS-binding protein, which subsequently binds to CD14. The LPS–LPS-binding protein–CD14 complex activates TLR-4, present on Kuffer cells triggering an essential inflammatory cascade, including stress-activated and mitogen-activated protein kinases, Jun N-terminal kinase, p38, interferon regulatory factor 3, and nuclear factor-kB pathway.[33,34] Because of the unique anatomic link between liver and gut, liver is constantly exposed to TLR ligands. Normal liver does not show the sign of inflammation because of low expression of TLR-4 and its adaptor molecules in the liver and ability to modulate TLR-4 signaling by liver tolerance. But under pathologic conditions because of bacterial overgrowth and intestinal permeability, altered TLR-4/LPS signaling plays an important role in the pathogenesis of chronic liver diseases including NAFLD.[35] Studies in mice have shown that a high-fat diet can lead to metabolic endotoxemia by a moderate increase in plasma LPS, which is 10 to 100 times lower than what is achieved during septicemia.[36]

Of all the 13 TLRs identified in mammals, TLR-2, TLR-4, its coreceptor CD14 and TLR-9 have been well studied in NAFLD. TLR-5 is expressed in gut mucosa, which helps defend against bacterial infections and is activated by bacterial flagellin. There is now evidence that transfer of the gut microbiota from TLR-5–deficient mice to WT GF mice can confer many features of metabolic syndrome.[37] TLR-2 recognizes components of gram-positive bacteria cell wall, such as peptidoglycan and lipoteichoic acid. Szabo and coworkers investigated the role of TLR-2 and TLR-4 polymorphism on liver damage and on cytokine induction in a methionine-choline deficient (MCD) diet-induced model of NASH.[38] They found that in TLR-2$^{-/-}$ mice there is an increase in liver injury associated with NASH and may suggest a protective role for TLR-2–mediated signals in liver injury.[38] Similarly, Rivera and colleagues[39] found that hepatocellular damage was notably more severe and TNF-α level was elevated by approximately threefold in TLR-2$^{-/-}$ mice. Possibly the TLR-2 deficiency exacerbates NASH by altering signaling via the TLR-4 pathway, whereas its presence may play a protective role against the induction of steatohepatitis. However, in an animal study Csak and colleagues[40] showed that there is a significant attenuation of steatohepatitis, serum alanine transaminase levels, oxidative stress, and protection from fibrosis in the presence of myeloid differentiation factor 2 and TLR-4 deficiency in TLR-4 knockout mice suggesting that the deficiency of TLR-4 attenuates the liver injury. In a human study by Brun and colleagues,[41] polymorphism at C (-159) T in the CD14 gene promoter region was found to be associated with increased risk of NASH. Their results showed that TT genotype of C (-159) T might enhance the sensitivity to intestinal LPS.[41] Recent reports have identified involvement of TLR-9 in the pathogenesis of NAFLD. The functional importance of TLR-9 signaling in NASH was confirmed in mice deficient in TLR-9, which showed protection from choline-deficient diet-induced liver steatosis, inflammation, injury, and fibrosis compared with wild animals.[42]

Another important contributor to microbiota dysbiosis, participating in the activation of lipid peroxidation and generation of reactive oxygen species, a mechanism in NAFLD/NASH progression, are the inflammasomes.[43] Inflammasomes are cytoplasmic multiprotein complexes composed of leucin-rich-repeat containing proteins and nucleotide-binding domains, which are sensors of PAMPs and DAMPs. Recently, Henao-Mejia and colleagues[44] showed that changes in gut microbiota associated with NLRP6 and NLRP3 inflammasome (subfamily of nucleotide-binding oligomerization domain receptors) deficiency were linked with exacerbated hepatic steatosis and enhanced TNF-α expression. Furthermore, cohousing inflammasome-deficient mice with WT mice transferred the phenotype, providing direct evidence that inflammasome-mediated dysbiosis is implicated in NASH progression.[44]

Impaired choline metabolism

Choline, a phospholipid component of cell membrane, plays an important role in the fat metabolism in the liver. It helps in the very-low-density lipoprotein assembly and lipid transport from the liver.[45] Deficiency of choline thus can lead to accumulation of fat in the liver as seen in choline-deficient animal models of hepatic steatosis. Gut microbiota can convert dietary choline into toxic methylamines (dimethylamine and trimethylamine), which can induce hepatic inflammation after absorption. Gut microbiota thus can lead to NAFLD by causing choline deficiency and by increasing toxic methylamines. It has also been shown that the host factors and gastrointestinal bacteria respond to dietary choline deficiency and the generation of bacterial biomarkers of fatty liver in such a situation provide evidence that gastrointestinal microbes have a role in NAFLD.[46] In a recent study, 15 female subjects were placed on well-controlled diets in which choline levels were manipulated. 16S ribosomal RNA bacterial genes were used to characterize microbiota in stool samples.[46] Subjects were genotyped for the *PEMT* promoter single-nucleotide polymorphism rs12325817 a single nucleotide polymorphism that affect choline levels. Hepatic fat was measured by magnetic resonance imaging at the beginning and end of the base-line diet, after 21 and 42 days of the low-choline diet. The authors found that the compositions of the gastrointestinal microbiota changed with choline levels of diets with each individual maintaining a distinct microbiome. Levels of Gammaproteobacteria and Erysipelotrichi were directly associated with changes in liver fat in each subject during choline depletion. Levels of Gammaproteobacteria and Erysipelotrichi, change in amount of liver fat, and the studied single nucleotide polymorphism accurately predicted the degree to which subjects developed fatty liver on a choline-deficient diet.[46]

Altered bile acid metabolism

Bile acids are regulators of hepatic lipid and glucose metabolism and have a strong bactericidal action because of the effect of bile acids on the bacterial cell membrane phospholipids.[47] Fat-rich diet can also affect the gut microbiota by changing the composition of bile acids. However, gut microbiota can also affect the bile acid metabolism through farsenoid X (FXR) receptor stimulation. FXR and its downstream signaling play an important role in the control of hepatic lipogenesis and the export of very-low-density lipoprotein from the liver.[47] The same signal pathways are also involved in the regulation of hepatic gluconeogenesis, glycogen synthesis, and insulin sensitivity. Dysregulation of bile acid transport and impaired receptor signaling may thus contribute to the pathogenesis and are promising drug targets for treatment of NAFLD. In a recent study, conventional (WT), conventional FXR knockout (FXR null), and GF mice were randomized to undergo either ileocecal resection or sham operation.[48] After the resection, WT mice showed significant increases in the expression of genes regulating bile acid transport but the induction of bile acid transport genes was absent or attenuated in FXR null and GF mice. The study suggests that the mice lacking microbiota (GF) or FXR are unable to increase the expression of bile acid transporter genes. By modifying bile acid metabolism and FXR/TGR5 signaling, gut flora could therefore contribute indirectly to the development of NAFLD.[48]

Endogenous ethanol

Except for the history of alcohol, the hepatic injury is usually indistinguishable between patients with alcoholic liver disease and NAFLD. Gut microbiota could be contributing to the liver injury in patients with NAFLD by producing the endogenous alcohol. Alcohol metabolism produces acetate and acetaldehyde leading to fatty acid synthesis and hepatic oxidative stress, respectively, the two hits in the pathogenesis of NAFLD/NASH. The endogenous alcohol could also affect the intestinal permeability leading to endotoxemia and its consequences including NAFLD/NASH. In a recent study from Buffalo, the relationship between gut microbiota and endogenous alcohol was studied by 16S ribosomal RNA pyrosequencing and peripheral blood ethanol concentration in nonalcoholic obese and healthy children.[49] Healthy subjects and obese children had different microbiome with abundance of alcohol-producing bacteria (Escherichia, a well-known ethanol producer) in NASH microbiome. Patients with NASH also had higher blood ethanol concentration than the healthy and obese non-NASH subjects suggesting a link between the gut microbiota, endogenous alcohol, and NASH.[49] Besides Escherichia other gut bacteria including Bacteroides, Bifidobacterium, and Clostridium are capable of producing alcohol, which also explains higher blood alcohol levels without increase in Escherichia in some of the patients with NASH.[50–52]

Probiotics, Antibiotics, and Prebiotics in Obesity and NAFLD

Probiotics are commensal microorganisms that provide health benefits to the host by preventing bacterial translocation and epithelial invasion, inhibiting mucosal adherence by bacteria, and by stimulating host immunity. Probiotics deliver anti-inflammatory mediators that downregulate proinflammatory cytokines including interferon-α and TNF-α by nuclear factor-Kβ pathway.[53] Antiobesity effect of probiotics in animal experiments have shown that *Lactobacillus casei* strains prevent obesity-associated metabolic abnormalities by improving insulin resistance.[54] Efficacy of probiotics in patients and animal models of NAFLD also suggests a link between the gut microbiota and NAFLD. In an animal study, treatment with VSL#3 given for 4 weeks in ob/ob mice fed with a high-fat diet improved liver histology, reduced hepatic total fatty acid content, and decreased serum alanine aminotransferase levels.[55] In another mice study, *Lactobaccilus casei* Shirota has been shown to protect against the fructose-induced NAFLD through mechanisms involving an attenuation of the TLR-4 signaling cascade in the liver.[56] In a MCD diet–induced mouse model of NASH, VSL#3 failed to prevent MCD-induced liver steatosis or inflammation.[57] There was upregulation of serum endotoxin and expression of the TLR-4 signaling even in the presence of VSL#3 but VSL#3 treatment reduced the hepatic fibrosis resulting in diminished accumulation of collagen and smooth muscle actin.[57] Data suggest that VSL#3 treatment modulates liver fibrosis but does not protect from inflammation and steatosis in NASH. Encouraging results have been observed in humans with probiotics where VSL#3 given for 2 to 3 months has been shown to improve the liver enzymes, cytokine profile, and oxidative stress in patients with NAFLD.[58] Although the Cochrane meta-analysis suggests the requirement of larger randomized studies with probiotics in patients with NAFLD, individual randomized controlled trials have found it to be useful.[59]

The positive effect of polymyxin B and metronidazole in reducing the severity of steatosis during total parenteral nutrition or after intestinal bypass in animal models and humans provides a reasonable prospect for use of antibiotics to treat NAFLD.[60,61]

Prebiotics are nondigestible oligosaccharides that act as fertilizers of colonic microbiota and increase the growth of beneficial commensal organisms (eg, Bifidobacterium and *Lactobacillus* spp) and have been shown to be beneficial in reducing adiposity.[62] In one of the studies involving 97 young adolescents, subjects who received the prebiotic supplement for 1 year had a smaller increase in body mass index and total fat mass compared with the control group.[63] In a pilot study, seven patients with NASH received either 16 g/day of oligofructose or placebo for 8 weeks and showed that compared with placebo, the prebiotic group had significant reduction in liver enzymes after 8 weeks and insulin levels after 4 weeks.[64]

SUMMARY

Gut–liver axis plays a central role in the pathogenesis of obesity and NAFLD, mainly through the crosstalk of the intestinal microbiota with the host immune system modulating inflammation, insulin resistance, and intestinal permeability. Gut microbiota is linked to obesity through increased energy harvesting and storage and to NAFLD though the systemic inflammation, cytokines, and insulin resistance secondary to endotoxemia resulting from SIBO and increased gut permeability.

REFERENCES

1. Neish AS. Microbes in gastrointestinal health and disease. Gastroenterology 2009;136:65–80.
2. Bäckhed F, Ding H, Wang T, et al. The gut microbiota as an environmental factor that regulates fat storage. Proc Natl Acad Sci U S A 2004;101:15718–23.
3. Tennyson CA, Friedman G. Microecology, obesity, and probiotics. Curr Opin Endocrinol Diabetes Obes 2008;15:422–7.

4. Hugenholtz P, Goebel BM, Pace NR. Impact of culture-independent studies on the emerging phylogenetic view of bacterial diversity. J Bacteriol 1998;180: 4765–74.

5. Eckburg PB, Bik EM, Bernstein CN, et al. Diversity of the human intestinal microbial flora. Science 2005;308:1635–8.

6. Nicholson JK, Holmes E, Wilson ID. Gut microorganisms, mammalian metabolism and personalized health care. Nat Rev Microbiol 2005;3:431–8.

7. Ogden CL, Carroll MD, Curtin LR, et al. Prevalence of overweight and obesity in the United States, 1999-2004. JAMA 2006;295:1549–55.

8. Ogden CL, Carroll MD, Kit BK, et al. Prevalence of obesity and trends in body mass index among US children and adolescents, 1999-2010. JAMA 2012;307:483–90.

9. Rychlik JL, May T. The effect of a methanogen, *Methanobrevibacter smithii*, on the growth rate, organic acid production, and specific ATP activity of three predominant ruminal cellulolytic bacteria. Curr Microbiol 2000;40:176–80.

10. Bäckhed F, Manchester JK, Semenkovich CF, et al. Mechanisms underlying the resistance to diet-induced obesity in germ-free mice. Proc Natl Acad Sci U S A 2007;104:979–84.

11. Turnbaugh PJ, Ley RE, Mahowald MA, et al. An obesity-associated gut microbiome with increased capacity for energy harvest. Nature 2006;444:1027–31.

12. Ley RE, Bäckhed F, Turnbaugh P, et al. Obesity alters gut microbial ecology. Proc Natl Acad Sci U S A 2005;102:11070–5.

13. Ley RE, Turnbaugh PJ, Klein S, et al. Microbial ecology: human gut microbes associated with obesity. Nature 2006;444:1022–3.

14. Kalliomäki M, Collado MC, Salminen S, et al. Early differences in fecal microbiota composition in children may predict overweight. Am J Clin Nutr 2008;87: 534–8.

15. Muccioli GG, Naslain D, Bäckhed F, et al. The endocannabinoid system links gut microbiota to adipogenesis. Mol Syst Biol 2010;6:392.

16. Duseja A, Das A, Das R, et al. The clinicopathological profile of Indian patients with nonalcoholic fatty liver disease (NAFLD) is different from that in the West. Dig Dis Sci 2007;52:2368–74.

17. Duseja A, Sharma B, Kumar A, et al. Nonalcoholic fatty liver in a developing country is responsible for significant liver disease. Hepatology 2010;52:2248–9.

18. Williams CD, Stengel J, Asike MI, et al. Prevalence of nonalcoholic fatty liver disease and nonalcoholic steatohepatitis among a largely middle-aged population utilizing ultrasound and liver biopsy: a prospective study. Gastroenterology 2011;140:124–31.

19. Machado M, Marques-Vidal P, Cortez-Pinto H. Hepatic histology in obese patients undergoing bariatric surgery. J Hepatol 2006;45:600–6.

20. Day CP, James OF. Steatohepatitis: a tale of two "hits"? Gastroenterology 1998; 114:842–5.

21. Dowman JK, Tomlinson JW, Newsome PN. Pathogenesis of non-alcoholic fatty liver disease. QJM 2010;103:71–83.

22. Duseja A, Das R, Nanda M, et al. Nonalcoholic steatohepatitis in Asian Indians is neither associated with iron overload nor with HFE gene mutations. World J Gastroenterol 2005;11:393–5.

23. Duseja A, Aggarwal R. APOC3 and PNPLA3 in non-alcoholic fatty liver disease: need to clear the air. J Gastroenterol Hepatol 2012;27:848–51.

24. Gäbele E, Dostert K, Hofmann C, et al. DSS induced colitis increases portal LPS levels and enhances hepatic inflammation and fibrogenesis in experimental NASH. J Hepatol 2011;55:1391–9.

25. Wigg AJ, Roberts-Thomson IC, Dymock RB, et al. The role of small intestinal bacterial overgrowth, intestinal permeability, endotoxaemia, and tumour necrosis factor alpha in the pathogenesis of non-alcoholic steatohepatitis. Gut 2001; 48:206–11.
26. Shanab AA, Scully P, Crosbie O, et al. Small intestinal bacterial overgrowth in nonalcoholic steatohepatitis: association with Toll-like receptor 4 expression and plasma levels of interleukin 8. Dig Dis Sci 2011;56:1524–34.
27. Miele L, Valenza V, La Torre G, et al. Increased intestinal permeability and tight junction alterations in nonalcoholic fatty liver disease. Hepatology 2009;49: 1877–87.
28. Amar J, Chabo C, Waget A, et al. Intestinal mucosal adherence and translocation of commensal bacteria at the early onset of type 2 diabetes: molecular mechanisms and probiotic treatment. EMBO Mol Med 2011;3:559–72.
29. Burcelin R, Garidou L, Pomié C. Immuno-microbiota cross and talk: the new paradigm of metabolic diseases. Semin Immunol 2012;24:67–74.
30. Takeda K, Akira S. Toll-like receptors in innate immunity. Int Immunol 2005; 17:1–14.
31. Rana D, Duseja A, Dhiman RK, et al. Maturation defective myeloid dendritic cells in nonalcoholic fatty liver disease patients release inflammatory cytokines in response to endotoxin. Hepatol Int 2013;7:562–9.
32. Aderem A, Ulevitch RJ. Toll-like receptors in the induction of the innate immune response. Nature 2000;406:782–7.
33. Ruiz AG, Casafont F, Crespo J, et al. Lipopolysaccharide-binding protein plasma levels and liver TNF-alpha gene expression in obese patients: evidence for the potential role of endotoxin in the pathogenesis of non-alcoholic steatohepatitis. Obes Surg 2007;17:1374–80.
34. Thuy S, Ladurner R, Volynets V, et al. Nonalcoholic fatty liver disease in humans is associated with increased plasma endotoxin and plasminogen activator inhibitor 1 concentrations and with fructose intake. J Nutr 2008;138:1452–5.
35. Miura K, Seki E, Ohnishi H, et al. Role of Toll-like receptors and their downstream molecules in the development of nonalcoholic Fatty liver disease. Gastroenterol Res Pract 2010;2010:362847.
36. Cani PD, Amar J, Iglesias MA, et al. Metabolic endotoxemia initiates obesity and insulin resistance. Diabetes 2007;56:1761–72.
37. Vijay-Kumar M, Aitken JD, Carvalho FA, et al. Metabolic syndrome and altered gut microbiota in mice lacking Toll-like receptor 5. Science 2010;328:228–31.
38. Szabo G, Velayudham A, Romics L Jr, et al. Modulation of non-alcoholic steatohepatitis by pattern recognition receptors in mice: the role of Toll-like receptors 2 and 4. Alcohol Clin Exp Res 2005;29(Suppl 11):140S–5S.
39. Rivera CA, Gaskin L, Allman M, et al. Toll-like receptor-2 deficiency enhances non-alcoholic steatohepatitis. BMC Gastroenterol 2010;10:52.
40. Csak T, Velayudham A, Hritz I, et al. Deficiency in myeloid differentiation factor-2 and Toll-like receptor 4 expression attenuates nonalcoholic steatohepatitis and fibrosis in mice. Am J Physiol Gastrointest Liver Physiol 2011;300: G433–41.
41. Brun P, Castagliuolo I, Floreani AR, et al. Increased risk of NASH in patients carrying the C(-159)T polymorphism in the CD14 gene promoter region. Gut 2006;55:1212.
42. Miura K, Kodama Y, Inokuchi S, et al. Toll-like receptor 9 promotes steatohepatitis by induction of interleukin-1beta in mice. Gastroenterology 2010;139: 323–34.

43. Robertson SJ, Rubino SJ, Geddes K, et al. Examining host-microbial interactions through the lens of NOD: from plants to mammals. Semin Immunol 2012; 24:9–16.
44. Henao-Mejia J, Elinav E, Jin C, et al. Inflammasome-mediated dysbiosis regulates progression of NAFLD and obesity. Nature 2012;482:179–85.
45. Vance DE. Role of phosphatidylcholine biosynthesis in the regulation of lipoprotein homeostasis. Curr Opin Lipidol 2008;19:229–34.
46. Spencer MD, Hamp TJ, Reid RW, et al. Association between composition of the human gastrointestinal microbiome and development of fatty liver with choline deficiency. Gastroenterology 2011;140:976–86.
47. Trauner M, Claudel T, Fickert P, et al. Bile acids as regulators of hepatic lipid and glucose metabolism. Dig Dis 2010;28:220–4.
48. Dekaney CM, von Allmen DC, Garrison AP, et al. Bacterial-dependent up-regulation of intestinal bile acid binding protein and transport is FXR-mediated following ileo-cecal resection. Surgery 2008;144:174–81.
49. Zhu L, Baker SS, Gill C, et al. Characterization of gut microbiomes in nonalcoholic steatohepatitis (NASH) patients: a connection between endogenous alcohol and NASH. Hepatology 2013;57:601–9.
50. Frantz JC, McCallum RE. Growth yields and fermentation balance of Bacteroides fragilis cultured in glucose-enriched medium. J Bacteriol 1979;137:1263–70.
51. Amaretti A, Bernardi T, Tamburini E, et al. Kinetics and metabolism of Bifidobacterium adolescentis MB 239 growing on glucose, galactose, lactose, and galactooligosaccharides. Appl Environ Microbiol 2007;73:3637–44.
52. Weimer PJ, Zeikus JG. Fermentation of cellulose and cellobiose by Clostridium thermocellum in the absence of Methanobacterium thermoautotrophicum. Appl Environ Microbiol 1977;33:289–97.
53. Nardone G, Rocco A. Probiotics: a potential target for the prevention and treatment of steatohepatitis. J Clin Gastroenterol 2004;38:S121–2.
54. Naito E, Yoshida Y, Makino K, et al. Beneficial effect of oral administration of Lactobacillus casei strain Shirota on insulin resistance in diet-induced obesity mice. J Appl Microbiol 2011;110:650–7.
55. Li Z, Yang S, Lin H, et al. Probiotics and antibodies to TNF inhibit inflammatory activity and improve nonalcoholic fatty liver disease. Hepatology 2003;37:343–50.
56. Wagnerberger S, Spruss A, Kanuri G, et al. Lactobaccilus casei Shirota protects from fructose-induced liver steatosis: a mouse model. J Nutr Biochem 2013;24:531–8.
57. Velayudham A, Dolganiuc A, Ellis M, et al. VSL#3 probiotic treatment attenuates fibrosis without changes in steatohepatitis in a diet-induced nonalcoholic steatohepatitis model in mice. Hepatology 2009;49:989–97.
58. Loguercio C, Federico A, Tuccillo C, et al. Beneficial effects of a probiotic VSL#3 on parameters of liver dysfunction in chronic liver diseases. J Clin Gastroenterol 2005;39:540–3.
59. Lirussi F, Mastropasqua E, Orando S, et al. Probiotics for non-alcoholic fatty liver disease and/or steatohepatitis. Cochrane Database Syst Rev 2007;(1):CD005165.
60. Pappo I, Becovier H, Berry EM, et al. Polymyxin B reduces cecal flora, TNF production and hepatic steatosis during total parenteral nutrition in the rat. J Surg Res 1991;51:106–12.
61. Drenick EJ, Fisler J, Johnson D. Hepatic steatosis after intestinal bypass–prevention and reversal by metronidazole, irrespective of protein-calorie malnutrition. Gastroenterology 1982;82:535–48.

62. Neyrinck AM, Delzenne NM. Potential interest of gut microbial changes induced by non-digestible carbohydrates of wheat in the management of obesity and related disorders. Curr Opin Clin Nutr Metab Care 2010;13:722–8.

63. Abrams SA, Griffin IJ, Hawthorne KM, et al. Effect of prebiotic supplementation and calcium intake on body mass index. J Pediatr 2007;151:293–8.

64. Daubioul CA, Horsmans Y, Lambert P, et al. Effects of oligofructose on glucose and lipid metabolism in patients with nonalcoholic steatohepatitis: results of a pilot study. Eur J Clin Nutr 2005;59:723–6.

The Role of Medications for the Management of Patients with NAFLD

Natalia Mazzella, MD[a], Laura M. Ricciardi, MD[b],
Arianna Mazzotti, MD[a], Giulio Marchesini, MD[c],*

KEYWORDS

- Nonalcoholic fatty liver disease • Drug treatment • Antioxidants • Insuin-sensitizers
- PPAR agonists • Anti-fibrotic agents

KEY POINTS

- There is a recognized clinical need for an effective treatment of nonalcoholic fatty liver disease (NAFLD); current approaches remain suboptimal and no drug has so far been approved by International Agencies.
- Several factors complicate the development of novel pharmacotherapies, particularly the imprecision of surrogate markers, making histologic assessment compulsory.
- Incretin mimetics, farnesoid x-receptor blockers, peroxisome proliferator activated receptor α/δ agonists, and lysyl oxidase-like-2 inhibitory monoclonal antibodies are currently under scrutiny in randomized controlled trials.
- Although indicated by clinical guidelines, a careful follow-up and treatment of NAFLD is not the rule in the community. If, when, and how long drug therapy should be instituted and continued to reduce the burden of disease are being researched.

INTRODUCTION

Lifestyle changes are a mandatory strategy for the prevention and treatment of nonalcoholic fatty liver disease (NAFLD), but the results depend on individual subjects and therefore are largely unpredictable. Also, subjects who achieve a marked reduction

Funding Sources: Prof Marchesini: Funding from the European Community's Seventh Framework Programme (FP7/2007–2013) under grant agreement no. HEALTH-F2-2009-241762 for the project FLIP.
Conflict of Interests: Prof Marchesini: Advisory board Sanofi; Speaker's fee from Merck-Sharp and Dome, Lilly, NOVO Nordisk, Boehringer Ingelheim, Sanofi. Dr Mazzella, Dr Ricciardi, Dr Mazzotti: No conflict of interest.
[a] Unit of Metabolic Diseases & Clinical Dietetics, Postgraduate School of Nutrition, S. Orsola-Malpighi Hospital, Alma Mater Studiorum University, Via Massarenti, 9, Bologna 40138, Italy; [b] Unit of Metabolic Diseases & Clinical Dietetics, S. Orsola-Malpighi Hospital, Via Massarenti, 9, Bologna 40138, Italy; [c] Unit of Metabolic Disease & Clinical Dietetics, S. Orsola-Malpighi Hospital, Alma Mater Studiorum University, Via Massarenti, 9, Bologna I-40138, Italy
* Corresponding author.
E-mail address: giulio.marchesini@unibo.it

Clin Liver Dis 18 (2014) 73–89
http://dx.doi.org/10.1016/j.cld.2013.09.005
1089-3261/14/$ – see front matter © 2014 Elsevier Inc. All rights reserved.
liver.theclinics.com

of body weight tend to regain weight along the years; in this case recurrence and/or progression of disease may be very likely. This finding stimulated intensive research on pharmacologic treatment strategies and several randomized controlled trials having histology as treatment outcome have been published.[1–11] Several classes of drugs have been tested in the last 10 years, acting at different levels along the sequence of events from pure fatty liver to advanced disease (**Fig. 1**), but no drug has been so far been approved for the treatment of NAFLD. This finding opens a series of challenging questions that may be summarized, such as if, when, and how long should treatment be instituted/continued, considering that also with drugs the results are far from optimal? The situation is similar to that observed in other metabolic disorders largely linked to unhealthy lifestyles, namely, type 2 diabetes and obesity. International guidelines on the treatment of type 2 diabetes have never reached a general consensus as to the need to institute immediate pharmacologic treatment—with well-defined, effective, and safe drugs—soon after diagnosis, unless at risk of acute complications. In obesity all guidelines recommend systematic behavior treatment of weight loss before drug therapy—and very few drugs are approved by International Agencies. Drug therapy may also be effectively superimposed to drugs to increase the final results.[12]

The current scientific evidence on the principal drugs tested so far in several randomized controlled trials, divided according to their prevalent mechanism of action, is presented in **Table 1** and is reviewed in this chapter.

INSULIN SENSITIZERS

As insulin resistance is the basis for liver fat accumulation, insulin sensitizers probably remain the best pharmacologic option for NAFLD treatment.

Metformin

Metformin is a biguanide used widely in clinical practice as a first-line treatment for patients with type 2 diabetes mellitus for over 50 years. Metformin reduces blood

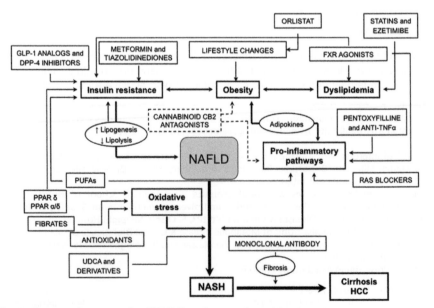

Fig. 1. The complex network of NAFLD pathogenesis and treatment.

Table 1
Principal randomized controlled trials of medication use in subjects with NAFLD

First Author,[Ref.] Year	Treatment	No. of Cases	Duration (mo)	Results (Comparison vs Control)
Lindor et al,[1] 2004	UDCA (13–15 mg/kg/d) vs PL	80/86	24	126 cases completed the 2-y treatment and had a second biopsy. No outcome difference between groups
Bugianesi et al,[2] 2005	MET (2 g) vs Vit. E (800 IU) or prescriptive diet	55/28/27	12	No difference between Vit. E and prescriptive diet, considered control group. ↓ALT and AST with metformin. Second biopsy only in 17 metformin cases: ↓steatosis, ↓necroinflammation and ↓fibrosis
Dufour et al,[3] 2006	UDCA (12–15 mg/kg) + Vit. E (400 IU) or UDCA/PL or PL/PL	15/18/15	24	↓AST and ALT with UDCA + Vit. E; ↓activity score with UDCA + Vit. E ($P<.05$), mostly as effect of ↓steatosis
Belfort et al,[4] 2006	PIO (45 mg) vs Placebo	26/26 with IGT/DM	6	↓ALT; Improved insulin sensitivity; ↓Steatosis ($P = .003$) and necroinflammation ($P = .001$); no difference in fibrosis ($P = .08$)
Ratziu et al,[5] 2008	ROSI (8 mg) vs Placebo	32/31	12	↓ALT; ↓Steatosis (no other improvement in histology)
Aithal et al,[6] 2008	PIO (30 mg) vs Placebo	37/37	12	↓ALT ($P = .009$); ↓γ-GT ($P = .002$); ↓Ferritin; second biopsy in 31/30 cases: ↓hepatocellular injury ($P = .005$), ↓Fibrosis ($P = .05$)
Haukeland et al,[7] 2009	MET (mean, 2.6 g) vs PL	24/24	6	No difference in liver biochemistry, insulin resistance, and histology between groups (second biopsy in 44 cases; 20 on metformin)
Leuschner et al,[8] 2010	UDCA (23–28 mg/kg) vs PL	91/94	18	↓ALT; second biopsy in 137 cases: ↓lobular inflammation, no difference in fibrosis ($P = .133$)
Sanyal et al,[9] 2010	PIO (30 mg) vs Vit. E (800 IU) vs PL	80/84/83	24	↓Steatohepatitis in the Vit. E arm ($P = .001$), not in the pioglitazone arm ($P = .04$); ↓lobular inflammation and steatosis with both treatment; no effect on fibrosis ($P = .12$ and $P = .24$, respectively)
Ratziu et al,[10] 2011	UDCA (28–35 mg/kg) vs PL	61/55	12	↓ALT; ↓Glycemia; ↓Insulin resistance; ↓Fibrotest ($P<.001$)
Torres et al,[11] 2011	ROSI (8 mg/d) vs ROSI (4 mg) + MET (500 mg) vs ROSI (4 mg) + Losartan (50 mg)	41/49/45	12	↓ALT in all groups, without differences; 108 cases had a second biopsy (31/37/40). Improvement in steatosis, necroinflammation, ballooning, and fibrosis in all groups ($P≤.001$), without differences between groups

Abbreviations: DM, diabetes mellitus; IGT, impaired glucose tolerance; MET, metformin; PIO, pioglitazone; PL, placebo; ROSI, rosiglitazone.
Data from Refs.[1-11]

glucose by decreasing hepatic gluconeogenesis, by stimulating glucose uptake in the muscle, and by increasing fatty acid oxidation in adipose tissue. The final effect is an improvement of peripheral insulin sensitivity.

Following a seminal study in 2001,[13] a few clinical trials have reported a beneficial effect of metformin in NAFLD, but limited data are available on histology; metformin led to some improvements in steatosis and necroinflammation, but not in fibrosis. In most studies the changes seen with metformin were not different from those in the control arm and a recent systematic review concluded for a negative effect of metformin on histology.[14] For this reason, the US Guidelines on NAFLD do not support metformin for the treatment of adult NAFLD.[15]

The potential role of metformin has also been examined in pediatric NAFLD patients with results similar to those observed in adults; metformin reduces liver enzymes and improves metabolic parameters, but not histologic features.[16,17]

Metformin treatment also promotes weight loss possibly via appetite control, which makes metformin the first-choice anti-diabetic medication for type 2 diabetes mellitus treatment in obese patients. However, it is unclear whether the benefits of metformin are greater than what might be achieved with weight loss from diet and exercise alone or with a weight loss medication that does not directly affect insulin sensitivity.[18]

The potential beneficial effects of metformin, however, extend outside liver fat. Metformin significantly decreases arterial stiffness, a marker of generalized atherosclerosis, associated with change in circulating adiponectin, a possible marker of the association between liver dysfunction and atherosclerotic vascular disease in patients with NAFLD. Furthermore, metformin has anticancer properties and is being tested to prevent primary cancer in several at-risk conditions. For all these reasons, metformin use might be re-evaluated in NAFLD.

Glitazones (Thiazolidinediones)

Thiazolidinediones (TZDs) have a significant effect on insulin sensitivity in insulin-resistant states and in type 2 diabetes mellitus, as well as in patients with fatty liver or nonalcoholic steatohepatitis (NASH).

TZDs (troglitazone, rosiglitazone, and pioglitazone) are a class of peroxisome proliferator activated receptor γ (PPAR-γ) agonists notable for the ability to cause differentiation of pluripotent stem cells into adipocytes. PPARs are predominantly expressed in adipose tissue, but are also present in muscle, liver, pancreas, heart, and spleen. TZDs treatment increases plasma adiponectin levels and has been shown in patients with type 2 diabetes and those with NASH. Patients with NASH have low plasma adiponectin levels, which are inversely related to insulin resistance and hepatic triglyceride content and are independent of the degree of obesity or glucose tolerance status; the increase in plasma adiponectin levels could mediate some of the insulin-sensitizing effects of PPAR-γ agonists,[19] adding to their anti-inflammatory effects in patients with NASH.

TZDs are probably the best pharmacologic option for subjects with NAFLD. Three large randomized controlled trials reported a beneficial effect of pioglitazone on liver histology, although the advantage was limited for fibrosis.[6,8,9] Rosiglitazone proved effective only on steatosis and liver enzymes, without an effect on necroinflammation and fibrosis.[7] Continuing use of TZDs does not further improve the effects on histology,[20] which are lost after treatment is stopped (**Box 1**).[21]

In conclusion, the efficacy of insulin sensitizers (particularly TZDs), strictly dependent on increased insulin sensitivity, is proven, although limited. Whether they need to be used in association with hepatoprotective agents in individual patients, to maximize the anti-inflammatory and antifibrotic activity, must be defined. There is now solid

---

Box 1
Insulin sensitizers—mechanism of action

Metformin

- Activation of adenosine monophosphate-activated protein kinase, a regulator of energy metabolism
- Reduced hepatic gluconeogenesis via inhibition of the sterol regulatory element-binding protein-1c (SREBP-1c)
- Adipokine synthesis or secretion

Tiazolidinediones

- Adipocyte differentiation and adipogenesis
- Modification of adipose tissue distribution, with decreased visceral fat, including hepatic fat, and increased peripheral adiposity associated with weight gain
- "Browning" of adipose tissue mitochondria
- Stimulation of fatty acid oxidation and inhibition of hepatic fatty acid synthesis
- Improved insulin signaling and increase in adiponectin levels

---

evidence for their use,[22] mitigated by undesired side effects (weight gain) and also adverse events.

LIPID-LOWERING DRUGS, ANTIOXIDANT AND HEPATOPROTECTIVE AGENTS

Several studies confirm a link between altered hepatocyte cholesterol metabolism and hepatic-free cholesterol accumulation and NAFLD development and progression. Dietary lipid intake is also an important cofactor in NAFLD development and progression,[23] as in some genetic variants linked with lipid metabolism, like the patatin-like phospholipase domain-containing protein 3,[24] supporting the concept that drugs used for lipid control may be an effective treatment of NAFLD.[25] Reducing lipid levels may also be important to reduce peroxidation, also achieved by different drugs.

The adipose tissue is considered a metabolically active endocrine organ producing pro-inflammatory cytokines, including tumor necrosis factor-α and interleukin-6 and -8, and there is evidence for the activation of other inflammatory pathways and oxidative stress, acting as a "second hit" in the transition between simple fatty liver and steatohepatitis (NASH). Excessive fat accumulation in the liver, whatever its cause, may increase the production of reactive oxygen species, leading to lipid peroxidation and immunologic dysfunction, which prompted testing the effectiveness of antioxidant and cytoprotective compounds, potentially stopping hepatocyte damage (**Box 2**).

Statins

By their activity on hydroxymethylglutaryl CO_2 reductase, statins effectively reduce cholesterol levels in NAFLD in a dose-dependent manner, but their effects are not limited to cholesterol concentrations. Statins reduce the cardiovascular risk, the main cause of death in NAFLD, and control the inflammatory mechanisms involved in NAFLD pathogenesis.[26,27]

The use of statins in NAFLD received additional attention after the publication of the GREACE study, the first randomized controlled trial showing therapeutic benefit on clinical endpoints in NAFLD.[23] In a post-hoc analysis, the use of statins in patients with high transaminase levels presumably due to NAFLD effectively reduced the

---

Box 2
Lipid-lowering drugs, antioxidant and hepatoprotective agents—mechanism of action

- Decreased lipotoxicity and improved insulin sensitivity (lipid-lowering drugs)
- PPAR-α activity (fibrates)
- Reduced lipid peroxidation and free radicals scavenging activity (antioxidants)
- Anti-inflammatory properties, including the inhibition of pro-inflammatory cytokine production, translating into reduced apoptosis (pentoxyfilline)
- Modulation of inflammation and fibrogenesis and interference with intrahepatic glycolysis and gluconeogenesis (sylibin)

---

cardiovascular risk. Atorvastatin was the most widely used drug; pharmacokinetic differences translate into different effectiveness in preventing fibrosis of necroinflammation in NAFLD[26] and also the absence of dyslipidemia.[26]

In NAFLD, statins improved liver enzyme levels,[27,28] without any alleged risk of hepatotoxicity.[27–29] Very few data are available on liver histology; in the only small randomized controlled trial with posttreatment histology, 1-year treatment with simvastatin had no significant effect.[23] Pitavastatin did not improve the severity of hepatic steatosis, whereas atorvastatin improved the grade of steatosis, without conflicting results on fibrosis.[24,27]

Ezetimibe

Ezetimibe reduces the absorption of the cholesterol and its target is the Niemann-Pick C1-like 1 protein. This protein is located in the brush border of the intestine and in the liver and is a sterol transporter that is important for the absorption of the cholesterol in the enterocytes and hepatocytes. The excessive amounts of cholesterol are lipotoxic through activation of the liver X receptor. Therefore, the inhibition of the Niemann-Pick C1-like 1 protein does not only lead to a reduced hepatic cholesterol accumulation, but also to decreased lipotoxicity.

Ezetimibe may be used without any restriction in patients with hepatic diseases. In subjects with NAFLD or NASH, ezetimibe reduced liver enzyme levels and the concentration of inflammatory markers[27,30,31]; in a few reports the histologic features of steatosis, ballooning, and the NAFLD activity score also improved.[27,31,32] As to fibrosis, there is good evidence for improvement in animal models, but more data are needed in humans.[31]

Fibrates

Fibrates (fenofibrate, bezafibrate, gemfibrozil) effectively lower serum triglycerides and moderately increase high-density lipoproteins through binding to and activation of PPAR-α.

PPAR-α, member of the PPAR nuclear receptor subfamily, is highly expressed in the hepatocytes, where it controls genes involved in lipid and lipoprotein metabolism, including the uptake and oxidation of free fatty acids, triglyceride hydrolysis, and up-regulation of reverse cholesterol transport, mediated by apolipoprotein A-I and A-II. Furthermore, fibrates improve insulin sensitivity, stimulate fatty acid oxidation, and inhibit vascular inflammation.

Fenofibrate is commonly used in clinical practice to treat hypertriglyceridemia; in NAFLD it increases the expression of enzymes involved in the catabolism of lipid peroxides and reduces hepatic lipid peroxide content.[33,34] Gemfibrozil decreases serum aminotransferase levels in patients with NAFLD, but no data are available on insulin resistance and liver histology.[35] Bezafibrate, a PPAR pan-agonist, reduces hepatic lipids and the formation of proinflammatory lipoperoxides; along this line it might be particularly effective in NASH.

In conclusion, fibrates might be effective in NAFLD, at least in subjects with fasting hypertriglyceridemia, preventing lipid accumulation in the liver, NASH, and fibrosis.

Polyunsaturated Fatty Acids

Polyunsaturated fatty acids (PUFA) are major constituents of cell membranes and are particularly susceptible to free radical-mediated oxidation. There is some evidence that a low intake of n-3 fatty acids may have a role in NAFLD pathogenesis, highlighting a potential therapeutic target.

When compared with controls, individuals with NAFLD have lower polyunsaturated fat intake. The composition of hepatic long chain fatty acids is characterized by a decrease in the relative levels of n-3 PUFA and an increase in the hepatic n-6/n-3 PUFA ratio,[36,37] associated with defective desaturation activity and dietary imbalance, resulting in hepatic steatosis.[38,39]

In humans, fish oil provides a convenient source of essential n-3 PUFA with few side effects and may directly reduce hepatic lipogenesis and steatosis, improving inflammation and hepatocyte injury. Given the well-recognized problems of adhering to lifestyle interventions and of achieving sustainable weight loss, and considering the side effects of pharmacologic agents, dietary fish oil supplementation represents a practical alternative therapy.[37,40]

In NAFLD, the dietary supplementation with long-chain n-3 PUFAs seems to reduce hepatic steatosis safely.[41–43] A recent meta-analysis reported a statistically significant effect of PUFA supplementation on liver fat in 6/7 studies, a significant improvement of alanine aminotransferase (ALT) levels in 2, while aspartate aminotransferase (AST) was unaffected by PUFA. In 5 studies, steatosis was reduced by n-3 PUFA supplementation in the absence of weight loss. Fibrosis, hepatocyte ballooning, and lobular inflammation were reduced in 85% of the patients.[43,44] Collectively, the data support a role for n-3 long-chain PUFA in NAFLD. The same results might be achieved by a diet rich in n-3 PUFA (fish, nuts, almonds, and other natural products).

Orlistat

Orlistat, a reversible inhibitor of gastric and pancreatic lipase, blocks the absorption of approximately 30% of dietary triglycerides. Orlistat improved AST/ALT, cholesterol, and triglyceride levels and reduced the grade of steatosis, inflammation, and fibrosis in an uncontrolled study. Two small trials in humans investigated the effect of orlistat in NAFLD, with negative results.[45,46] Therefore, orlistat might be an effective treatment of NASH only in the setting of significant weight loss, possibly enhanced by a lifestyle program.[47]

Vitamin E

Vitamin E is the most widely used antioxidant in biomedical research studies, but it is also linked to a greater risk of cardiovascular disease in epidemiologic studies.

Several studies have examined the role of supplemental vitamin E in liver disease. Despite the encouraging in vitro work, results from clinical studies are conflicting. At doses of 400 to 1200 IU daily, the administration of vitamin E reduces serum aminotransferases and alkaline phosphatase, both in monotherapy and as add-on to ursodeoxycholic acid (UDCA), and improves NASH, steatosis, and lobular inflammation, but not fibrosis scores, which are only improved by the association with vitamin C.[9,48–50] The recent US Guidelines recommend vitamin E and conclude that

"Vitamin E administered at daily dose of 800 IU/day improves liver histology in non-diabetic adults with biopsy-proven NASH."[15]

Pentoxifylline

Pentoxifylline (PTX) is a methylxanthine derivative and a nonselective phosphodiesterase inhibitor with well-known hemorheologic activity and anti-inflammatory properties; it acts as a free radical scavenger, inhibits pro-inflammatory cytokine production, namely, tumor necrosis factor-α (TNF-α), and reduces apoptosis.

In patients with NASH, PTX treatment for greater than 1 year versus placebo resulted in a statistically significant normalization or improvement of 30% or more in ALT but not in AST.[51,52] In a systematic review including 6 trials, PTX treatment at a dose of 800 mg to 1600 mg per day for 3 to 6 months improved liver enzymes; histology was only improved after 12 months of follow-up.[53] The positive effects on liver fibrosis might be the consequence of reduced oxidized lipid products. The overall methodological quality of the published studies is however relatively weak and larger studies are needed for additional validation.[54]

Sylibin

Silybin is a potent antioxidant representing about 50% to 70% of the silymarin extract of Silybum marianum (milk thistle). Silybin modulates inflammation and fibrogenesis and interferes with intrahepatic glycolysis and gluconeogenesis. As with other flavolignans, limitations of silybin use include low water solubility, low bioavailability, and poor intestinal absorption, but derivatives with improved solubility may overcome these pharmacologic limitations.

Silybin treatment attenuated liver damage and diabetes in animal models of NASH. The synthetic derivative in use in clinical practice is the silybin phytosome complex (silybin plus phosphatidylcholine), coformulated with vitamin E, with much higher bioavailability.

In animal models silybin administration reduces insulin resistance and liver enzymes, as well as hepatic and myocardial damage, at doses similar to those used in humans. Considering the good tolerability of sylibin and its positive effects, further investigation is warranted.

BILE ACIDS AND DERIVATIVES
Ursodeoxycholic Acid (UDCA)

The rationale for using UDCA (a tertiary bile acid) as a broad hepatoprotective agent is based on a large body of preclinical data[55] and on controlled trials (**Box 3**). The

---

Box 3
Bile acids and derivatives—mechanism of action

- Hepatoprotective effect (UDCA)
- Anti-inflammatory action, mediated by decreased transcription of tumor necrosis factor-α (UDCA)
- Improved insulin sensitivity in muscle tissue and in the liver
- Down-regulation of lipogenic and apoptotic pathways (Nor-UDCA), favoring increased cholesterol efflux
- Protection against bile-salt-induced cellular toxicity (Tauro-UDCA)
- Anti-inflammatory and lipid-lowering activity (UDCA-LPE)

histologic efficacy remains controversial but there is strong evidence of biochemical effectiveness (on ALT), arguing in favor of a broader hepatoprotective effect of UDCA.

Between 1994 and 2008, 4 studies on UDCA treatment were published on NASH. At doses of 12 to 15 mg/kg/d UDCA monotherapy did not produce any significant effect on liver enzyme levels and histology[1]; the combination of UDCA and vitamin E resulted in significant effects on histology.[3] High-dose UDCA (28–35 mg/kg/d) versus placebo improved liver enzymes, glucose, and insulin levels,[8,11] but the UDCA-treated group lost on average 3% of original body weight, possibly contributing to the favorable results.

Although UDCA monotherapy will not be further tested in NASH, UDCA derivatives have shown promising efficacy stronger than UDCA in preclinical models. In a genetic model of NASH, nor-ursodeoxycholic acid, a C23 homolog of UDCA, improved steatohepatitis by down-regulating lipogenic and apoptotic pathways while increasing hepatic cholesterol efflux. Tauro-ursodeoxycholic acid, a hydrophilic conjugate of UDCA, was able to block apoptosis, thus resulting in improved insulin resistance. Finally, a synthetic bile acid-phospholipid conjugate ursodeoxycholyl-lysophosphatidylethanolamide (UDCA-LPE) was designed to target phosphatidyl-choline to hepatocytes by means of the bile acid transport systems. In in vivo models of NASH, it reduced hepatic fat overload and inhibited de novo lipogenesis, also reducing proinflammatory pathways and liver enzyme levels.

A recent study confirmed that UDCA-LPE ameliorates hepatic injury in different stages of NAFLD, such as steatosis and advanced steatohepatitis. For the excellent anti-inflammatory and lipid-lowering properties, and inhibition of disease progression, UDCA-LPE represents a promising compound suitable for the treatment of NAFLD.[56]

NEW AREAS OF RESEARCH

Several new areas of research are being exploited or old areas are receiving new interest and developments, to provide more effective and safer drugs for NAFLD treatment (**Box 4**).

Box 4
New areas of research—mechanism of action of new drugs

- Stimulation of the farnesoid X receptor-α that regulates glucose and lipid metabolism (OCA)

- Immunomodulatory and anti-inflammatory action, mediated by the inhibition of nuclear factor-kB and down-regulation of inducible nitric oxide synthase (OCA)

- Increased hepatic insulin signaling and sensitivity (GLP-1 agonists)

- Decreased hepatic lipogenesis and liver triglyceride content (GLP-1 agonists)

- GLP-1 agonist- and DPP-4 inhibitor-mediated protection of pancreatic β-cells from endoplasmic reticulum stress and apoptosis

- Insulin-sensitizing activity in the liver (PPAR-δ agonists)

- Reduced food intake (Endocannabinoid CB2 agonists)

- Improved insulin sensitivity and block of the hepatic recruitment of inflammatory cells and the development of fibrosis (ARB)

- Direct inhibition or even reversal of hepatic fibrosis (Lysyl oxidase-like-2 inhibitory monoclonal antibody)

Obeticholic Acid and Farnesoid X Receptor Agonists

Bile acids are critical regulators of hepatic lipid and glucose metabolism through 2 major receptor pathways: farnesoid X receptor (FXR), a member of the nuclear hormone receptor superfamily, and G protein-coupled bile acid receptor 1 (GPBAR1). FXRs are mainly found in the liver, kidney, and intestines, and overall inhibit hepatic bile acid production.

FXR knockout mice have high plasma triglyceride and cholesterol levels as well as a hepatic phenotype similar to NASH patients,[57] including the possible development of hepatocellular carcinoma (HCC).[58] Signaling through FXR and GPBAR1 modulates metabolic pathways, regulating not only bile acid synthesis and their enterohepatic recirculation but also triglyceride, cholesterol and glucose levels, energy homeostasis, and immune responses.

Obeticholic acid (OCA, INT-747, 6α-ethyl-chenodeoxycholic acid), a semisynthetic derivative of chenodeoxycholic acid, is a natural agonist of the FXR-α nuclear hormone receptor that regulates glucose and lipid metabolism. In animal models, OCA decreases insulin resistance and hepatic steatosis and displays immunomodulatory and anti-inflammatory properties.[59] In a phase 2 trial, OCA administration for 6 weeks was well tolerated, increased insulin sensitivity, and reduced liver enzymes and the markers of liver inflammation and fibrosis in patients with type 2 diabetes and NAFLD.[60] A large US multicenter, 18-month phase IIb study of OCA in NASH patients is currently ongoing. Overall, adverse events were not different in patients on treatment or on placebo.

Incretin Mimetics

The rationale for the use of the glucagon-like peptide-1 analogues (GLP-1a) and the dipeptidyl peptidase-4 inhibitors (DPP-4i) in NAFLD does not only derive from their insulin-sensitizing activity but also from the evidence of a reduced activity of the incretin system in NASH patients. The expression of GLP-1 receptors in liver or hepatocytes is inconsistent in different laboratories, but the expression in the biopsies from NASH patients is generally lower compared with control biopsies,[61] and DPP-4 activity is 30% increased.[62] Notably, both the serum activity and the intensity of DPP-4 immunostaining in the liver are associated with the intensity of fatty infiltration and histologic grading of NASH, providing a rationale for the use of DPP-4i to slow the progression of hepatic steatosis and inflammation.[63] GLP-1a and DPP-4i are also likely to improve NAFLD through improved insulin sensitivity.[64]

The protective effects of incretin-mimetic agents on hepatic steatosis were found in diet-induced obese mice treated with GLP-1 analogues and with DPP-IV inhibitors (in linagliptin-treated diet-induced obese mice liver fat content was reduced by up to 30%),[64–68] but data were not confirmed in patients treated with exenatide.[69] More research is needed to explore the mechanism and the possibility of using incretin-mimetic agents as therapy for NAFLD.[70] Notably, clinical studies have provided evidence that DPP-4i can be used safely without any risk of hypoglycemia even in nondiabetic patients.[63]

PPAR-δ Agonists

The function of PPAR-δ has long been unrecognized. Now PPAR-δ seems to be the most promising of all PPAR targets for its specific action on the liver, muscle, and fat. The liver was only recently identified as a major PPAR-δ-responsive tissue, able to burn large amounts of glucose, thus reducing hyperglycemia and improving insulin sensitivity. PPAR-δ also regulates the catabolism and/or the β-oxidation of lipids in adipose tissue and muscle, increases the production of mono-unsaturated fatty acids, and may protect the liver from free fatty acid-mediated lipotoxicity and inflammatory response.[71,72]

The lipogenic activity of PPAR-δ has also been observed in human studies.[73] Ligands for PPAR-δ have been proposed to act as insulin sensitizers, based on improvements in standard glucose-tolerance tests. Studies based on long-term ligand treatment regimens show a significant weight loss and a decreased fat mass, conditions potentially responsible for increased insulin sensitivity. Along this line, the PPAR-δ agonist GW0742 was reported to reduce hepatic steatosis and hyperglycemia.[72] In mice fed the steatogenic metionine-choline-deficient diet, the PPAR-δ agonist GW501516 improved hepatic steatosis and reduced inflammation.[74,75] Thus, PPAR-δ might be helpful in NASH,[76] but no selective PPAR-δ agonists are clinically available at present.

PPAR-α/δ Agonists

GFT505 and its main active metabolites are PPAR modulators with preferential activity on human PPAR-α in vitro (half-maximal effective concentration) and with additional activity on human PPAR-δ. After oral administration, it accumulates predominantly in the liver, with concomitant repression of pro-inflammatory and profibrotic genes. Preclinical and clinical data demonstrated that GFT505 treatment improves several metabolic parameters, including fasting plasma glucose and insulin sensitivity (homeostasis model of assessment-insulin resistance) in abdominally obese patients.[77] This improvement in metabolic parameters supports its use in the treatment of hepatic steatosis and the results seem promising. GFT505 treatment decreased plasma concentrations of liver enzymes and had a protective effect on steatosis, inflammation, and fibrosis.[78,79] A randomized, double-blind, placebo-controlled, 1-year phase IIb study (ClinicalTrial.gov identifier NCT01694849) is currently ongoing and will assess the efficacy and safety of GFT505 in patients with histologically proven NASH. No serious adverse events have so far been reported.

Endocannabinoids (Cannabinoid Receptor Blockers Type 1 and Type 2 (CB1 and CB2))

The endocannabinoid system, involved in the regulation of food intake and body weight, represents a target for NASH therapy.[80] Rimonabant was the first selective CB1 receptor blocker introduced into clinical practice. CB1 antagonism also improved obesity-associated dyslipidemia and insulin resistance to a greater extent than expected from weight loss. For this reason, different studies were planned in NAFLD, supported by studies in experimental animals. Unfortunately, the alarming incidence of central side effects, including severe depression,[81] led to rimonabant withdrawal. Contrary to CB1, highly expressed in the brain, CB2 receptors are mainly expressed in the periphery, predominantly by immune cells, and play a key role in inflammatory processes possibly involved in the pathogenesis of obesity-associated insulin resistance and the progression of fatty liver to NASH.[81] Modulation of CB2 receptors is thus emerging as a potential therapeutic strategy, and the development of peripherally acting CB1/CB2 antagonists remains an area of intense research.[82]

Drugs Modulating the Renin-Angiotensin System (RAS)

In the liver, chronic injury up-regulates the local tissue renin-angiotensin system, which contributes to the recruitment of inflammatory cells and the development of fibrosis. Angiotensin receptor blockers (ARBs) might reduce oxidative stress, attenuating the progression of hepatic fibrosis. In human studies, 2 ARBs (losartan and valsartan) reduced transaminase levels[11,83]; one reduced the grade of liver steatosis, fibrosis, and ballooning, but ARB use never did reach the clinical stage. Nonetheless, they are widely used, with a well-characterized safety profile, in the presence of comorbidities.

Lysyl Oxidase-Like-2 Inhibitory Monoclonal Antibody

Fibroblasts constitute the major cell type of the stromal compartment and contribute to tumor growth, angiogenesis, and fibrotic disease through paracrine signaling. The matrix enzyme lysyl oxidase-like-2 has an important role in the creation and maintenance of the pathologic microenvironment in cancer and fibrotic diseases. The inhibition of this enzyme by a lysyl oxidase-like-2 inhibitor monoclonal antibody (sintuzumab, GS-6624; Gilead Sciences, Foster City, CA, USA) is associated with reduced tumor volume in a mice model, probably due to a reduction of cross-linked collagenous matrix and activated fibroblasts. The use of this monoclonal antibody is also associated with the inhibition of transfer growth factor-β signaling in fibroblasts and reduced porto-portal and porto-central fibrosis. This evidence is the basis for the development of a new class of drugs to be tested in several hepatic diseases characterized by advanced fibrosis/cirrhosis, to reduce directly the progression to fibrotic stage and/or to reverse stable fibrosis.[84] At least 2 phase IIb trials are at present recruiting participants for studies in advanced NASH with/without cirrhosis by the use of GS-6624, infused every 2 weeks for 96 weeks. Outcome results are expected by August 2015.

SUMMARY

There is a definite clinical need for an effective treatment of NAFLD, but current approaches remain suboptimal. Several factors will complicate the development of novel pharmacotherapies, including: (1) the multifactorial pathogenesis of NAFLD, (2) the heterogeneity of the patient population, (3) the imprecision of current disease staging techniques, (4) ill-validated surrogate markers, making histologic assessment compulsory, (5) the slowly progressive nature of NASH and the tendency of a proportion of cases to show spontaneous disease regression, likely related to the improvement of metabolic control.[85]

At present, no drugs have been approved with specific indications for NAFLD; there is however general consensus that continuing clinical research is needed on hard end points (ie, improvement or resolution of NASH), with no worsening of fibrosis and/or improvement of steatosis (quantitatively assessed) and sustained normalization of liver enzymes.[86] Although indicated by clinical guidelines, a careful follow-up and treatment of NAFLD are not the rule in the community. Four questions remain unanswered: (1) Should drug therapy be initiated independently of lifestyle changes? (2) Which drug, if any, in individual patients, according to age, comorbidities, and disease severity? Which drug for NAFLD patients with diabetes, where most putative drugs are already in use, and in normal-weight NAFLD? (3) Should treatment be continued life-long, in the absence of significant lifestyle changes?

Efforts should be made to close the gap and reduce the future burden of NAFLD and its complications.[87]

REFERENCES

1. Lindor KD, Kowdley KV, Heathcote EJ, et al. Ursodeoxycholic acid for treatment of nonalcoholic steatohepatitis: results of a randomized trial. Hepatology 2004; 39:770–8.

2. Bugianesi E, Gentilcore E, Manini R, et al. A randomized controlled trial of met-formin versus vitamin E or prescriptive diet in nonalcoholic fatty liver disease. Am J Gastroenterol 2005;100:1082–90.
3. Dufour JF, Oneta CM, Gonvers JJ, et al. Randomized placebo-controlled trial of ursodeoxycholic acid with vitamin E in nonalcoholic steatohepatitis. Clin Gastroenterol Hepatol 2006;4:1537–43.
4. Belfort R, Harrison SA, Brown K, et al. A placebo-controlled trial of pioglitazone in subjects with nonalcoholic steatohepatitis. N Engl J Med 2006;355:2297–307.
5. Ratziu V, Giral P, Jacqueminet S, et al. Rosiglitazone for nonalcoholic steatohepatitis: one-year results of the randomized placebo-controlled Fatty Liver Improvement with Rosiglitazone Therapy (FLIRT) Trial. Gastroenterology 2008;135:100–10.
6. Aithal GP, Thomas JA, Kaye PV, et al. Randomized, placebo-controlled trial of pioglitazone in nondiabetic subjects with nonalcoholic steatohepatitis. Gastroenterology 2008;135:1176–84.
7. Haukeland JW, Konopski Z, Eggesbo HB, et al. Metformin in patients with nonalcoholic fatty liver disease: a randomized, controlled trial. Scand J Gastroenterol 2009;44:853–60.
8. Leuschner UF, Lindenthal B, Herrmann G, et al. High-dose ursodeoxycholic acid therapy for nonalcoholic steatohepatitis: a double-blind, randomized, placebo-controlled trial. Hepatology 2010;52:472–9.
9. Sanyal AJ, Chalasani N, Kowdley KV, et al. Pioglitazone, vitamin E, or placebo for nonalcoholic steatohepatitis. N Engl J Med 2010;362:1675–85.
10. Ratziu V, de Ledinghen V, Oberti F, et al. A randomized controlled trial of high-dose ursodesoxycholic acid for nonalcoholic steatohepatitis. J Hepatol 2011;54:1011–9.
11. Torres DM, Jones FJ, Shaw JC, et al. Rosiglitazone versus rosiglitazone and metformin versus rosiglitazone and losartan in the treatment of nonalcoholic steatohepatitis in humans: a 12-month randomized, prospective, open-label trial. Hepatology 2011;54:1631–9.
12. Wadden TA, Berkowitz RI, Womble LG, et al. Randomized trial of lifestyle modification and pharmacotherapy for obesity. N Engl J Med 2005;353:2111–20.
13. Marchesini G, Brizi M, Bianchi G, et al. Metformin in non-alcoholic steatohepatitis. Lancet 2001;358:893–4.
14. Vernon G, Baranova A, Younossi ZM. Systematic review: the epidemiology and natural history of non-alcoholic fatty liver disease and non-alcoholic steatohepatitis in adults. Aliment Pharmacol Ther 2011;34:274–85.
15. Chalasani N, Younossi Z, Lavine JE, et al. The diagnosis and management of non-alcoholic fatty liver disease: practice guideline by the American Gastroenterological Association, American Association for the Study of Liver Diseases, and American College of Gastroenterology. Gastroenterology 2012;142:1592–609.
16. Mazza A, Fruci B, Garinis GA, et al. The role of metformin in the management of NAFLD. Exp Diabetes Res 2012;2012:716404.
17. Shyangdan D, Clar C, Ghouri N, et al. Insulin sensitisers in the treatment of non-alcoholic fatty liver disease: a systematic review. Health Technol Assess 2011;15:1–110.
18. Loomba R, Lutchman G, Kleiner DE, et al. Clinical trial: pilot study of metformin for the treatment of non-alcoholic steatohepatitis. Aliment Pharmacol Ther 2009;29:172–82.

19. Gastaldelli A, Harrison S, Belfort-Aguiar R, et al. Pioglitazone in the treatment of NASH: the role of adiponectin. Aliment Pharmacol Ther 2010;32:769–75.
20. Ratziu V, Charlotte F, Bernhardt C, et al. Long-term efficacy of rosiglitazone in nonalcoholic steatohepatitis: results of the fatty liver improvement by rosiglitazone therapy (FLIRT 2) extension trial. Hepatology 2010;51:445–53.
21. Lutchman G, Modi A, Kleiner DE, et al. The effects of discontinuing pioglitazone in patients with nonalcoholic steatohepatitis. Hepatology 2007;46:424–9.
22. Ratziu V, Caldwell S, Neuschwander-Tetri BA. Therapeutic trials in nonalcoholic steatohepatitis: insulin sensitizers and related methodological issues. Hepatology 2010;52:2206–15.
23. Musso G, Cassader M, Gambino R. Cholesterol-lowering therapy for the treatment of nonalcoholic fatty liver disease: an update. Curr Opin Lipidol 2011;22: 489–96.
24. Schattenberg JM, Schuppan D. Nonalcoholic steatohepatitis: the therapeutic challenge of a global epidemic. Curr Opin Lipidol 2011;22:479–88.
25. Foster T, Budoff MJ, Saab S, et al. Atorvastatin and antioxidants for the treatment of nonalcoholic fatty liver disease: the St Francis Heart Study randomized clinical trial. Am J Gastroenterol 2011;106:71–7.
26. Dima A, Marinescu AG, Dima AC. Non-alcoholic fatty liver disease and the statins treatment. Rom J Intern Med 2012;50:19–25.
27. Nseir W, Mograbi J, Ghali M. Lipid-lowering agents in nonalcoholic fatty liver disease and steatohepatitis: human studies. Dig Dis Sci 2012;57:1773–81.
28. Tzefos M, Olin JL. 3-hydroxyl-3-methylglutaryl coenzyme A reductase inhibitor use in chronic liver disease: a therapeutic controversy. J Clin Lipidol 2011;5: 450–9.
29. Chatrath H, Vuppalanchi R, Chalasani N. Dyslipidemia in patients with nonalcoholic fatty liver disease. Semin Liver Dis 2012;32:22–9.
30. Chan DC, Watts GF, Gan SK, et al. Effect of ezetimibe on hepatic fat, inflammatory markers, and apolipoprotein B-100 kinetics in insulin-resistant obese subjects on a weight loss diet. Diabetes Care 2010;33:1134–9.
31. Filippatos TD, Elisaf MS. Role of ezetimibe in non-alcoholic fatty liver disease. World J Hepatol 2011;3:265–7.
32. Park H, Hasegawa G, Shima T, et al. The fatty acid composition of plasma cholesteryl esters and estimated desaturase activities in patients with nonalcoholic fatty liver disease and the effect of long-term ezetimibe therapy on these levels. Clin Chim Acta 2010;411:1735–40.
33. Fernandez-Miranda C, Perez-Carreras M, Colina F, et al. A pilot trial of fenofibrate for the treatment of non-alcoholic fatty liver disease. Dig Liver Dis 2008; 40:200–5.
34. Fabbrini E, Mohammed BS, Korenblat KM, et al. Effect of fenofibrate and niacin on intrahepatic triglyceride content, very low-density lipoprotein kinetics, and insulin action in obese subjects with nonalcoholic fatty liver disease. J Clin Endocrinol Metab 2010;95:2727–35.
35. Basaranoglu M, Acbay O, Sonsuz A. A controlled trial of gemfibrozil in the treatment of patients with nonalcoholic steatohepatitis. J Hepatol 1999;31:384.
36. Zelber-Sagi S, Nitzan-Kaluski D, Goldsmith R, et al. Long term nutritional intake and the risk for non-alcoholic fatty liver disease (NAFLD): a population based study. J Hepatol 2007;47:711–7.
37. Parker HM, Johnson NA, Burdon CA, et al. Omega-3 supplementation and non-alcoholic fatty liver disease: a systematic review and meta-analysis. J Hepatol 2013;56:944–51.

38. Valenzuela R, Espinosa A, Gonzalez-Manan D, et al. N-3 long-chain polyunsaturated fatty acid supplementation significantly reduces liver oxidative stress in high fat induced steatosis. PLoS One 2012;7:e46400.
39. Araya J, Rodrigo R, Pettinelli P, et al. Decreased liver fatty acid delta-6 and delta-5 desaturase activity in obese patients. Obesity (Silver Spring) 2010;18:1460–3.
40. Zhu FS, Liu S, Chen XM, et al. Effects of n-3 polyunsaturated fatty acids from seal oils on nonalcoholic fatty liver disease associated with hyperlipidemia. World J Gastroenterol 2008;14:6395–400.
41. Shapiro H, Tehilla M, Attal-Singer J, et al. The therapeutic potential of long-chain omega-3 fatty acids in nonalcoholic fatty liver disease. Clin Nutr 2011;30:6–19.
42. Capanni M, Calella F, Biagini MR, et al. Prolonged n-3 polyunsaturated fatty acid supplementation ameliorates hepatic steatosis in patients with non-alcoholic fatty liver disease: a pilot study. Aliment Pharmacol Ther 2006;23:1143–51.
43. Spadaro L, Magliocco O, Spampinato D, et al. Effects of n-3 polyunsaturated fatty acids in subjects with nonalcoholic fatty liver disease. Dig Liver Dis 2008;40:194–9.
44. Tanaka N, Sano K, Horiuchi A, et al. Highly purified eicosapentaenoic acid treatment improves nonalcoholic steatohepatitis. J Clin Gastroenterol 2008;42:413–8.
45. Zelber-Sagi S, Kessler A, Brazowsky E, et al. A double-blind randomized placebo-controlled trial of orlistat for the treatment of nonalcoholic fatty liver disease. Clin Gastroenterol Hepatol 2006;4:639–44.
46. Harrison SA, Fecht W, Brunt EM, et al. Orlistat for overweight subjects with nonalcoholic steatohepatitis: a randomized, prospective trial. Hepatology 2009;49:80–6.
47. Peng L, Wang J, Li F. Weight reduction for non-alcoholic fatty liver disease. Cochrane Database Syst Rev 2011;(6):CD003619.
48. Pietu F, Guillaud O, Walter T, et al. Ursodeoxycholic acid with vitamin E in patients with nonalcoholic steatohepatitis: long-term results. Clin Res Hepatol Gastroenterol 2012;36:146–55.
49. Lavine JE, Schwimmer JB, Molleston JP, et al. Treatment of nonalcoholic fatty liver disease in children: TONIC trial design. Contemp Clin Trials 2010;31:62–70.
50. Harrison SA, Torgerson S, Hayashi P, et al. Vitamin E and vitamin C treatment improves fibrosis in patients with nonalcoholic steatohepatitis. Am J Gastroenterol 2003;98:2485–90.
51. Zein CO, Yerian LM, Gogate P, et al. Pentoxifylline improves nonalcoholic steatohepatitis: a randomized placebo-controlled trial. Hepatology 2011;54:1610–9.
52. Satapathy SK, Sakhuja P, Malhotra V, et al. Beneficial effects of pentoxifylline on hepatic steatosis, fibrosis and necroinflammation in patients with non-alcoholic steatohepatitis. J Gastroenterol Hepatol 2007;22:634–8.
53. Lee YM, Sutedja DS, Wai CT, et al. A randomized controlled pilot study of Pentoxifylline in patients with non-alcoholic steatohepatitis (NASH). Hepatol Int 2008;2:196–201.
54. Zein CO, Lopez R, Fu X, et al. Pentoxifylline decreases oxidized lipid products in nonalcoholic steatohepatitis: new evidence on the potential therapeutic mechanism. Hepatology 2012;56:1291–9.
55. Ratziu V. Treatment of NASH with ursodeoxycholic acid: pro. Clin Res Hepatol Gastroenterol 2012;36(Suppl 1):S41–5.
56. Pathil A, Mueller J, Warth A, et al. Ursodeoxycholyl lysophosphatidylethanolamide improves steatosis and inflammation in murine models of nonalcoholic fatty liver disease. Hepatology 2012;55:1369–78.

57. Kong B, Luyendyk JP, Tawfik O, et al. Farnesoid X receptor deficiency induces nonalcoholic steatohepatitis in low-density lipoprotein receptor-knockout mice fed a high-fat diet. J Pharmacol Exp Ther 2009;328:116–22.
58. Zhang Y, Edwards PA. FXR signaling in metabolic disease. FEBS Lett 2008;582: 10–8.
59. Adorini L, Pruzanski M, Shapiro D. Farnesoid X receptor targeting to treat nonalcoholic steatohepatitis. Drug Discov Today 2012;17:988–97.
60. Mudaliar S, Henry RR, Sanyal AJ, et al. Efficacy and safety of the farnesoid X receptor agonist obeticholic acid in patients with type 2 diabetes and nonalcoholic fatty liver disease. Gastroenterology 2013;145(3):574–82.e1.
61. Pedersen J, Holst JJ. Glucagon like-peptide 1 receptor and the liver. Liver Int 2011;31:1243–5.
62. Balaban YH, Korkusuz P, Simsek H, et al. Dipeptidyl peptidase IV (DDP IV) in NASH patients. Ann Hepatol 2007;6:242–50.
63. Yilmaz Y, Atug O, Yonal O, et al. Dipeptidyl peptidase IV inhibitors: therapeutic potential in nonalcoholic fatty liver disease. Med Sci Monit 2009;15:HY1–5.
64. Kern M, Kloting N, Niessen HG, et al. Linagliptin improves insulin sensitivity and hepatic steatosis in diet-induced obesity. PLoS One 2012;7:e38744.
65. Ding X, Saxena NK, Lin S, et al. Exendin-4, a glucagon-like protein-1 (GLP-1) receptor agonist, reverses hepatic steatosis in ob/ob mice. Hepatology 2006; 43:173–81.
66. Son JP, Son MK, Jun SW, et al. Effects of a new sustained-release microsphere formulation of exenatide, DA-3091, on obese and non-alcoholic fatty liver disease mice. Pharmazie 2013;68:58–62.
67. Mells JE, Fu PP, Sharma S, et al. Glp-1 analog, liraglutide, ameliorates hepatic steatosis and cardiac hypertrophy in C57BL/6J mice fed a Western diet. Am J Physiol Gastrointest Liver Physiol 2012;302:G225–35.
68. Shirakawa J, Fujii H, Ohnuma K, et al. Diet-induced adipose tissue inflammation and liver steatosis are prevented by DPP-4 inhibition in diabetic mice. Diabetes 2011;60:1246–57.
69. Kenny PR, Brady DE, Torres DM, et al. Exenatide in the treatment of diabetic patients with non-alcoholic steatohepatitis: a case series. Am J Gastroenterol 2010;105:2707–9.
70. Lee J, Hong SW, Rhee EJ, et al. GLP-1 receptor agonist and non-alcoholic fatty liver disease. Diabetes Metab J 2012;36:262–7.
71. Liu S, Hatano B, Zhao M, et al. Role of peroxisome proliferator-activated receptor {delta}/{beta} in hepatic metabolic regulation. J Biol Chem 2011;286: 1237–47.
72. Lee MY, Choi R, Kim HM, et al. Peroxisome proliferator-activated receptor delta agonist attenuates hepatic steatosis by anti-inflammatory mechanism. Exp Mol Med 2012;44:578–85.
73. Riserus U, Sprecher D, Johnson T, et al. Activation of peroxisome proliferator-activated receptor (PPAR)delta promotes reversal of multiple metabolic abnormalities, reduces oxidative stress, and increases fatty acid oxidation in moderately obese men. Diabetes 2008;57:332–9.
74. Iwaisako K, Haimerl M, Paik YH, et al. Protection from liver fibrosis by a peroxisome proliferator-activated receptor delta agonist. Proc Natl Acad Sci U S A 2012;109:E1369–76.
75. Nagasawa T, Inada Y, Nakano S, et al. Effects of bezafibrate, PPAR pan-agonist, and GW501516, PPARdelta agonist, on development of steatohepatitis in mice fed a methionine- and choline-deficient diet. Eur J Pharmacol 2006;536:182–91.

76. Wu HT, Chen CT, Cheng KC, et al. Pharmacological activation of peroxisome proliferator-activated receptor delta improves insulin resistance and hepatic steatosis in high fat diet-induced diabetic mice. Horm Metab Res 2011;43: 631–5.
77. Cariou B, Zair Y, Staels B, et al. Effects of the new dual PPAR alpha/delta agonist GFT505 on lipid and glucose homeostasis in abdominally obese patients with combined dyslipidemia or impaired glucose metabolism. Diabetes Care 2011; 34:2008–14.
78. Cariou B, Hanf R, Lambert-Porcheron S, et al. Dual peroxisome proliferator-activated receptor alpha/delta agonist GFT505 improves hepatic and peripheral insulin sensitivity in abdominally obese subjects. Diabetes Care 2013;36: 2923–30.
79. Staels B, Rubenstrunk A, Noel B, et al. Hepato-protective effects of the dual PPARalpha/delta agonist GFT505 in rodent models of NAFLD/NASH. Hepatology 2013. [Epub ahead of print].
80. Kashi MR, Torres DM, Harrison SA. Current and emerging therapies in nonalcoholic fatty liver disease. Semin Liver Dis 2008;28:396–406.
81. Mallat A, Lotersztajn S. Endocannabinoids and their role in fatty liver disease. Dig Dis 2010;28:261–6.
82. Durazzo M, Belci P, Collo A, et al. Focus on therapeutic strategies of nonalcoholic fatty liver disease. Int J Hepatol 2012;2012:464706.
83. Yokohama S, Yoneda M, Haneda M, et al. Therapeutic efficacy of an angiotensin II receptor antagonist in patients with nonalcoholic steatohepatitis. Hepatology 2004;40:1222–5.
84. Barry-Hamilton V, Spangler R, Marshall D, et al. Allosteric inhibition of lysyl oxidase-like-2 impedes the development of a pathologic microenvironment. Nat Med 2010;16:1009–17.
85. Schuppan D, Gorrell MD, Klein T, et al. The challenge of developing novel pharmacological therapies for non-alcoholic steatohepatitis. Liver Int 2010;30: 795–808.
86. Sanyal AJ, Brunt EM, Kleiner DE, et al. Endpoints and clinical trial design for nonalcoholic steatohepatitis. Hepatology 2011;54:344–53.
87. Nascimbeni F, Pais R, Bellentani S, et al. From NAFLD in clinical practice to answers from guidelines. J Hepatol 2013;59:859–71.

The Role of Diet and Nutritional Intervention for the Management of Patients with NAFLD

Francisco Barrera, MD[a,b], Jacob George, PhD, FRACP[a],*

KEYWORDS

- Nonalcoholic fatty liver • Macronutrients • Lifestyle intervention • Steatohepatitis
- Mediterranean diet • Weight loss • Insulin resistance

KEY POINTS

- Diet and nutrition are intimately involved in the pathogenesis of nonalcoholic fatty liver disease (NAFLD), and nutritional counseling is a mainstay of therapy. However, well-designed, adequately powered studies to test the roles of weight reduction and dietary macronutrient and micronutrient composition on liver histology and liver disease outcomes is lacking.
- The aim of nutritional counseling is to reduce body weight by 7% or more; this is associated with a reduction in steatosis, hepatocyte ballooning, and inflammation.
- Increasing evidence supports the notion of weight-independent benefits of several macronutrients, including increasing omega-3 and monounsaturated fatty acid intake and reducing carbohydrates, particularly fructose.
- Preliminary reports suggest a role for micronutrient and nutritional supplements as adjuncts for NAFLD therapy, but the results of ongoing larger clinical trials are awaited.
- Reduced long-term adherence to nutritional and behavioral aspects of NAFLD management compromises the effectiveness of these therapies. The development and implementation of strategies to increase adherence and compliance should remain a focus of research.

INTRODUCTION

Human nutrition has undergone revolutionary changes over the last few decades in affluent societies. New technologies and industrialization have multiplied food production capacity and, combined with reduced physical activity and leisure time, has

Conflicts of Interest: The authors disclose no conflicts.
Funding: Robert W. Storr Bequest to The Sydney Medical Foundation, University of Sydney, and National Health and Medical Research Council (NHMRC 632630 and 1049857).
[a] Storr Liver Unit, Westmead Millennium Institute, Westmead Hospital, University of Sydney, Darcy Road, Westmead, New South Wales 2145, Australia; [b] Department of Gastroenterology, Pontificia Universidad Católica de Chile, Marcoleta 367, Santiago 8330024, Chile
* Corresponding author. Storr Liver Unit, Department of Medicine, Westmead Hospital, Darcy Road, Westmead, New South Wales 2145, Australia.
E-mail address: jacob.george@sydney.edu.au

Clin Liver Dis 18 (2014) 91–112
http://dx.doi.org/10.1016/j.cld.2013.09.009
1089-3261/14/$ – see front matter © 2014 Elsevier Inc. All rights reserved.
liver.theclinics.com

resulted in a marked imbalance between energy consumption and expenditure. Thus, food intake has increasingly evolved toward high energy density, nutrient imbalanced, fast-food formats, while multiple environmental lifestyle-associated factors have contributed to a significant increase in the net population energy intake. This energetic imbalance has translated into a dramatic increase in obesity and insulin resistance. Worldwide, it is estimated that there are 1.5 billion overweight and 500 million obese adults[1]; with this, the incidence and prevalence of metabolic syndrome (MS), diabetes, hypertension, and cardiovascular disease has increased proportionally. Obesity-related noncommunicable disease complications are a major health and economic concern that accounts for approximately 10% of the national health budget in countries like the United States.

Nonalcoholic fatty liver disease (NAFLD), considered the hepatic manifestation of the MS, is defined by the presence of macrovesicular in more than 5% of the hepatocytes in the absence of significant alcohol intake (arbitrarily defined as ≤30 g/d in men and ≤20 g/d in women) or other causes of secondary hepatic fat accumulation. Currently, NAFLD is the principal cause of chronic liver disease in most countries of the world, with an estimated prevalence of 20% to 30% in affluent nations. This prevalence increases to 50% in patients with diabetes and 70% in obese individuals. The term *NAFLD*, at the histologic level, comprises a spectrum of liver damage including, in its common form, simple steatosis and nonalcoholic steatohepatitis (NASH), a potentially progressive form defined by the presence of hepatocyte ballooning, inflammation, and variable degrees of fibrosis. Importantly, the presence of obesity at least doubles the prevalence of NASH and its progression to cirrhosis, liver failure, and hepatocellular carcinoma.[2] In this regard, it is important to note that NASH can complicate and accelerate other liver disease progression, including from chronic hepatitis C and B infection.

Several studies have demonstrated a positive impact of dietary interventions in treating obesity, insulin resistance, and NAFLD (**Table 1**). As an initial approach, nutritional intervention seems simple, cost-effective, and safe; however, long-term success rates have been disappointing. These results in term are a consequence of several practical limitations, at an individual and societal level, to implementation. These limitations include time scarcity, low availability of healthy foods, nonhunger cues for eating, low physical activity environments and sociocultural behaviors that adversely influence patients' acceptance of lifestyle measures, and the poor long-term adherence to such strategies. In this review, the authors summarize the evidence for diet and nutritional interventions in NAFLD and describe strategies to optimize their efficacy in clinical practice.

WEIGHT LOSS: THE MAIN TARGET OF DIET INTERVENTION

A dysregulated interaction between adipose tissue and hepatocytes is one of the primary and sentinel events in NAFLD pathogenesis. Adipose tissue expansion is associated with a decreased response to insulin and, consequently, increased lipolysis and free fatty acids (FA) production. In addition, because of the close association between adipocytes and inflammatory cells, increasing adiposity results in chronic low-grade systemic inflammation. The result is that obesity creates the perfect milieu for NASH development, including increased FA flux to the liver for lipogenesis, insulin resistance, de novo hepatocyte lipid synthesis, an increase in systemic production of proinflammatory mediators (leptin, tumor necrosis factor α [TNF-α], monocyte chemoattractant protein-1), and a reduction in antiinflammatory mediators, such as adiponectin and interleukin 10.[2] Lipid and cholesterol accumulation in the liver further generates local injury and inflammatory cascades that ultimately result in the develop-ment of liver cell injury, inflammation and liver fibrosis. On the other hand, it should also be remembered that NAFLD is independently associated with an increased risk of dia-betes mellitus (T2DM) (2-fold increase) and cardiovascular disease (CVD) (1.4- to 2.0-fold increase) (**Fig. 1**).[3] Fortunately, at least in the early stages, all of these metabolic processes are reversible because weight loss can regress adipose tissue inflamma-tion and lipolysis and, thus, normalize the metabolic disturbance.[4]

The benefits of weight loss in NAFLD have been demonstrated in several clinical tri-als (see **Table 1**). Ueno and colleagues[5] randomized 25 patients with NAFLD to a 3-month intervention based on a hypocaloric diet and physical activity (n = 15) or to a control group (n = 10). The active intervention group obtained a 10% reduction in body mass index (BMI) and a significant decrease in aminotransferases and hepatic steatosis. In a pilot study, Huang and colleagues[6] likewise evaluated liver histology af-ter 1 year of intensive dietary counseling in 23 patients with biopsy-proven NASH at baseline. Overall, there was no significant improvement in the liver biopsy at 12 months (n = 15). However, in a separate subanalysis of patients with histologic improvement (n = 9), the investigators demonstrated that these individuals had achieved signifi-cantly higher weight loss compared with patients without histologic improvement (n = 6) (7% reduction vs 3% increase in BMI). In another randomized trial, Harrison and colleagues[7] compared the effects of a lifestyle intervention and vitamin E (800 IU/d) with or without orlistat (120 mg 3 times a day) in 50 patients with NAFLD. In this report, histologic improvement was directly associated with the magnitude of weight loss. Thus, more than 5% weight loss was associated with steatosis reduction, whereas more than 9% weight loss was associated with a reduction in ballooning, inflammation, and the NAFLD activity score (NAS) at the 9-month follow-up. Promrat and colleagues[8] consolidated the concept of dose-dependent weight-loss benefits in perhaps the most rigorous randomized controlled trial, albeit with low numbers (n = 31). Although reductions in steatosis and an improvement in liver tests were achieved by all patients in the intervention arm, only those with 7% or more weight loss (regardless of treatment allocation) obtained a significant reduction in liver inflam-mation and hepatocyte ballooning on biopsy. Thus, from these small studies, weight loss of 7% or more seems to be a critical component of any dietary intervention for NAFLD. At a practical clinical level, one needs to be cognizant of the results from a meta-analysis of lifestyle interventions that suggest that the average weight loss 2 to 3 years after a lifestyle intervention was approximately 3.5 kg, less than the opti-mum required for improvements in liver histology.[9]

Several strategies have been suggested for improving weight reduction and subse-quent weight maintenance. A meta-analysis of 12 studies suggests that very-low-calorie diets (800 kcal/d) can induce higher rates of weight loss at 1 year (17 kg vs 7 kg) and weight-loss maintenance at a 4-year follow-up (7 kg vs 2 kg).[10] These results were based mainly on observational reports. A subsequent meta-analysis that excluded these studies did not demonstrate significant differences.[11] In addition, rapid weight reduction can be associated with NAFLD progression and even acute or subacute liver failure as reported following bariatric surgery (biliopancreatic diversion).[12] Hence, most guidelines recommend a moderately low-calorie diet (500–1000 calories less than the daily requirement, equivalent to approximately 1000–1200 calories per day for women and 1200–1600 calories per day for men), aim-ing for weight loss of 0.5 to 1.0 kg/wk (**Table 2**).[13–15]

Different nutrient compositions and various commercial diets have been attempted to optimize weight loss. The very-low-carbohydrate (CHO) diet (based on ≤10% of the total calorie intake from CHO in the induction phase and then gradually increasing to

Table 1
Summary of studies assessing lifestyle intervention effects on liver histopathology in NAFLD

Author	Patients (n)	Study Type	Intervention	Duration	Outcomes
Tendler et al,[97] 2007	5 (Age 35.6 y, BMI 36.4 kg/m²)	Prospective single-arm pilot	Diet: very-low-CH diet (<20 g/d) normocaloric diet plus nutritional supplement; PA: not described; Follow-up: biweekly 0–3 mo, monthly 3–6 mo	6 mo	Weight loss: −11%; Histology (available for all patients): reduction of liver steatosis and inflammation; Others: reduction in blood pressure and total cholesterol/HDL ratio; no significant change in AST, ALT, insulin, or glucose
Huang et al,[6] 2005	23 (Age 47.8 y, BMI 33.8 kg/m²)	Prospective single-arm pilot	Diet: hypocaloric (total calories not specified, 40%–45% CH, 30–35 fat); PA: not specified; Follow-up: weekly 0–3 mo, biweekly 3–6 mo, monthly 6–12 mo	12 mo	Weight loss: −3%; Histology (available for 15/23): no significant histologic changes were observed; Other: no significant changes in ALT, AST, HOMA, triglycerides, or HDL
Ueno et al,[5] 1997	25 (Age 45 y, BMI 30 kg/m²)	Randomized controlled (15 intervention, 10 control)	Groups: LI intervention and control; Diet: hypocaloric (25 kcal/kg, 50% CH, 30% fat); PA: walk 10,000 steps/d or 20-min jog twice/d; Follow-up: not specified, first mo was in-hospital intervention; total 3 mo	3 mo	Weight loss: intervention group: −10%, control group: +3.4%; Histology (available for all patients): steatosis (−1) was significantly reduced in intervention group (P = .05), no significant changes in inflammation or fibrosis observed; no significant changes observed in control group; Other: reduction in ALT, AST, glucose, and cholesterol in intervention group

| Harrison et al,[7] 2009 | 50 (Age 47 y, BMI 36.4 kg/m^2) | Randomized controlled trial (1:1) | Groups: intervention: LI + vitamin E (800 IU/d) + Orlistat (120 mg TID) vs control: LI + vitamin E
LI was the same for both groups
Diet: hypocaloric diet (1400 kcal/d)
PA: no specific recommendation
Follow-up: not specified | 36 wk | Weight loss: LI + vitamin E group: −6%; LI + vitamin E + orlistat group: −8.3% ($P = .36$)
Histology (available for 18/25 in control group and 23/25 in intervention group): no significant differences in steatosis, inflammation, and ballooning observed between groups
In subanalysis: weight loss >5% associated with steatosis reduction and >9% with reductions in inflammation and hepatocyte ballooning
Other: both groups similarly reduced AST and ALT; intervention group reduced significantly more LDL |
| Promrat et al,[8] 2010 | 31 (Age 48 y, BMI 34 kg/m^2) | Randomized placebo-controlled trial (21 intervention, 10 control) | Groups: LI intervention and control
Diet: moderate hypocaloric, 25% fat diet vs control
PA: 200 min/wk (unsupervised)
Follow-up: weekly 0–6 mo, biweekly 6–12 mo | 48 wk | Weight loss: intervention group: −9%; control group: 0.2%, ($P<.01$)
Histology (available for 10/10 in control group, and 18/21 in intervention group): higher NAS reduction in intervention group (−2.4 vs −1.4 $P<.01$); patients with >7% weight loss reduced more steatosis (−0.9), inflammation (−0.6), ballooning (−0.7) score than patients with <7% weight loss, regardless of treatment allocation
Other: reduced ALT and Waist circumference (WC), no differences in glucose, insulin, or HOMA |

Data are presented as means.

Abbreviations: ALT, alanine aminotransferase; AST, aspartate aminotransferase; BMI, body mass index; CHO, carbohydrates; HDL, high-density lipoprotein; HOMA, homeostasis model assessment index; LI, lifestyle intervention; NAS, NAFLD activity score; PA, physical activity.

Data from Refs.[5–8,97]

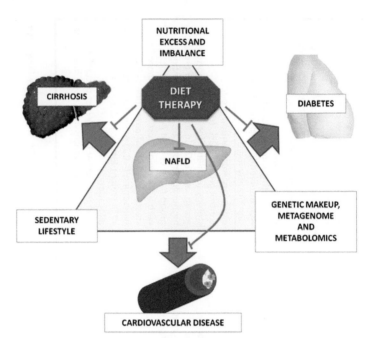

Fig. 1. Multidisciplinary approach to NAFLD. NAFLD is the hepatic manifestation of a severe systemic metabolic disturbance. Its presence is not only associated with an increased risk for liver-related complications but also for diabetes and CVD. Treating NAFLD require a multidisciplinary approach, including interventions aiming to reduce liver damage, CVD, and insulin resistance.

an average of 34%) was associated with a marginal but significant decrease in weight, compared with a low-fat diet (mean −0.9 kg at the end of the intervention) in a meta-analysis of 13 randomized controlled trials (n = 1415; mean follow-up 15 months).[16] However, this difference is of limited metabolic impact, and the adherence to this degree of restriction in CHO is difficult to maintain.[17] A meal replacement–based diet (based on replacing 2 meals by specifically designed soups, energy bars, or drinks) is another reported strategy that has been associated with increased weight loss (average −4 kg) at the 6- and 12-month follow-up.[11] This approach could represent an attractive alternative for patients who have previously failed standard diet interventions.

As discussed, strategies and interventions that seek to achieve weight loss are critical to NAFLD management. However, recent data suggest that the decision to undertake a diet intervention in NAFLD should not be based solely on its weight-loss efficacy. Rather, consideration should also be given to the weight-independent beneficial effects of nutrients, personal preference, and long-term feasibility. These aspects of NAFLD management are discussed in the next section.

MACRONUTRIENT EFFECTS IN NAFLD
Low-CHO Versus a Low-Fat Diet

It is now increasingly recognized that specific macronutrient combinations might benefit NAFLD independent of weight loss. Several studies postulate that CHO restriction can improve insulin resistance by reducing glycemic load and beta cell insulin

Table 2
Recommended nutritional intervention for patients with NAFLD

Dietary Recommendation	Do	Do not
1. Dietary restriction of calories (500–1000 kcal/d deficit)	• Vegetables (3–5 servings/d) • Whole grains (half of daily intake)	• Fast food (least possible) • Oversized food servings • Empty calories (cakes, cookies, ice cream, candies)
2. Choose between low fat (<30%) or low carbohydrate (<40%) according to patient preferences and nature of metabolic disturbances	• Fruits (2–4 servings/d) • Nuts (4 servings/wk) • Yogurts • Olive oil • Oily fish (tuna, salmon mackerel, and sardines) (3.5-oz serving at least 2/wk)	• Potato chips (least possible) • Potatoes • Sugar-sweetened beverages (least possible) • Unprocessed red meats (>300 g/wk)
3. If low-carbohydrate diet is decided, replace calories with PUFA, MUFA, and proteins derived from fish, poultry, nuts, and legumes	• Legumes (4 servings/wk) • Low-fat dairy products • Wine (<1 small glass/d) • Coffee	• Processed meats (>2/wk) • Salt
4. If low-fat diet is decided, replace calories with low–glycemic index foods and proteins derived from fish, poultry, nuts, and legumes		
5. Reduce intake of trans FA (<1%), saturated fats (<7%), and cholesterol (<200 mg/d), particularly in the presence of hypercholesterolemia		
6. Increase the intake of cereal-derived nonsoluble fiber (whole grain) (25 g/d)		

Adapted from US Department of Agriculture. Available at: www.choosemyplate.gov; American Heart Association. Available at: www.heart.org; and World Cancer Research Fund/American Institute for Cancer Research. Available at: http://www.dietandcancerreport.org. Accessed July 19, 2013.

secretion.[18] Low-CHO diets have also been associated with reductions in serum triglycerides, insulin, and glucose and increases in high-density lipoprotein (HDL).[19] Regarding NAFLD, in a recent epidemiologic cross-sectional study (n = 19,479), aminotransferase levels (a surrogate measure of NAFLD at a population level) increased in direct relation to CHO intake after adjusting for age, BMI, and energy intake. Higher aminotransferases were particularly observed in patients in whom the CHO intake was greater than 60% of the total calories.[20] In another report, a post hoc analysis of 52 obese insulin-resistant patients submitted to a hypocaloric diet based on a low-CHO/high-fat diet (40% and 45% total calories per day, respectively) or a high-CHO/low-fat diet (60% and 25%, respectively) observed a significantly greater decrease in alanine transaminase (ALT) and serum insulin in the patients allocated to the low CHO, after adjusting by weight loss.[21] Likewise, in a randomized study of 22 obese patients comparing a low-CHO (<50 g/d) versus a high-CHO (>180 g/d) hypocaloric diet, a greater reduction in liver glucose production and in hepatic steatosis at 48 hours was observed in patients on the low-CHO diet.[22] However, the differences in liver steatosis disappeared after achieving more than 7% weight loss, regardless of the CHO composition of the diet.[22] This data suggest that although there is an early weight-independent effect of low-CHO diets on liver steatosis and insulin resistance, this effect is surpassed by significant weight loss. In line with this, another study randomized 170 obese or overweight patients to a hypocaloric low-CHO diet (>1200 calories restriction per day, <90 g CHO per day, and >30% calories per day from fat) or a hypocaloric low-fat diet (<20% of total calorie intake). At the 6-month follow-up, a similar reduction in weight (7.4%), fat mass, visceral adipose mass, insulin resistance, and liver fat (~40% reduction by magnetic resonance spectroscopy [MRS]) was observed among the patients who completed the protocol (n = 102).[23] None of these studies provided histology assessment. Thus, although moderate CHO restriction seems to have no additional effect on liver steatosis in patients with significant weight loss (≥7%), its impact on liver inflammation and fibrosis and its utility in patients without significant weight loss remains to be elucidated.

Glycemic Index and Fructose

Glycemic index (GI) is defined as the proportion of food converted and absorbed as glucose, and it is expressed as a percentage. Hence, glycemic load refers to the absolute amount of glucose in grams that is provided by the food group concerned. High-glycemic-load foods (including those rich in simple sugars, such as chocolates, candies, cookies, and starches, such as potato, pasta, bread, and rice) increase postprandial glycemia and insulinemia, particularly in patients with insulin resistance.[24] Most studies on diets based on the GI have been from the endocrine and diabetes literature. Pertaining to the overall efficacy of dietary regimens based on the GI, a recent meta-analysis concluded that higher glucose and insulin exposure was associated with long-term complications, such as type 2 diabetes mellitus and CVD.[25,26] Likewise, a Cochrane meta-analysis of 6 trials with a follow-up between 1 and 6 months (n = 202) concluded that a diet based on low-GI products induced significantly higher weight loss (−1.1 kg) and fat mass reduction.[27] In a cross-sectional analysis of 257 healthy subjects, Valtueña and colleagues[28] described an association between high-GI food intake and the presence of liver steatosis as assessed by ultrasound. However, to the authors' knowledge, the effects of such diets on NAFLD and, in particular, on hepatic inflammation have not been specifically addressed in longitudinal prospective studies and should be explored.

Fructose intake has increased markedly during the last decades mainly derived from sucrose (table sugar, 50% glucose and 50% fructose) and corn syrup (~55% fructose and 45% glucose).[29] In the United States, fructose composes 10% of the total caloric intake, and one-third of this is derived from sugar-sweetened beverages.[30] Fructose has several metabolic characteristics that differ from glucose: (1) It has a reduced satiating effect caused by reduced postprandial insulin and leptin secretion and ghrelin inhibition.[31] (2) After entering the circulation, most fructose is taken up by the liver through its specific GLUT 5 transporter (glucose transporter type 5). (3) Within the liver, fructose is converted into triose phosphate and uric acid by enzymes (fructokinase and aldolase B) in an ATP-consuming manner not regulated by insulin or hepatocyte energy status. (4) Part of the excess of triose phosphate can be used for lipogenesis and increase very-low-density lipoprotein (VLDL) export and hepatocyte steatosis. Fructose metabolism is associated with increased lipogenesis, reduced lipid oxidation (by inhibition of CPT1 through its metabolite malonyl coenzyme A), increased free radical oxygen species production, increased gut permeability, bacterial overgrowth, and elevated serum lipopolysaccharide levels.[32,33] In animal studies, some of these mechanisms have been considered to play a role in NASH and insulin resistance pathogenesis.

Looking at longitudinal epidemiologic data, an analysis of the Framingham study database (n = 6039) demonstrated that the consumption of 1 or more soft drinks per day was associated with an increased risk of obesity (odds ratio [OR]: 1.31, 95% confidence interval [CI] = 1.02–1.68) and MS (OR: 1.44, 95% CI = 1.20–1.74), including all of its components (impaired fasting glucose, high blood pressure, hyper-triglyceridemia, and low HDL).[34] A further cross-sectional analysis of 427 patients with biopsy-proven NAFLD from the US NASH clinical research network database demonstrated that the intake of 7 or more sugar-sweetened drinks per week was associated with significantly higher fibrosis and inflammation (all patients) and in hepatocyte ballooning (patients aged >48 years) after controlling for confounding factors (age, sex, BMI, and total calorie intake).[35] A recent study in 47 overweight patients submitted to a daily intake of 1 L of sugar-sweetened soft drinks per day for 6 months presented a significant increase in liver fat (150%), muscle fat (200%), visceral adipose tissue fat (25%), serum triglycerides (32.7%), and cholesterol (11.4%).[36]

Importantly, there is debate regarding whether this effect is specific for an excess intake of fructose or is only a consequence of calorie excess. Meta-analyses have not demonstrated significant effects of increased fructose intake on weight,[37–39] and increased fasting triglycerides are only observed in normal individuals with a high intake of fructose ($\geq$100 g/d, average US intake 55 g/d).[40] In a recent study, 55 healthy subjects were exposed either to a high-fructose (1.5, 3.0, or 4.0 g/kg/d, n = 7, 17, and 11, respectively), high-glucose (3 g/kg/d, n = 10), or high-saturated-fat diet (30% of total calorie intake, n = 10). A significant increase in liver steatosis (assessed by MRS) was observed only in patients exposed to 3 g/kg/d or more of fructose, and this was higher compared with the glucose group (60%, $P<.05$) and similar to the saturated-fat exposed groups (90%, P = nonsignificant).[41] Significant decreases in liver insulin sensitivity were observed in the high fructose and glucose groups.[41] Even though a direct role of fructose in human NAFLD pathogenesis remains to be demonstrated, patients should be advised to restrict fructose-rich food and beverage intake until further studies are available.

Lipids: the Good, the Bad, and the Ugly

Polyunsaturated FA (PUFA) have been extensively studied in NAFLD. Omega 3 (ω-3) FA, particularly docosahexaenoic acid and eicosapentaenoic acid, induce a reduction in liver steatosis by upregulation of peroxisome proliferator-activated receptor α and a consequent increase in FA oxidation and reduced lipogenesis.[42] In addition, ω-3 FAs possess potent antiinflammatory and insulin sensitizing effects through actions on the G protein-coupled receptor 120 (GPR120) and GPR40 and inflammasome regulation in macrophages.[43] Concomitantly, a cross-sectional analysis has reported a reduction in ω-3 FAs and in the ω-3/ω-6 ratio in patients with NAFLD compared with controls.[44] Epidemiologic studies further suggest that increased fish intake (major source of ω-3 FAs) may be associated with a reduced risk of hepatocellular carcinoma and CVD.[45,46] A recent meta-analysis based on 9 intervention studies demonstrated that patients who received an average of 4 g/d of ω-3 supplementation in the form of capsules or oil had a significant reduction in liver steatosis as assessed by MRS or liver ultrasound. However, no significant effect was observed on liver function tests.[47] Currently there are 9 registered trials evaluating ω-3 supplements treatment in NAFLD of which 5 are already completed, and their results should be available soon.

Meta-analyses suggest that a higher monounsaturated FA (MUFA) intake is associated with greater HDL and lower triglycerides and improved glycemic control in patients with diabetes.[48] Animal models suggest that MUFAs have a positive impact on fat distribution, favoring the deposition of fat in adipose tissues rather than the liver.[49] In this regard, a recent randomized study of 45 patients with diabetes comparing a high-CHO/low-GI/high-fiber diet (CHO 52% of total calorie intake and 28 g of fiber) with a high MUFA diet (28% of total calorie intake) for 8 weeks demonstrated significantly greater steatosis reduction in the high-MUFA-diet group (−27% vs 5%, $P<.05$).[50] Although the data on PUFA and MUFA are promising, future randomized controlled trials including histology outcomes are needed to confirm any benefits from these interventions in NAFLD. For the hepatologist, such studies will also inform the treatment of NASH and its potential to reduce the rate of liver disease progression to clinical end points.

Trans FA and saturated FA have been associated with increments in LDL, decreases in HDL, and an elevated cardiovascular risk.[51,52] In contrast, scarce evidence is available about their effects in NAFLD. In a cross-sectional case control trial, Musso and colleagues[53] compared 7-day alimentary records of 25 patients with NASH and 25 matched controls. Patients with NAFLD had higher saturated fat and cholesterol intake and lower consumption of PUFA, fiber, and vitamin C and E. In animal models, exposure to high fat (63.33% of total calories per day), high-trans-FA diet (28.5% of total calorie intake) increases body weight, aminotransferase levels, serum FA, liver steatosis, lipogenesis, and inflammatory mediators.[54] However, it should be borne in mind that the trans-FA intake in this diet represents at least twice as much as normal human consumption (3.5%–12.5%).[55]

Lipidomics analysis has demonstrated a significant increase in free cholesterol in the livers of patients with NASH. Consistent with this, an adverse role for dietary cholesterol on liver disease outcomes has been reported from a large epidemiologic study. In this cohort of 9221 adult patients who participated in the National Health and Nutrition Examination Survey I, a high-cholesterol intake (>500 mg/d) was associated with a significantly increased risk of cirrhosis and liver cancer.[56] At the experimental level, high-cholesterol diets (1%–2% w/w) in animal models have been reported to increase hepatocyte-free cholesterol accumulation in mitochondria and to result in glutathione depletion, increased susceptibility to TNF-α- and FAS (TNF receptor superfamily, member 6)-mediated apoptosis, macrophages recruitment, and liver fibrosis.[57] Thus, even though no prospective study in humans has demonstrated a liver-specific effect, considering their association with increased cardiovascular risk, excessive saturated fats, trans FA, and cholesterol intake should be reduced in patients with NAFLD, particularly in patients with hypercholesterolemia.

Is a High-Protein Diet Good for NAFLD?

As demonstrated in the multicenter randomized Diogenes study (n = 773 overweight adults), a modest increase in protein intake (+5.4% of total calorie intake) combined with a low-GI diet, is associated with improved weight-loss maintenance assessed 26 weeks after the weight-loss phase.[58] This finding may relate to the satiating effect and increased energy expenditure associated with protein metabolism. However, it is important to consider the long-term effects of this type of diets. In 2 long-term follow-up cohorts (n = 129,716 and 10–16 years of follow-up[59]; n = 38,094 with 10 years of follow-up[60]), an increased intake of animal-derived protein was associated with a significantly increased incidence of diabetes (hazard ratio [HR] 2.23, $P<.01$) and cardiovascular mortality (HR 1.14, $P = .03$) in the whole sample and cancer-related mortality in men (HR 1.45, $P<.01$). A subsequent meta-analysis (n = 1,280,380) reported that the association with diabetes and CVD was only significant for processed meat (relative risk [RR] 1.42, 95% CI = 1.1–1.9 for coronary heart disease and RR 1.19, 95% CI = 1.1–1.3 for diabetes per 50-g serving per day).[61] Moreover, a further analysis of one of these cohorts (Nurse Health Study) suggested that nuts, low-fat diary, fish, and poultry actually reduce cardiovascular risk.[62] These studies suggest that high-protein diets can be an alternative for weight maintenance but caution should be taken with the protein source, prioritizing fish, poultry, nuts, and legume-derived protein.

ROLE OF MICRONUTRIENTS, ANTIOXIDANTS, AND FIBER

Because of their antioxidant properties, different micronutrient supplements have been attempted for NAFLD therapy (**Table 3**). Among these, the most validated intervention is vitamin E supplementation. In the Pioglitazone versus Vitamin E versus Placebo for the Treatment of Nondiabetic Patients with Nonalcoholic Steatohepatitis (PIVENS) trial, 247 patients with biopsy-proven NASH were randomized into 3 groups: vitamin E (α-tocopherol) 800 IU/d, pioglitazone 30 mg/d, or placebo. Vitamin E and pioglitazone treatments were associated with a significant reduction in transaminases, hepatic steatosis, and inflammation, although pioglitazone did not reach the predetermined significant P value that was required based on the multiple comparisons.[63] In the Treatment of NAFLD in Children (TONIC) trial, 173 children (aged 8–17 years) were randomized to vitamin E supplementation (800 IU/d), metformin (500 mg twice a day) or placebo for 96 weeks. Although no significant differences in the primary outcome (ALT) or histologic features were observed between the groups after the intervention, the vitamin E group had a significant improvement in the NAFLD activity score (mainly reduced hepatocyte ballooning) and a higher rate of NASH resolution.[64] Although caution should be exercised, considering the reports of increased all-cause mortality and hemorrhagic stroke,[65] vitamin E supplementation is currently recommended as the first-line pharmacotherapy for NAFLD in nondiabetic patients (level of evidence 1B).[66] A subsequent analysis suggested that this intervention was cost-effective only in patients with a high risk of developing cirrhosis (fibrosis stage $\geq$3).[67]

The antioxidant properties of vitamin C were assessed in a prior randomized placebo-controlled trial that included 45 patients with biopsy-proven NAFLD submitted to a combination of vitamin E (1000 IU/d) and vitamin C (1000 mg/d). Although the active intervention group demonstrated a significant improvement in liver histology compared with the baseline, this improvement was not significantly superior to that of the placebo group.[68]

Resveratrol, a polyphenolic antioxidant compound present in red wine, mulberries, peanuts, and grapes, reduces insulin resistance and promotes weight loss through a Sirtuin 1–dependent mechanism.[69] In a preliminary randomized, double-blind, crossover study in 11 obese men, 150 mg/d of resveratrol supplementation for 30 days was associated with a significant increase in muscle mitochondrial function and energy expenditure and a reduction in liver fat, blood pressure, serum glucose, triglycerides, ALT, inflammatory markers, and postprandial FA.[70] It is hoped that the results of an ongoing randomized controlled trial will give further support to the benefit of this therapy in NAFLD (NCT01464801).

Vitamin D deficiency has been shown to have pleiotropic effects and has increasingly been associated with NAFLD and hepatic inflammation.[71] This association is not unexpected considering their common risk factors, including obesity and a sedentary lifestyle. Vitamin D also has direct antiinflammatory actions on macrophages and B and T helper cells, increases adiponectin secretion, and reduces stellate cells

Table 3
Summary of prospective randomized studies assessing micronutrient intervention effects on NAFLD

Author	Supplement	Patients (n)	Study Type	Intervention	Duration and Follow-up	Outcomes
Sanyal et al,[63] 2010 (PIVENS)	Vitamin E	247 nondiabetic patients biopsy-proven patients with NAFLD (age 46 y, BMI 35 kg/m²)	Randomized controlled double-blind Analysis: ITT	Group 1: vitamin E 800 IU/d (RRR-α-tocopherol) Group 2: pioglitazone 30 mg/d Group 3: placebo	Duration: 96 wk Discontinue treatment: placebo 14%, vitamin E 7%, pioglitazone 18% End of study biopsy assessment: placebo 87%, vitamin E 95%, pioglitazone 86%	Histology: Higher NAS score improvement rates in vitamin E group compared with placebo (43% vs 19%, $P = .001$); pioglitazone group did not reach the predetermined significant P value compared with placebo (34%, $P = .04$) Others: significant reductions in ALT and AST ($P<.001$), steatosis ($P<.01$), and inflammation ($P<.05$) for vitamin E and pioglitazone group compared with placebo Adverse effects: weight gain in pioglitazone group (+4.7 kg)
Lavine et al,[64] 2011 (TONIC)	Vitamin E	173 patients with biopsy-proven NAFLD (age 13 y, BMI 34 kg/m²)	Randomized controlled double-blind Analysis: ITT for ALT not for histology	Group 1: vitamin E 800 IU/d (RRR-α-tocopherol) Group 2: metformin 500 mg BID Group 3: placebo	Duration: 96 wk Discontinue treatment: placebo 1%, vitamin E 1%, metformin 4% End of study biopsy assessment: placebo 81%, vitamin E 86%, metformin 88%	Histology: significant decrease in hepatocyte ballooning ($P<.01$), NAS score ($P<.05$), and rates of NASH resolution ($P<.01$) in vitamin E group compared with placebo; significant decrease only in hepatocyte ballooning for metformin group compared with placebo ($P<.04$) Other: no significant differences in ALT change between groups Adverse effects: no significant differences between groups

Study	Intervention	Population	Study design	Intervention details	Duration/Assessment	Results
Harrison et al,[68] 2003	Vitamin E and C	49 patients with biopsy-proven NAFLD (age 51 y, BMI 33 kg/m²)	Randomized controlled double-blind Analysis: not ITT	Group 1: vitamin E 1000 IU/d and vitamin C 1000 mg/d Group 2: placebo	Duration: 6 mo Discontinue treatment: intervention 8%, placebo 8% End of study biopsy assessment: intervention 92%, placebo 92%	Histology: no significant differences between groups; intervention group presented significant improvement in fibrosis respect baseline ($P<.01$) Other: significant reduction of ALT ($P<.01$) and weight ($P<.05$) in placebo group, not in intervention group Adverse effects: not reported
Timmers et al,[70] 2011	Resveratrol	11 healthy obese, nondiabetic patients (age 53 y, BMI 32 kg/m²)	Randomized controlled double-blind crossover	Resveratrol 150 mg/d or placebo (4 wk); wash-out period (4 wk); crossover to resveratrol 150 mg/d or placebo (4 wk), respectively	Duration: 4 wk per intervention Discontinue treatment: 0% End of study MRS assessment: 82%	Histology: not assessed Others: reduced lipid content in liver ($P<.05$), and increased in muscle ($P<.05$) (assessed by MRS and biopsy respectively); reduction in serum glucose, insulin, HOMA, ALT, leptin, and TNF-α ($P<.05$) Adverse effects: nil
Abdelmalek et al,[77] 2009	Betaine	55 patients with biopsy-proven NAFLD (age 46 y, BMI 35 kg/m²)	Randomized double-blind controlled trial Analysis: ITT	Group 1: betaine 10 g BID Group 2: placebo	Duration: 12 mo Discontinue treatment: intervention 35%, placebo 38% End of study biopsy assessment: intervention 59%, placebo 64%	Histology: higher reduction of steatosis (-0.47 vs 0.67, $P<.01$); no differences in NAS score reduction between groups (-0.2 vs 1.0, $P = NS$) Other: no differences in ALT, AST, or weight change observed between groups Adverse effects: higher nausea, vomiting, bloating, and diarrhea in betaine group ($P<.05$)

(continued on next page)

Table 3
(continued)

Author	Supplement	Patients (n)	Study Type	Intervention	Duration and Follow-up	Outcomes
Malaguarnera et al,[78] 2010	L-Carnitine	74 patients with biopsy-proven NAFLD (age 48 y, BMI 27 kg/m²)	Randomized double-blind controlled Analysis: ITT	Group1: L-carnitine 1 g BID Group 2: placebo	Duration: 24 wk Discontinue treatment: 0% End of study biopsy assessment: intervention 100%, placebo 100%	Histology: Lower end of study score in steatosis (0.9 vs 1.7, $P<.001$), portal inflammation (1.3 vs 1.8, $P<.05$) and fibrosis (1.9 vs 1.6, $P<.05$) in intervention group; lower end of study lobular inflammation score in placebo group (1.4 vs 1.9, $P<.001$) Others: Higher reduction in AST, ALT, GGT, glucose, HOMA, total cholesterol, PCR, and TNF-α in intervention group Adverse effects: no significant differences between study groups

Data are presented as means.
Abbreviations: ALT, alanine aminotransferase; AST, aspartate aminotransferase; GGT, gamma glutamyl transpeptidase; HOMA, homeostasis model assessment index; ITT, intention to treat; NS, nonsignificant; PCR, polymerase chain reaction.
Data from Refs.[63,64,68,70,77,78]

proliferation.[72] Likewise in animal models of NAFLD, treatment with phototherapy to increase active vitamin D was associated with a significant decrease in hepatocyte apoptosis, inflammation, and fibrosis.[73] Further human studies are required to assess vitamin D efficacy in NAFLD.

Fiber has been linked to several beneficial metabolic effects, including increased satiety, increased incretin secretion, reduced absorption rate of CHO and proteins, modulation of gut microbiota, and increased fermentation products, such as butyrate.[74] A meta-analysis suggested that whole-grain intake was significantly associated with reduced CVD (RR 0.79, 95% CI = 0.7–0.9) and T2DM risk (RR 0.74, 95% CI = 0.7–0.8).[75] This approach has not been studied in patients with NAFLD.

Choline (present in red meat, eggs, and dairy products) is of major relevance for mitochondrial membrane stabilization and VLDL production. Betaine, a compound derived from choline oxidation, has been used for reducing liver steatosis and hepatocyte apoptosis in initial open-label trials.[76] A subsequent randomized controlled trial of 55 patients failed to demonstrate a significant benefit of this therapy (see **Table 3**).[77] L-carnitine, a quaternary amine derived from lysine and methionine is involved in mitochondrial lipid oxidation. In a randomized placebo-controlled trial of 74 patients with biopsy-proven NASH, L-carnitine 2 g/d supplementation for 24 weeks was associated with a significant reduction in steatosis, inflammation, and fibrosis compared with placebo.[78] However, it is important to consider the recently reported association between increased cardiovascular events and trimethylamine N-oxide concentrations, a metabolite derived from L-carnitine and choline metabolism by human gut microbiota in future studies.[79,80]

The benefit of coffee and alcohol intake has been studied in relation to NAFLD. Coffee and caffeine consumption is associated with a reduction in NAFLD, liver fibrosis, and hepatocellular carcinoma risk.[81–83] Although alcohol intake in excess results in enhanced liver damage, moderate alcohol intake has been consistently associated with a reduction in liver steatosis and NASH risk. As an example, 2 cross-sectional analyses have associated moderate alcohol consumption ($\leq$20 g/d) with a reduction in liver steatosis (assessed by ultrasound)[84] and NASH risk (assessed by biopsy).[85] However, promoting moderate alcohol intake in nondrinking patients with NAFLD is currently not recommended (level of evidence 1B).[66]

PRACTICAL APPROACHES TO NUTRITIONAL INTERVENTION IN NAFLD

The typical Western diet pattern abundant in red meat, trans FA, high-fructose-containing soft drinks, and high-GI CHO and low in PUFA, MUFA, vegetable-derived proteins, and fiber provides an ominous mixture of nutrients for the liver and for metabolic processes. This point was nicely illustrated by Kechagias and colleagues[86] who submitted 16 healthy young patients to a highcalorie, fast food–based diet (>2 fast food–based meals per day) for 4 weeks. This practice resulted in a significant increase in weight (mean +6.5 kg) and ALT (70% of patients increased their ALT to abnormal values) and a doubling of the liver fat content. From a management perspective, the detection and correction of the elements of this markedly unbalanced diet, together with increases in incidental and leisure time physical activity, lies at the core of effective management of patients with NAFLD. However, most patients with NAFLD have more subtle dietary abnormalities; every patient should be individually assessed, with a tailored intervention designed and adequately supported.

Food-oriented nutritional recommendations have several advantages, including a more practical approach, the synergistic beneficial effects of nutrient combinations, reduced portion sizes and caloric content, effects on satiety, and displacement of other foods or beverages. In a prospective analysis of 120,877 patients followed for between 12 and 20 years, potato chips, potatoes, sugar-sweetened beverages, unprocessed red meats, and processed meats were identified as food groups associated with weight gain; vegetables, whole grains, fruits, nuts, and yogurts were associated with weight reduction.[87] Recently in a randomized crossover trial, a Mediterranean diet based on olive oil, nuts, fruits, vegetables, fish, legumes, dairy products, and wine was compared with a low-fat/high-CHO diet for 6 weeks in 12 biopsy-proven patients with NAFLD. At the end of the active intervention, patients demonstrated a significant reduction in hepatic steatosis (−39% vs −7% assessed by MRS) and insulin resistance.[88] The Mediterranean diet has also been demonstrated to be associated with a reduction in T2DM risk, CVD, cancer, and all-cause mortality.[89,90] These trials illustrate specific food groups that should be promoted in patients with NAFLD. A summary of the recommendations is provided in **Table 2**.

Lifestyle interventions should always aim to enable long-term change in dietary and physical activity habits not just a temporary change. After the initial weight-loss phase, the weight-maintenance phase is key for preventing long-term complications. This objective demands different strategies to educate patients to adopt specific habits in their diet that are easy to follow and maintain. Cognitive behavioral therapy has been used in most of the interventions for weight loss. This therapy is aimed at changing behaviors or the cognitive processes underlying the alimentary habits in order to increase adherence to the intervention. Two studies have demonstrated that monthly behavioral therapy sessions for 2.0 to 2.5 years including behavioral methods like goal setting, problem solving, relapse prevention, self-monitoring, and daily self-weighing produce a moderate but significant decrease in weight regain (1.5 and 2.2 kg).[91,92] In addition, the intensity of intervention is relevant. The authors' group, for example, demonstrated that moderate-intensity counseling (6 sessions in 10 weeks) was significantly more effective in achieving weight loss compared with low-intensity (3 sessions in 4 weeks) lifestyle interventions.[93] Although beyond the scope of this review, physical activity has also demonstrated increased weight-loss maintenance and a reduction in hepatic steatosis.[94] Environmental interventions, including family or worksite interventions, are also associated with a moderate increase in weight maintenance.[95] At a practical level, for benefits at a population level, such initiatives require backing by governmental strategic policy initiatives. Finally, a recent meta-analysis showed a potential benefit for Web-based support in weight maintenance; nevertheless, because of the heterogeneity of the studies, the investigators abstained from drawing a conclusion.[96]

SUMMARY

NAFLD is the most prevalent chronic liver disease in many countries; on a global scale, this noncommunicable chronic disease will pose an ever-increasing health burden. Pharmacologic interventions remain few, with limited efficacy and significant potential adverse effects. Thus, lifestyle intervention is, at present, a mainstay of therapy. Weight loss induces a significant reduction in hepatic steatosis and inflammation, particularly in patients achieving a 7% or more reduction in weight. A sustained and gradual reduction in body weight can be achieved by a moderate restriction in daily caloric intake (500–1000 kcal/d deficit). However, strategies to enhance long-term adherence are crucial to optimize current lifestyle-intervention therapies.

Increasing evidence supports a role for the weight-independent effects on steatosis, liver tests, and insulin resistance of diets rich in MUFA and PUFA and low in CHO, particularly fructose. Moreover, because NAFLD is the hepatic manifestation of a systemic metabolic disturbance, interventions should focus toward prevention of the 4 major associated consequences: liver disease progression, diabetes mellitus and its complications, CVD, and cancer. Importantly, interventions, such as the Mediterranean diet, reductions of high-GI foods, and reductions in trans FA diets and saturated fats have been associated with a reduction in diabetes mellitus and CVD. Considering these facts, the authors propose that these specific recommendations should be included in NAFLD therapy even before definitive histology-based supportive evidence becomes available (see **Table 2**). Strategies to enhance long-term adherence to lifestyle interventions, including a multidisciplinary approach, behavioral therapy, environmental modifications, and changes to government policy, should be included. Finally, further research is required to determine the effectiveness of specific nutrient interventions on liver histology and the utility of nutritional supplements; there is a need to develop new tools for increasing long-term compliance.

REFERENCES

1. Swinburn BA, Sacks G, Hall KD, et al. The global obesity pandemic: shaped by global drivers and local environments. Lancet 2011;378(9793):804–14.
2. Barrera F, George J. Non-alcoholic fatty liver disease: more than just ectopic fat accumulation. Drug Discov Today Dis Mech 2013;10(1–2):e47–54.
3. Musso G, Gambino R, Cassader M. Need for a three-focused approach to nonalcoholic fatty liver disease. Hepatology 2011;53(5):1773 [author reply: 1774].
4. Bird L. Macrophages yo-yo during weight loss. Nat Rev Immunol 2010;10(11): 750.
5. Ueno T, Sugawara H, Sujaku K, et al. Therapeutic effects of restricted diet and exercise in obese patients with fatty liver. J Hepatol 1997;27(1):103–7.
6. Huang MA, Greenson JK, Chao C, et al. One-year intense nutritional counseling results in histological improvement in patients with non-alcoholic steatohepatitis: a pilot study. Am J Gastroenterol 2005;100(5):1072–81.
7. Harrison SA, Fecht W, Brunt EM, et al. Orlistat for overweight subjects with nonalcoholic steatohepatitis: a randomized, prospective trial. Hepatology 2009;49(1): 80–6.
8. Promrat K, Kleiner DE, Niemeier HM, et al. Randomized controlled trial testing the effects of weight loss on nonalcoholic steatohepatitis. Hepatology 2010; 51(1):121–9.
9. Douketis JD, Macie C, Thabane L, et al. Systematic review of long-term weight loss studies in obese adults: clinical significance and applicability to clinical practice. Int J Obes (Lond) 2005;29(10):1153–67.
10. Anderson JW, Konz EC, Frederich RC, et al. Long-term weight-loss maintenance: a meta-analysis of US studies. Am J Clin Nutr 2001;74(5):579–84.
11. Franz MJ, VanWormer JJ, Crain AL, et al. Weight-loss outcomes: a systematic review and meta-analysis of weight-loss clinical trials with a minimum 1-year follow-up. J Am Diet Assoc 2007;107(10):1755–67.
12. D'Albuquerque LA, Gonzalez AM, Wahle RC, et al. Liver transplantation for subacute hepatocellular failure due to massive steatohepatitis after bariatric surgery. Liver Transpl 2008;14(6):881–5.
13. Eckel RH. Clinical practice. Nonsurgical management of obesity in adults. N Engl J Med 2008;358(18):1941–50.
14. Rosenzweig JL, Ferrannini E, Grundy SM, et al. Primary prevention of cardiovascular disease and type 2 diabetes in patients at metabolic risk: an endocrine society clinical practice guideline. J Clin Endocrinol Metab 2008;93(10):3671–89.

15. Grundy SM, Cleeman JI, Daniels SR, et al. Diagnosis and management of the metabolic syndrome: an American Heart Association/National Heart, Lung, and Blood Institute scientific statement. Circulation 2005;112(17):2735–52.
16. Bueno NB, de Melo IS, de Oliveira SL, et al. Very-low-carbohydrate ketogenic diet v. low-fat diet for long-term weight loss: a meta-analysis of randomised controlled trials. Br J Nutr 2013 Oct;110(7):1178–87.
17. Hu T, Mills KT, Yao L, et al. Effects of low-carbohydrate diets versus low-fat diets on metabolic risk factors: a meta-analysis of randomized controlled clinical trials. Am J Epidemiol 2012;176(Suppl 7):S44–54.
18. Ebbeling CB, Swain JF, Feldman HA, et al. Effects of dietary composition on energy expenditure during weight-loss maintenance. JAMA 2012;307(24): 2627–34.
19. Santos FL, Esteves SS, da Costa Pereira A, et al. Systematic review and meta-analysis of clinical trials of the effects of low carbohydrate diets on cardiovascular risk factors. Obes Rev 2012;13(11):1048–66.
20. Kwon OW, Jun DW, Lee SM, et al. Carbohydrate but not fat is associated with elevated aminotransferases. Aliment Pharmacol Ther 2012;35:1064–72.
21. Ryan MC, Abbasi F, Lamendola C, et al. Serum alanine aminotransferase levels decrease further with carbohydrate than fat restriction in insulin-resistant adults. Diabetes Care 2007;30(5):1075–80.
22. Kirk E, Reeds DN, Finck BN, et al. Dietary fat and carbohydrates differentially alter insulin sensitivity during caloric restriction. Gastroenterology 2009;136(5): 1552–60.
23. Haufe S, Engeli S, Kast P, et al. Randomized comparison of reduced fat and reduced carbohydrate hypocaloric diets on intrahepatic fat in overweight and obese human subjects. Hepatology 2011;53(5):1504–14.
24. Thomas T, Pfeiffer AF. Foods for the prevention of diabetes: how do they work? Diabetes Metab Res Rev 2012;28(1):25–49.
25. Livesey G, Taylor R, Livesey H, et al. Is there a dose-response relation of dietary glycemic load to risk of type 2 diabetes? Meta-analysis of prospective cohort studies. Am J Clin Nutr 2013;97(3):584–96.
26. Ma XY, Liu JP, Song ZY. Glycemic load, glycemic index and risk of cardiovascular diseases: meta-analyses of prospective studies. Atherosclerosis 2012; 223(2):491–6.
27. Thomas DE, Elliott EJ, Baur L. Low glycaemic index or low glycaemic load diets for overweight and obesity. Cochrane Database Syst Rev 2007;(3):CD005105.
28. Valtueña S, Pellegrini N, Ardigo D, et al. Dietary glycemic index and liver steatosis. Am J Clin Nutr 2006;84(1):136–42 [quiz: 268–9].
29. Tappy L, Le KA. Metabolic effects of fructose and the worldwide increase in obesity. Physiol Rev 2010;90(1):23–46.
30. Vos MB, Kimmons JE, Gillespie C, et al. Dietary fructose consumption among US children and adults: the Third National Health and Nutrition Examination Survey. Medscape J Med 2008;10(7):160.
31. Teff KL, Elliott SS, Tschop M, et al. Dietary fructose reduces circulating insulin and leptin, attenuates postprandial suppression of ghrelin, and increases triglycerides in women. J Clin Endocrinol Metab 2004;89(6):2963–72.
32. Lim JS, Mietus-Snyder M, Valente A, et al. The role of fructose in the pathogenesis of NAFLD and the metabolic syndrome. Nat Rev Gastroenterol Hepatol 2010;7(5):251–64.
33. Vos MB, Lavine JE. Dietary fructose in nonalcoholic fatty liver disease. Hepatology 2013;57(6):2525–31.

34. Dhingra R, Sullivan L, Jacques PF, et al. Soft drink consumption and risk of developing cardiometabolic risk factors and the metabolic syndrome in middle-aged adults in the community. Circulation 2007;116(5):480–8.
35. Abdelmalek MF, Suzuki A, Guy C, et al. Increased fructose consumption is associated with fibrosis severity in patients with nonalcoholic fatty liver disease. Hepatology 2010;51(6):1961–71.
36. Maersk M, Belza A, Stodkilde-Jorgensen H, et al. Sucrose-sweetened beverages increase fat storage in the liver, muscle, and visceral fat depot: a 6-mo randomized intervention study. Am J Clin Nutr 2012;95(2):283–9.
37. Sievenpiper JL, de Souza RJ, Mirrahimi A, et al. Effect of fructose on body weight in controlled feeding trials: a systematic review and meta-analysis. Ann Intern Med 2012;156(4):291–304.
38. Ha V, Sievenpiper JL, de Souza RJ, et al. Effect of fructose on blood pressure: a systematic review and meta-analysis of controlled feeding trials. Hypertension 2012;59(4):787–95.
39. Wang DD, Sievenpiper JL, de Souza RJ, et al. The effects of fructose intake on serum uric acid vary among controlled dietary trials. J Nutr 2012;142(5):916–23.
40. Tappy L. Q&A: 'toxic' effects of sugar: should we be afraid of fructose? BMC Biol 2012;10:42.
41. Lecoultre V, Egli L, Carrel G, et al. Effects of fructose and glucose overfeeding on hepatic insulin sensitivity and intrahepatic lipids in healthy humans. Obesity (Silver Spring) 2013;21(4):782–5.
42. Pettinelli P, Del Pozo T, Araya J, et al. Enhancement in liver SREBP-1c/PPAR-alpha ratio and steatosis in obese patients: correlations with insulin resistance and n-3 long-chain polyunsaturated fatty acid depletion. Biochim Biophys Acta 2009;1792(11):1080–6.
43. Yan Y, Jiang W, Spinetti T, et al. Omega-3 fatty acids prevent inflammation and metabolic disorder through inhibition of NLRP3 inflammasome activation. Immunity 2013;38(6):1154–63.
44. Elizondo A, Araya J, Rodrigo R, et al. Polyunsaturated fatty acid pattern in liver and erythrocyte phospholipids from obese patients. Obesity (Silver Spring) 2007;15(1):24–31.
45. Joensen AM, Overvad K, Dethlefsen C, et al. Marine n-3 polyunsaturated fatty acids in adipose tissue and the risk of acute coronary syndrome. Circulation 2011;124(11):1232–8.
46. Sawada N, Inoue M, Iwasaki M, et al. Consumption of n-3 fatty acids and fish reduces risk of hepatocellular carcinoma. Gastroenterology 2012;142(7):1468–75.
47. Parker HM, Johnson NA, Burdon CA, et al. Omega-3 supplementation and nonalcoholic fatty liver disease: a systematic review and meta-analysis. J Hepatol 2012;56(4):944–51.
48. Schwingshackl L, Hoffmann G. Monounsaturated fatty acids and risk of cardiovascular disease: synopsis of the evidence available from systematic reviews and meta-analyses. Nutrients 2012;4(12):1989–2007.
49. Bessesen DH, Vensor SH, Jackman MR. Trafficking of dietary oleic, linolenic, and stearic acids in fasted or fed lean rats. Am J Physiol Endocrinol Metab 2000;278(6):E1124–32.
50. Bozzetto L, Prinster A, Annuzzi G, et al. Liver fat is reduced by an isoenergetic MUFA diet in a controlled randomized study in type 2 diabetic patients. Diabetes Care 2012;35(7):1429–35.
51. Sun Q, Ma J, Campos H, et al. A prospective study of trans fatty acids in erythrocytes and risk of coronary heart disease. Circulation 2007;115(14):1858–65.

52. Mozaffarian D, Micha R, Wallace S. Effects on coronary heart disease of increasing polyunsaturated fat in place of saturated fat: a systematic review and meta-analysis of randomized controlled trials. PLoS Med 2010;7(3): e1000252.
53. Musso G, Gambino R, De Michieli F, et al. Dietary habits and their relations to insulin resistance and postprandial lipemia in nonalcoholic steatohepatitis. Hepatology 2003;37(4):909–16.
54. Obara N, Fukushima K, Ueno Y, et al. Possible involvement and the mechanisms of excess trans-fatty acid consumption in severe NAFLD in mice. J Hepatol 2010;53(2):326–34.
55. Kris-Etherton PM, Lefevre M, Mensink RP, et al. Trans fatty acid intakes and food sources in the U.S. population: NHANES 1999-2002. Lipids 2012;47(10): 931–40.
56. Ioannou GN, Morrow OB, Connole ML, et al. Association between dietary nutrient composition and the incidence of cirrhosis or liver cancer in the United States population. Hepatology 2009;50(1):175–84.
57. Van Rooyen DM, Larter CZ, Haigh WG, et al. Hepatic free cholesterol accumulates in obese, diabetic mice and causes nonalcoholic steatohepatitis. Gastroenterology 2011;141(4):1393–403, 1403.e1–5.
58. Larsen TM, Dalskov SM, van Baak M, et al. Diets with high or low protein content and glycemic index for weight-loss maintenance. N Engl J Med 2010;363(22): 2102–13.
59. Fung TT, van Dam RM, Hankinson SE, et al. Low-carbohydrate diets and all-cause and cause-specific mortality: two cohort studies. Ann Intern Med 2010; 153(5):289–98.
60. Sluijs I, Beulens JW, van der AD, et al. Dietary intake of total, animal, and vegetable protein and risk of type 2 diabetes in the European Prospective Investigation into Cancer and Nutrition (EPIC)-NL study. Diabetes Care 2010;33(1):43–8.
61. Bryan NS. Letter by Bryan regarding article, "red and processed meat consumption and risk of incident coronary heart disease, stroke, and diabetes mellitus: a systematic review and meta-analysis". Circulation 2011;123(3):e16 [author reply: e17].
62. Bernstein AM, Sun Q, Hu FB, et al. Major dietary protein sources and risk of coronary heart disease in women. Circulation 2010;122(9):876–83.
63. Sanyal AJ, Chalasani N, Kowdley KV, et al. Pioglitazone, vitamin E, or placebo for nonalcoholic steatohepatitis. N Engl J Med 2010;362(18):1675–85.
64. Lavine JE, Schwimmer JB, Van Natta ML, et al. Effect of vitamin E or metformin for treatment of nonalcoholic fatty liver disease in children and adolescents: the TONIC randomized controlled trial. JAMA 2011;305(16):1659–68.
65. Guallar E, Hanley DF, Miller ER 3rd. An editorial update: annus horribilis for vitamin E. Ann Intern Med 2005;143(2):143–5.
66. Chalasani N, Younossi Z, Lavine JE, et al. The diagnosis and management of non-alcoholic fatty liver disease: practice guideline by the American Association for the Study of Liver Diseases, American College of Gastroenterology, and the American Gastroenterological Association. Hepatology 2012;55(6):2005–23.
67. Mahady SE, Wong G, Craig JC, et al. Pioglitazone and vitamin E for nonalcoholic steatohepatitis: a cost utility analysis. Hepatology 2012;56(6):2172–9.
68. Harrison SA, Torgerson S, Hayashi P, et al. Vitamin E and vitamin C treatment improves fibrosis in patients with nonalcoholic steatohepatitis. Am J Gastroenterol 2003;98(11):2485–90.

69. Sun C, Zhang F, Ge X, et al. SIRT1 improves insulin sensitivity under insulin-resistant conditions by repressing PTP1B. Cell Metab 2007;6(4):307–19.
70. Timmers S, Konings E, Bilet L, et al. Calorie restriction-like effects of 30 days of resveratrol supplementation on energy metabolism and metabolic profile in obese humans. Cell Metab 2011;14(5):612–22.
71. Targher G, Bertolini L, Scala L, et al. Associations between serum 25-hydroxy-vitamin D3 concentrations and liver histology in patients with non-alcoholic fatty liver disease. Nutr Metab Cardiovasc Dis 2007;17(7):517–24.
72. Kwok RM, Torres DM, Harrison SA. Vitamin D and NAFLD: is it more than just an association? Hepatology 2013;58(3):1166–74.
73. Nakano T, Cheng YF, Lai CY, et al. Impact of artificial sunlight therapy on the progress of non-alcoholic fatty liver disease in rats. J Hepatol 2011;55(2):415–25.
74. Papathanasopoulos A, Camilleri M. Dietary fiber supplements: effects in obesity and metabolic syndrome and relationship to gastrointestinal functions. Gastroenterology 2010;138(1):65–72.e1–2.
75. Ye EQ, Chacko SA, Chou EL, et al. Greater whole-grain intake is associated with lower risk of type 2 diabetes, cardiovascular disease, and weight gain. J Nutr 2012;142(7):1304–13.
76. Abdelmalek MF, Angulo P, Jorgensen RA, et al. Betaine, a promising new agent for patients with nonalcoholic steatohepatitis: results of a pilot study. Am J Gastroenterol 2001;96(9):2711–7.
77. Abdelmalek MF, Sanderson SO, Angulo P, et al. Betaine for nonalcoholic fatty liver disease: results of a randomized placebo-controlled trial. Hepatology 2009;50(6):1818–26.
78. Malaguarnera M, Gargante MP, Russo C, et al. L-carnitine supplementation to diet: a new tool in treatment of nonalcoholic steatohepatitis–a randomized and controlled clinical trial. Am J Gastroenterol 2010;105(6):1338–45.
79. Koeth RA, Wang Z, Levison BS, et al. Intestinal microbiota metabolism of L-carnitine, a nutrient in red meat, promotes atherosclerosis. Nat Med 2013;19(5):576–85.
80. Tang WH, Wang Z, Levison BS, et al. Intestinal microbial metabolism of phosphatidylcholine and cardiovascular risk. N Engl J Med 2013;368(17):1575–84.
81. Birerdinc A, Stepanova M, Pawloski L, et al. Caffeine is protective in patients with non-alcoholic fatty liver disease. Aliment Pharmacol Ther 2012;35(1):76–82.
82. Anty R, Marjoux S, Iannelli A, et al. Regular coffee but not espresso drinking is protective against fibrosis in a cohort mainly composed of morbidly obese European women with NAFLD undergoing bariatric surgery. J Hepatol 2012;57(5):1090–6.
83. Bravi F, Bosetti C, Tavani A, et al. Coffee reduces risk for hepatocellular carcinoma: an updated meta-analysis. Clin Gastroenterol Hepatol 2013. [Epub ahead of print]. http://dx.doi.org/10.1016/j.cgh.2013.04.039.
84. Moriya A, Iwasaki Y, Ohguchi S, et al. Alcohol consumption appears to protect against non-alcoholic fatty liver disease. Aliment Pharmacol Ther 2011;33(3):378–88.
85. Dunn W, Sanyal AJ, Brunt EM, et al. Modest alcohol consumption is associated with decreased prevalence of steatohepatitis in patients with non-alcoholic fatty liver disease (NAFLD). J Hepatol 2012;57(2):384–91.
86. Kechagias S, Ernersson A, Dahlqvist O, et al. Fast-food-based hyperalimentation can induce rapid and profound elevation of serum alanine aminotransferase in healthy subjects. Gut 2008;57(5):649–54.

87. Mozaffarian D, Hao T, Rimm EB, et al. Changes in diet and lifestyle and long-term weight gain in women and men. N Engl J Med 2011;364(25):2392–404.

88. Ryan MC, Itsiopoulos C, Thodis T, et al. The Mediterranean diet improves hepatic steatosis and insulin sensitivity in individuals with non-alcoholic fatty liver disease. J Hepatol 2013;59(1):138–43.

89. Sofi F, Cesari F, Abbate R, et al. Adherence to Mediterranean diet and health status: meta-analysis. BMJ 2008;337:a1344.

90. Estruch R, Ros E, Salas-Salvado J, et al. Primary prevention of cardiovascular disease with a Mediterranean diet. N Engl J Med 2013;368(14):1279–90.

91. Svetkey LP, Stevens VJ, Brantley PJ, et al. Comparison of strategies for sustaining weight loss: the weight loss maintenance randomized controlled trial. JAMA 2008;299(10):1139–48.

92. Wing RR, Tate DF, Gorin AA, et al. A self-regulation program for maintenance of weight loss. N Engl J Med 2006;355(15):1563–71.

93. St George A, Bauman A, Johnston A, et al. Effect of a lifestyle intervention in patients with abnormal liver enzymes and metabolic risk factors. J Gastroenterol Hepatol 2009;24(3):399–407.

94. Keating SE, Hackett DA, George J, et al. Exercise and non-alcoholic fatty liver disease: a systematic review and meta-analysis. J Hepatol 2012;57(1):157–66.

95. Verweij LM, Coffeng J, van Mechelen W, et al. Meta-analyses of workplace physical activity and dietary behaviour interventions on weight outcomes. Obes Rev 2011;12(6):406–29.

96. Neve M, Morgan PJ, Jones PR, et al. Effectiveness of web-based interventions in achieving weight loss and weight loss maintenance in overweight and obese adults: a systematic review with meta-analysis. Obes Rev 2010;11(4):306–21.

97. Tendler D, Lin S, Yancy WS Jr, et al. The effect of a low-carbohydrate, ketogenic diet on nonalcoholic fatty liver disease: a pilot study. Dig Dis Sci 2007;52: 589–93.

Role of Exercise in Optimizing the Functional Status of Patients with Nonalcoholic Fatty Liver Disease

Lynn H. Gerber, MD[a],*, Ali Weinstein, PhD[b], Lisa Pawloski, PhD[b]

KEYWORDS

- Exercise • Diet • Adherence • Behavior • Function • NAFLD

KEY POINTS

- Exercise promotes health.
- Exercise improves metabolic status and function.
- Exercise is useful in maintaining weight loss.
- Exercise has been shown to reduce visceral fat.
- The American College of Sports Medicine recommendations for exercise are appropriate for people with NAFLD.

INTRODUCTION

The rapid increase in the prevalence of obesity in the United States, and now worldwide,[1] has caught many of us by surprise. In addition, this weighty problem has had important negative effects on organ system health as well as whole person function.

At the organ system level, much has been written about the influence of fat on liver health. It is believed to be a toxic substance that can initiate and perpetuate a cascade of inflammation and end organ damage leading to fibrosis, cirrhosis, and possibly hepatocellular carcinoma.[1–5]

There has been a significant effort to understand the relationship between obesity, fatty liver, and untoward effects on organs.[6,7] Only a few studies have addressed the effect on whole person function.[8–11] Identifying the causal factor or factors for functional compromise is likely to lead to corrective actions that could be used to reverse the trend or mitigate its effect. Despite the conceptual and practical challenges of studying and treating problems of function, this is an area in need of investigation and clinical trials. It is of utmost interest and importance to patients; and those with obesity and nonalcoholic fatty liver disease (NAFLD) stand to benefit from promoting research and dialogue about clinical findings.

[a] Department of Medicine, Inova Fairfax Hospital, 3300 Gallows Road, Falls Church, VA 22042, USA; [b] George Mason University, 4400 University Drive, Fairfax, VA 22030, USA
* Corresponding author.
E-mail address: lynn.gerber@inova.org

Clin Liver Dis 18 (2014) 113–127
http://dx.doi.org/10.1016/j.cld.2013.09.016
1089-3261/14/$ – see front matter © 2014 Elsevier Inc. All rights reserved.

Published literature on this topic has supported the idea that the change in shape and weight of our population is multifactorial.[12] Important factors affecting obesity are likely to include macronutritional changes in diet with increased portion sizes[1]; decreased daily activity level and exercise; and possibly delayed treatment or inadequate treatment of cardiovascular and metabolic abnormalities. Data from 2005 indicate that less than half (49.1%) of US adults met the Centers for Disease Control/ American College of Sports Medicine physical activity recommendation (http:// apps.nccd.cdc.gov/brfss/index.asp/Trends/TrendData.asp).[13,14] Because of the complexity of the problem, a simple pill or silver bullet is unlikely to prevent or cure it. Nonetheless, exercise is a powerful contributor for successful management of cardiovascular and metabolic abnormalities.

Recognition of the importance of changing activity and exercise patterns has been recent. This lifestyle change has profound effects on health and affects multiple domains: mood and sleep, hormonal balance, and cardiovascular health.[15–17] Published work has shown that the institution of even small amounts of activity have been beneficial in improving biological and behavioral aspects of health.[16,18,19]

In the United States, patients with NAFLD follow the national trends of a sedentary lifestyle and are increasingly at risk for hypertension, cardiovascular disease, and components of metabolic syndrome.[20]

DEFINITIONS: FUNCTION, ACTIVITY, AND EXERCISE

Function is the word used to describe the sum of routines and behaviors that individuals expect to be able to perform in order to carry out needed and desirable life activities. Physical, emotional, and cognitive components contribute to function. There are objective measures of function, such as activities of daily living (ADL) assessments. These traditionally include self-care skills and ambulatory ability. Instrumental activities of daily living (IADL) refer to those activities that require more cognitive components of daily routines. Examples of IADLs include check writing, using the telephone, making appointments, shopping, and so forth. One's functional status is often a mixture of the necessary (ADL, IADL) and desired (leisure activities, hobbies, social, and so forth) activities in which individuals engage. Many have suggested that quality of life (QoL) is a mixture of both needed and desirable, and may represent the difference between only being able to perform needed activities and being able to also perform desired activities. Operationally, it is believed to be a measure of satisfaction, happiness, and well-being. The publication, *Healthy People 2010* (US Department of Health and Human Services, 2000; http://healthypeople.gov/2020/default. aspx) identifies QoL as an important health indicator.

Activity is defined as "any bodily movement produced by skeletal muscles requiring energy expenditure" (WHO). It is implied that this energy expenditure exceeds what is required for sedentary behavior. Energy expenditure is defined in terms of metabolic equivalents (METS). It is the amount of energy produced per unit surface area for an average person at rest. One MET is equivalent to 58.2 W/m^2, or 1 kcal/kg/h. This is a convention that was adopted to provide an index of intensity of exercise that is not dependent on body mass (weight). Examples of MET expenditures, which are activity dependent and not dependent on an individual's weight, are as follows: sleeping, 0.9; computing, 1.8; walking 4.8 km/h (3 miles/h), 3; jogging 6.4 to 8 km/h (4–5 miles/h), 7. These measures serve as a basis of determining the caloric needs for performing these activities and for assessing the energy expenditures for daily activities.

Exercise, in contrast with activity, is a structured, planned form of physical activity. There are several forms of exercise: aerobic or endurance, resistance or strengthening, and stretching/flexibility. All exercise is classified in terms of intensity (amount of energy expended during the exercise in METs is the common measure); duration, usually in number of minutes; and frequency, or how often is the exercise performed during a given period of time, usually a week. Intensity is usually measured in METS: light, 1.1 to 2.9; moderate, 3.0 to 5.9; and vigorous, 6.0 or greater. Not all patients would, left to their own choice, select the same types of exercise programs. Some prefer aerobic and others resistance or flexibility (stretching) activities. The use of METs applies to all.[21]

In addition, there is another rating system for intensity. It is a relative scale and depends on an individual's perceived level of exertion or effort. This is important in initiating and sustaining programs of activity and exercise. The relative level of effort expended may influence motivation to participate and adherence to a program. These measures, such as the rating of perceived exertion (RPE), also referred to as the Borg rating,[22] have shown a high correlation to cardiac status in a population of patients with cardiac disease. However, not all patient populations show strong correlations between the disease being studied and RPE. Some conditions have abnormalities of energy production and/or utilization, and have more metabolic disruption. NAFLD may be one of these. This is an important consideration in selecting exercise regimens for patients with NAFLD. If the perceived effort exceeds the tolerance level, most people will have short-lived adherence to the regimen.

There is general consensus about the importance of activity and exercise for cardiovascular health.[19,23,24] In addition, published works support benefit to cardiovascular, metabolic, musculoskeletal, and psychological health.[14,25]

People who engage in a high level of physical activity are likely to have a reduced risk for hyperglycemia, hyperlipidemia, and hypertension.[26] Others have shown that even a modest increase in physical activity produces benefits in waist circumference, metabolic markers, and fitness level, as reported by greater distance walked.[27]

Health benefits of physical activity have been established[28] and have been shown to improve function, specifically balance and reduction in the risk of falls, as well ADLs.[29] Recommendations are for 5 sessions and 150 minutes of moderate activity or 75 minutes of vigorous activity per week (**Box 1**).

FUNCTION AND NAFLD

NAFLD has been called the liver manifestation of the metabolic syndrome.[30] Much of the functional impact may result from metabolic factors, obesity, cardiovascular disease, and osteoarthritis, which frequently accompany NAFLD. Because obesity is such a common correlate of NAFLD, is present in approximately two-thirds of obese individuals and 90% of the morbidly obese,[31] for the purposes of this discussion, the functional impact of obesity is included as part of NAFLD.

Regardless of the cause or mechanism of developing steatosis, most people with NAFLD have metabolic abnormalities that are likely to interfere with participation in physical activity and affect function. David and colleagues[32] found the individuals with NAFLD had worse physical and mental health scores compared with the healthy US population without illness as measured by the Short Form 36.[33]

Functional compromise has been reported in NAFLD, affects many domains of life, and is experienced as significant (**Table 1**). The following have been identified: physical

---

Box 1
Benefits of exercise: WHO summary

A. Strong evidence for association with lower incidence:

   1. All-cause mortality

   2. Coronary heart disease

   3. High blood pressure

   4. Stroke

   5. Type 2 diabetes

   6. Metabolic syndrome

   7. Colon and breast cancer

   8. Depression

B. Moderate to strong evidence:

   1. Likely to have less risk of a hip or vertebral fracture

   2. Exhibit a higher level of cardiorespiratory and muscular fitness

   3. Are more likely to achieve weight maintenance

   4. Have a healthier body mass and composition

From World Health Organization. Physical activity and adults. Available at: http://www.who.int/dietphysicalactivity/factsheet_adults/en/index.html. Accessed September 4, 2013.

ADL (self-care, physical activity)[34]; increased risk for falls[29]; association with decreased physical performance as measured by SF36[32]; increased prevalence of depression and anxiety.[35] Additional analyses of data pertaining to function in this population indicates that the presence of fatigue, cognitive difficulties (memory, attention, concentration, forgetfulness, word finding abilities, and confusion) and orthostatic grading all correlate with functional status.[34,36]

Fatigue is one of the most prevalent and pervasive symptoms in people with NAFLD. Increasing fatigue, autonomic dysfunction, cognitive symptoms, and advancing age were found to be associated with a lower level of self-reported function.[8] A multivariate analysis showed increased cognitive difficulty, age, fatigue, lower albumin, and bilirubin were all independently associated with functional

---

Table 1
Findings associated with NAFLD likely to influence function

Findings	Functional Impact
1. Obstructive sleep apnea	Somnolence, headache Decreased physical activity Fatigue, cardiovascular disease
2. Osteoarthritis knee	Pain, decreased mobility
3. Depression	Decreased physical activity Decreased motivation
4. Balance	Falls
5. Weakness	Decreased mobility, balance, and stamina
6. Cognitive deficits	Memory loss

difficulty in patients with NAFLD. The characteristics and possible causes of this fatigue and its natural history are poorly understood. There are a variety of possible causes. Patients with NAFLD are less physically active and less fit.[10,37] NAFLD is associated with increased levels of inflammatory cytokines.[30] Recent studies have confirmed the presence of autonomic nervous system dysfunction in those with early stages of NAFLD.[36]

Fatigue is clinically important, prevalent, and often of sufficient magnitude to interfere with daily routines (function) and desired activities, including work, school, social, household, and leisure activity. The fatigue that is associated with chronic illness is usually not remediable with rest, and can be out of proportion to the disease severity.[37] For this reason, the evaluation of fatigue needs to include the likely contributors: cardiovascular status, pulmonary status, anemia, hormonal status, nutritional status, sleep patterns, neuromusculoskeletal status, medication, and cognition. These potential contributors should be evaluated before prescribing an exercise plan because they are likely to influence the exercise prescription and contribute to whether an individual will respond to exercise.

EXERCISE FOR NAFLD

Exercise has long been known to be the antidote for a substantial number of functional problems. The most established and accepted explanations for improved function have included improvement in aerobic fitness and exercise tolerance. This has been demonstrated in many disease processes as determined by improved measures of cardiac output and Vo_2 max, visceral fat reduction,[31,38] improvement in insulin sensitivity,[39] lipid reduction,[40] and in maintenance of weight loss.[41] The mechanism seems to be through the activation of adenosine monophosphate (AMP) protein kinase.[42,43] Data on its effect on people with NAFLD is less well established, but what has been published supports its effectiveness for a variety of physiologic abnormalities.

In addition to the high prevalence of obesity and metabolic syndrome in people with NAFLD, they have been shown to be less active and less aerobically fit that people without NAFLD.[44,45]

Exercise tolerance and function are, in part, an issue of the efficiency of glucose uptake. Achieving a level of 120 minutes of aerobic exercise (eg, running or swimming) per week is associated with improved glucose uptake and decreased insulin resistance. Improvement is believed to be mediated through AMP protein kinase, which is known to increase free fatty acid oxidation in the liver.[42] Skeletal muscle plays an important role in the development and mitigation of the metabolic syndrome, independent of total body fat. Exercise is the most effective treatment available for muscle function. The mechanism by which exercise promotes glucose transport and insulin sensitivity[46] and lipolysis[47] is by muscle contraction. Muscle contraction causes mechanical stress to muscle cells and induces intracellular signaling that releases hormones, growth factors, and produces oxidative stress.

However, the improved glucose uptake seems to be both insulin dependent and independent. It may be mediated through myokines, which are mediators of inflammation, which can help regulate various functions of other organs.[48] This regulation partially determines the benefits of exercise. Muscle-derived interleukin (IL)-6 is a myokine that is markedly increased in muscle and secreted into plasma following muscle contraction. It is believed that this may be responsible for the exercise-induced metabolic changes and antiinflammatory effects in other organs such as the liver, adipose tissue, and blood vessels.[49,50]

One possible insulin-independent effect of exercise is its impact on skeletal mass and preservation of muscle cells. Exercise increases protein synthesis and reduces muscle degradation, which is seen commonly in people who have limb immobilization and who are sedentary. Increased lean mass (fat-free mass) is known to increase glucose uptake and helps protect against NAFLD.

Several studies and systematic reviews have been conducted to assess the impact of exercise on the amount of fat in the liver. Data support the effectiveness of aerobic exercise in reducing hepatic fat.[51–54] This research does not necessarily establish that hepatic fat reduction is the primary cause of functional improvement. Nonetheless, this article has attempted to create a logic stream showing that people with NAFLD are likely to have several contributors to low functional level. These are due to cardiovascular and metabolic abnormalities that respond to exercise.

The specific exercise prescriptions used in the published studies referenced earlier were predominantly aerobic exercise targeting heart rates of 45% to 85% for exercise sessions of 2 to 6 times per week and for 2 to 24 weeks. There were variations in exercise prescriptions of sufficient magnitude to raise questions about the generalizability of the effect. For example, to see an aerobic effect and an increase in maximal oxygen consumption, the heart rate target should be 80% of maximum, calculated as $(220 - age) \times 0.80$. The American College of Sports Medicine recommends 3 to 5 sessions per week, 35 to 40 minutes of the recommended intensity after warm up and followed by cool down. Most studies report that aerobic benefits require 8 to 10 weeks of intervention.[55]

In an excellent systematic review[56] 12 randomized controlled trials are analyzed and the data pooled to perform a meta-analysis to support the view that exercise is effective in reducing hepatic fat but not alanine aminotransferase. The effect size for exercise was 0.37. Difficulties in performing this systematic review are not only the small numbers of participants in these trials but the variety of treatments and the use of different methods for measuring liver fat. These included computerized tomography, ultrasonography, and magnetic resonance spectroscopy.

Most therapeutic interventions include aerobic training. However, several small studies have recently reported possible benefits with resistance training.[54,57] The Shah study also included caloric restrictions to achieve weight loss.

Based on these studies, exercise is recommended for reduction of hepatic fat. At the present time, there is no consensus on the specific exercise prescriptions with regard to frequency, duration, intensity; combination with resistance exercise; and addition of caloric restriction. It is important to develop specific recommendations for exercise interventions both to maximize therapeutic outcomes (function, metabolic, and cardiovascular health) and to increase the likelihood of adherence and long-lasting behavioral change. Therefore, many recommend following the American College of Sports Medicine guidelines.[55]

To address the fundamental question of this article, what role does exercise have for the restoration of functional loss in people with NAFLD, there remain important unanswered questions. The outcome measures most frequently used are physiologic (metabolic syndrome, cardiovascular measures) and health status, rather than function.

Function, as described earlier, is a multidimensional construct. Little published information is available to answer whether any of our interventions improve function; and if they do, how this is accomplished. Function is complex, influenced by behavior, physiology, and lifestyle. Exercise is 1 potential contributor to functional outcome but is unlikely to be the sole contributor, or even the most important. Clearly, diet is an important contributor to good exercise outcomes as is behavioral change.

DIET AND EXERCISE

Dietary considerations include macronutrients (carbohydrate, protein, fat) and micronutrients (vitamins, minerals, supplements) and total caloric intake.

The major nutritional consideration of NAFLD is weight loss and obesity prevention. It is important to understand dietary contributions to weight management. Considerable research has examined the effect of both exercise and diet on weight loss, such that it is clear that both increased energy expenditure and reduction in caloric intake lead to weight loss. This article focuses on the impact of exercise in optimizing the functional status of patients with NAFLD, but the role that diet may play in optimizing exercise performance needs to be examined as well as the importance of including both dietary regulation and exercise to improve health outcomes for those with NAFLD.

There is an increasing amount of literature concerning weight loss in general among obese individuals and the independent effects of exercise and diet. Wu and colleagues[58] conducted a meta-analysis in which 18 randomized trials were examined to look at the independent effects of diet and exercise on overall weight loss. They found that the combination of diet and exercise produced more sustained weight loss compared with groups who only restricted diet. Furthermore, greater weight maintenance occurred with combined interventions that lasted more than 1 year.[58] Other studies[59] have looked at the impact of diet restriction only on indicators of cardiovascular diseases including inflammatory markers and found little conclusive evidence that there are independent or even combined benefits. However, although further research is still needed, much of the literature suggests a combined intervention of diet restriction and exercise is more effective in promoting weight loss, which has been shown to be an effective treatment for NAFLD.

Thus, as diet and exercise modification are both critical to controlling NAFLD, might certain dietary interventions be used to optimize exercise performance? There is relevant published literature concerning dietary approaches to improving exercise performance.

Within the fitness and exercise performance industries, there are hundreds if not thousands of dietary supplements targeted at improving exercise performance, often focused on resistance training and weight lifting but also to improve endurance and assist in the recovery and prevention of muscle breakdown. Much of the literature on supplements and exercise performance concerns athlete populations, and it is important to emphasize that small performance changes for athletes might not translate well into benefits to improve and/or prevent NAFLD.

In general, there are multiple nutritional strategies to improve exercise performance. During the training stage, the aim is often to make changes within the muscle tissue by altering protein synthesis and breakdown and ultimately maintain or increase lean body mass. There is a general belief that high carbohydrate diets are effective for endurance events and high protein intake is effective for strength and resistance events. However, for all athletes, there is an increased need for protein and endurance athletes have increased protein needs as they use amino acids for energy.

The use of protein supplements including protein bars and protein shakes have become popular among nonathletes with the idea that such supplements produce greater muscle mass and improve overall exercise performance. However, the literature is not so clear that such dietary interventions can enhance performance for a nonathlete and ultimately lead to weight loss and improve the metabolic markers that may assist in NAFLD maintenance. Even among athlete populations, there is still much to understand about the benefits of protein supplementation. In general, most of the literature has shown that some protein as well as amino acid supplementation can improve strength and physical performance as well as other exercise outcomes. Tieland and colleagues[60] conducted a randomized, double-blind, placebo-controlled trial among frail elderly individuals and concluded that although added protein supplementation did not increase bone or muscle mass, those who received the protein supplements showed better physical performance. However, there still is no clarity on how much protein is needed, when protein should be consumed (for recovery for instance), and in what form (ie, amino acids, whey, meat, and so forth).

Too much protein can be an issue, particularly as many with fatty liver disease are obese and may be at risk of kidney complications from prediabetes or diabetes symptoms. The average adult requires about 0.8 g of protein per kilogram of body weight per day. Those with chronic liver disease may require a bit more because of alterations in protein synthesis and metabolism (1.2–1.5 g of protein per kilogram of body weight). This added protein may not enhance exercise performance because it is the daily requirement for normal metabolic needs.

Another study showed that the protein requirement for individuals performing resistance training is higher than that for sedentary individuals.[57] The daily recommended protein intake is estimated to be 1.4 to 1.8 g/kg for those performing resistance exercise who have a normal intake of calories and carbohydrates,[61] and it is recommended that eating protein soon after exercise is important for protein synthesis and the efficient building of muscle. It is important to recognize that patients with NAFLD should be careful when trying new supplements aimed at weight loss or improving exercise performance.

There are a growing number of studies investigating other kinds of nutritional supplementation and improved exercise performance. Antioxidant supplementation has shown little or no effect on exercise performance. Electrolytes, such as those found in sports drinks, are a concern for more extreme athletic events in which individuals are at risk of severe dehydration, but for the average individual, sports drinks only add unnecessary additional calories (defeating the purpose of weight loss) and water is more highly recommended. Caffeine, one of the most well-known aids to enhancing exercise performance, has been shown to be protective against developing NAFLD. Birerdinc and colleagues[62] found that consuming 2 cups of caffeinated coffee daily was protective against NAFLD using data collected from the National Health and Nutrition Examination Survey. Moderate amounts of caffeine are acceptable for those with NAFLD.

Many new dietary supplements aimed at improving exercise function and weight loss being marketed every day and may be of great concern. Most supplements are not regulated by the US Food and Drug Administration and are typically only regulated when a safety issue occurs. Many supplements are produced outside the United States where there is also little oversight and regulation. Some supplements that contain mixtures of herbs may also contain added toxins such as heavy metals that could create stress on the liver. Recently, in a prospective randomized intervention study, a combination of vitamin C (1000 mg/d) and vitamin E (400 IU/d) inhibited improved insulin sensitivity and may counter the effects of exercise.[63] Mostly, such supplements may just be a waste of money, but some may cause complications in the long-term in those with NAFLD because they may lead to stress on organs that filter toxins including the liver and kidneys.[64]

BEHAVIORAL CONSIDERATIONS SUPPORTING ADOPTION OF THERAPEUTIC EXERCISE AND HEALTHY EATING

The usefulness of exercise is highly dependent on participation and adherence to a prescribed program. Data on the reversibility of its salubrious effects is surprising.

Box 2
Behavioral strategies to promote adoption of exercise participation

1. Motivation. Determine the motivating factor for the individual. Each person is motivated by different factors.[69] For example, 1 person may want to avoid medication, whereas another wants to lose weight to be more attractive. It is imperative to identify factors that motivate the specific individual.

2. Attainable. Individuals are not disappointed when they exceed a goal that they have established. A common mistake is to create goals that are not reasonably achieved. When these goals are not achieved, motivation is severely impacted.[70] Therefore, it is essential to create goals that are achievable so that the individuals can be successful.

3. Measurable. The goals identified need to be achievable; this means that they must be quantifiable.[71] The attainment of the goal must be identifiable in a way that perception is not a component of the goals. Therefore, a goal of "I want to be more fit" does not reach the measurable requirement. Instead, the goal could be "I want to be able to walk around my block without getting breathless."

4. Memory. Habits are a major component of individuals' days and relatively little thought is given to activities that constitute daily routines. However, the key is switching a new behavior to a habit. Therefore, memory cues can be a powerful tool to remind an individual to engage in the new behavior.[72] For example, placing eating plans on the refrigerator or walking shoes by the front door.

5. Positive thoughts. Negative self-talk can be a huge detriment to motivation.[73] Individuals can be encouraged to monitor thoughts and replace negative thoughts with positive thoughts. Instead of "I will never be able to maintain an exercise routine" think "I know it is difficult but I will try my best to engage in exercise today."

6. Reinforcement. It is important for individuals to reward themselves when goals have been achieved.[74] The reward can be something tangible (such as going to see a movie) or can be as simple as getting praise from significant others. Reinforcement is most effective when the reward is given in close proximity to the achievement being rewarded.[75]

7. Environmental support. A focus on the physical environment can also be important because physical factors (such as availability of safe walking paths) can help enhance behavioral change.[76] Individuals may not have complete control over their physical environment, but they can exercise control over certain factors. For example, if a person wants to improve their diet, they can remove all of the junk food from their house.

8. Stress management. Stress is a common barrier to achieving a health goal.[77] As individuals report increased stress levels, the engagement in health behaviors is usually reduced.[78] Therefore, trying to keep stress levels down (there are various techniques, including deep breathing) can improve the chance of successful behavioral change.

9. Social support. This actually may be the most important factor in successful behavioral change.[79] Social support can take many forms, including family members, health professionals, and friends. Supportive social support persons and/or systems are essential components of any behavioral change strategy.

10. Problem solve. It usually takes multiple attempts to successfully achieve a goal. It can be useful to explore what might have gone wrong in previous attempts to strategize ways to overcome them if encountered again. In addition, identifying potential barriers and potential solutions before these barriers are ever actually faced is a useful tool in behavioral change. In other words, creating backup plans to enhance the chance of success (sometimes termed relapse prevention).[80]

Box 3
Exercise prescriptions for patients with NAFLD

Key Points:

1. Prescription must be compatible with age and medical status
2. Instructions must be clear and understandable so that the likelihood of adherence is maximized
3. Goals must be attainable
4. Outcomes should be measurable and provide examples of success and reinforcement for continued participation

The American College of Sports Medicine has published the following exercise guidelines:

Cardiorespiratory Exercise

- Adults should get at least 150 minutes of moderate-intensity exercise per week
- Exercise recommendations can be met through 30 to 60 minutes of moderate-intensity exercise (5 days per week) or 20 to 60 minutes of vigorous-intensity exercise (3 days per week)
- One continuous session and multiple shorter sessions (of at least 10 minutes) are both acceptable to accumulate the desired amount of daily exercise
- Gradual progression of exercise time, frequency, and intensity is recommended for best adherence and least injury risk
- People unable to meet these minimums can still benefit from some activity

Resistance Exercise

- Adults should train each major muscle group 2 or 3 days each week using a variety of exercises and equipment
- Very light or light intensity is best for older persons or previously sedentary adults starting exercise
- Two to 4 sets of each exercise will help adults improve strength and power
- For each exercise, 8 to 12 repetitions improve strength and power, 10 to 15 repetitions improve strength in middle-age and older persons starting exercise, and 15 to 20 repetitions improve muscular endurance
- Adults should wait at least 48 hours between resistance training sessions

Flexibility Exercise

- Adults should do flexibility exercises at least 2 or 3 days each week to improve range of motion
- Each stretch should be held for 10 to 30 seconds to the point of tightness or slight discomfort
- Repeat each stretch 2 to 4 times, accumulating 60 seconds per stretch
- Static, dynamic, ballistic, and proprioceptive neuromuscular facilitation stretches are all effective
- Flexibility exercise is most effective when the muscle is warm; try light aerobic activity or a hot bath to warm the muscles before stretching

Neuromotor Exercise

- Neuromotor exercise (sometimes called functional fitness training) is recommended for 2 or 3 days per week
- Exercises should involve motor skills (balance, agility, coordination, and gait), proprioceptive exercise training, and multifaceted activities (tai ji and yoga) to improve physical function and prevent falls in older adults
- 20 to 30 minutes per day is appropriate for neuromotor exercise

From Garber CE, Blissmer B, Deschenes MR, et al. Quantity and quality of exercise for developing and maintaining cardiorespiratory, musculoskeletal, and neuromotor fitness in apparently healthy adults: guidance for prescribing exercise. Med Sci Sports Exerc 2011;43:1334–59; with permission.

Inactivity and bed rest are associated with significant loss of lean mass and associated functional loss. This is true of normal healthy people and is more significant among the elderly. Significant protein loss from muscle is seen within 2 days of relative immobilization. Insulin-facilitated glucose uptake by muscle is also reduced within days, thereby resulting in a rapid reversal of normal synthetic processes and potential gains from exercise.[41]

Based on these data, and the understanding of the importance of patient engagement and participation in exercise, the clinician should be aware of the critical contribution of using successful approaches to achieving sustained behavioral change. Research has demonstrated that simply providing information about the benefits of exercise and proper nutrition is rarely sufficient to produce enduring behavioral change.[65] However, providing information on how to change behavior more systematically has demonstrated more efficacy in motivating individuals to initiate behavior change.[65] And an even more effective approach would be a structured, multiple-component intervention that used a variety of strategies.[66] Human motivation is a complex process and when layered with behavioral change, the complexity is infinitely increased. Therefore, a strategy that incorporates multiple components has a greater chance of being successful, because it will hit on a larger variety of potential intervention targets. Haber[67] provided a framework that can promote successful behavioral change in an individual. Ten points of intervention and focus were identified.[67] These areas are presented in **Box 2** and include the following key factors: motivation, attainability of goals, measurable outcomes, memory, positive thoughts, reinforcement, environmental support, stress management, social support, and problem solving.

Behavioral change, especially dietary and exercise behaviors, is difficult for most individuals. A multicomponent comprehensive approach is essential for increasing the probability of successful achievement of behavioral change. An individualized and complex approach that uses well-researched strategies is more efficacious to encourage individuals to change their behavior.[68]

SUMMARY AND RECOMMENDATIONS

Exercise should be an integral part of the management of NAFLD. It promotes health and well-being and there is level A evidence on its effectiveness for improving metabolic status and function. It is useful in maintaining weight loss and has been shown to reduce visceral fat. Exercise prescriptions should be specific and aimed at meeting treatment goals. Aerobic conditioning is recommended for cardiovascular and metabolic health, resistance training as an adjunct to these, and flexibility for functional and leisure activity. Physical activity has been shown to improve some aspects of performance and health. The authors recommend following the American College of Sports Medicine guidelines presented in **Box 3** for exercise/activity recommendations for people with NAFLD.

REFERENCES

1. Manson JE, Skerrett PJ, Greenland P, et al. The escalating pandemics of obesity and sedentary lifestyle. A call to action for clinicians. Arch Intern Med 2004;164: 249–58.
2. Bhala N, Angulo P, van der Poorten D, et al. The natural history of nonalcoholic fatty liver disease with advanced fibrosis or cirrhosis: an international collaborative study. Hepatology 2011;54:1208–16.
3. Clark JM. The epidemiology of non-alcoholic liver disease in adults. J Clin Gastroenterol 2006;40(Suppl 1):S5–10.

4. Teli MR, James OF, Burt AD, et al. The natural history of nonalcoholic fatty liver: a follow-up study. Hepatology 1995;22:1714–9.
5. Lazo M, Clark JM. The epidemiology of nonalcoholic fatty liver disease: a global perspective. Semin Liver Dis 2008;28:339–50.
6. Bellentani S, Saccoccio G, Masutti F, et al. Prevalence of and risk factors for hepatic steatosis in Northern Italy. Ann Intern Med 2000;132:112–7.
7. Targher G, Day C, Bonora E. Risk of cardiovascular disease in patients with nonalcoholic fatty liver disease current concepts. N Engl J Med 2010;363:1341–50.
8. Newton JL. Systemic symptoms in non-alcoholic fatty liver disease. Dig Dis 2010;28:214–9.
9. Harrison S, Day C. Benefits of lifestyle modifications in NAFLD. Gut 2007;56:1760–9.
10. Price JK, Srivastava R, Bai C, et al. Comparison of activity level among patients with chronic liver disease. Disabil Rehabil 2013;35:907–12.
11. Afendy A, Kallman JB, Stepanova M, et al. Predictors of health-related quality of life in patients with chronic liver disease. Aliment Pharmacol Ther 2009;30:469–76.
12. Fabbrini E, Sullivan S, Klein S. Obesity and nonalcoholic fatty liver disease: biochemical, metabolic, and clinical implications. Hepatology 2010;51:679–89.
13. Booth FW, Laye MJ, Lees SJ, et al. Reduced physical activity and risk of chronic disease: the biology behind the consequences. Eur J Appl Physiol 2008;102:381–90.
14. Blair SN, Kohl HW, Gordon NF, et al. How much physical activity is good for health? Annu Rev Public Health 1992;13:99–126.
15. Zelber-Sagi S, Nitzan-Kaluski D, Goldsmith R, et al. Role of leisure-time physical activity in nonalcoholic fatty liver disease: a population-based study. Hepatology 2008;48:1791–8.
16. Thomas C, Day CP, Trenell MI. Lifestyle interventions for the treatment of nonalcoholic fatty liver disease in adults: a systematic review. J Hepatol 2012;56:255–66.
17. Church TS, Kuk JL, Ross R, et al. Association of cardiorespiratory fitness, body mass index, and waist circumference to nonalcoholic fatty liver disease. Gastroenterology 2006;130:2023.
18. Hickman IJ, Jonsson JR, Prins JB, et al. Modest weight loss and physical activity in overweight patients with chronic liver disease results in sustained improvements in alanine aminotransferase, fasting insulin, and quality of life. Gut 2004;53:413–9.
19. Helmrich SP, Ragland DR, Leung RW, et al. Physical activity and reduced occurrence of non-insulin-dependent diabetes mellitus. N Engl J Med 1991;325:147–52.
20. Park Y, Zhu S, Palaniappan L, et al. The metabolic syndrome: prevalence and associated risk factor findings in the us population from the Third National Health and Nutrition Examination Survey, 1988-1994. Arch Intern Med 2003;163:427–36.
21. Jetté M, Sidney K, Blümchen G. Metabolic equivalents (METS) in exercise testing, exercise prescription, and evaluation of functional capacity. Clin Cardiol 1990;13:555–65.
22. Borg G, Linderholm H. Perceived exertion and pulse rate during graded exercise in various age groups. Acta Med Scand 1967;(Suppl 472):194.

23. Berlin JA, Colditz GJ. A meta-analysis of physical activity in the prevention of coronary heart disease. Am J Epidemiol 1990;132:612–28.
24. Nelson ME, Rejeski WJ, Blair SN, et al. Physical activity and public health in older adults: recommendation from the American College of Sports Medicine and the American Heart Association. Med Sci Sports Exerc 2007;8:1435–45.
25. Burchfiel CM, Sharp DS, Curb JD, et al. Physical activity and incidence of diabetes: the Honolulu Heart Program. Am J Epidemiol 1995;141:360–8.
26. Bauman AE. Updating the evidence that physical activity is good for health: an epidemiological review 2000-2003. J Sci Med Sport 2004;7:6–19.
27. St George A, Bauman A, Johnston A, et al. Independent effects of physical activity in patients with nonalcoholic fatty liver disease. Hepatology 2009;50: 68–76.
28. Armstrong T, Bauman A, Davies J. Physical activity patterns of Australian adults. Results of the 1999 National Physical Activity Survey. Canberra (Australia): Australian Institute of Health and Welfare; 2000.
29. Frith J, Kerr S, Robinson L, et al. Falls and fall-related injury are common in older people with chronic liver disease. Dig Dis Sci 2012;57:2697–702.
30. Tarantino G, Savastano S, Colao A. Hepatic steatosis, low-grade chronic inflammation and hormone/growth factor/adipokine imbalance. World J Gastroenterol 2010;16:4773–83.
31. Lazo M, Solga SF, Horska A, et al. Effect of a 12-month intensive lifestyle intervention on hepatic steatosis in adults with type 2 diabetes. Diabetes Care 2010; 10:2156–63.
32. David K, Kowdley KV, Unalp A, et al, The NASH CRN Group. Quality of life in adults with nonalcoholic fatty liver disease: baseline data from the NASH CRN group. Hepatology 2009;49:1904–12.
33. Ware J, Kosinski M, Dewey J. How to score version two of the SF36 health survey. Lincoln (RI): Quality Metric; 2000.
34. Elliott C, Frith J, Day CP, et al. Functional impairment in alcoholic liver disease and non-alcoholic fatty liver disease is significant and persists over 3 years of follow-up. Dig Dis Sci 2013;58:2383–91.
35. Elwing JE, Lustman PJ, Wang HL, et al. Depression, anxiety, and nonalcoholic steatohepatitis. Psychosom Med 2006;68:563–9.
36. Newton JL, Pairman J, Wilton K, et al. Fatigue and autonomic dysfunction in non-alcoholic fatty liver disease. Clin Auton Res 2009;19:319–26.
37. Newton JL, Jones DE, Henderson E, et al. Fatigue in non-alcoholic fatty liver disease (NAFLD) is significant and associates with inactivity and excessive daytime sleepiness but not with liver disease severity or insulin resistance. Gut 2008;57:807–13.
38. Johnson NA, Sachinwalla T, Walton DW, et al. Aerobic exercise training reduces hepatic and visceral lipids in obese individuals without weight loss. Hepatology 2009;50:1105–12.
39. Frank LL, Sorensen BE, Yasui Y, et al. Effects of exercise on metabolic risk variables in overweight postmenopausal women: a randomized clinical trial. Obes Res 2005;13:615–25.
40. Sullivan S, Kirk EP, Mittendorfer B, et al. Randomized trial of exercise effect on intrahepatic triglyceride content and lipid kinetics in nonalcoholic fatty liver disease. Hepatology 2012;55:1738–45.
41. Aoi W, Naito Y, Yoshikawa T. Dietary exercise as a novel strategy for the prevention and treatment of metabolic syndrome: effects on skeletal muscle function. J Nutr Metab 2011;2011:676208.

42. Yap F, Craddock L, Yang J. Mechanism of AMPK suppression of LXR-dependent Sreb-1c transcription. Int J Biol Sci 2011;7:645–50.
43. Mirza MS. Obesity, visceral fat and NAFLD: querying the role of adipokines in the progression of non-alcoholic fatty liver disease. ISRN Gastroenterol 2011; 2011:592404.
44. Perseghin G, Lattuada G, De Cobelli F, et al. Habitual physical activity is associated with intrahepatic fat content in humans. Diabetes Care 2007;30:683–8.
45. Kantartzis K, Thamer C, Peter A, et al. High cardiorespiratory fitness is an independent predictor of the reduction in liver fat during a lifestyle intervention in non-alcoholic fatty liver disease. Gut 2009;58:1281–8.
46. Goodyear LJ, Kahn BB. Exercise, glucose transport, and insulin sensitivity. Annu Rev Med 1998;49:235–61.
47. Greiwe JS, Holloszy JO, Semenkovich CF. Exercise induces lipoprotein lipase and GLUT-4 protein in muscle independent of adrenergic-receptor signaling. J Appl Phys 2000;89:176–81.
48. Gielen S, Adams V, Möbius-Winkler S, et al. Anti inflammatory effects of exercise training in the skeletal muscle of patients with chronic heart failure. J Am Coll Cardiol 2003;42:861–8.
49. Pedersen BK, Fischer CP. Beneficial health effects of exercise—the role of IL-6 as a myokine. Trends Pharmacol Sci 2007;28:152–6.
50. Pedersen BK, Edward F. Adolph distinguished lecture: muscle as an endocrine organ: IL-6 and other myokines. J Appl Phys 2009;107:1006–14.
51. Bonekamp S, Barone BB, Clark J, et al. The effect of an exercise training intervention on hepatic steatosis. Hepatology 2008;48:1119.
52. Chen SM, Liu CY, Li SR, et al. Effects of therapeutic lifestyle program on ultrasound-diagnosed nonalcoholic fatty liver disease. J Chin Med Assoc 2008;71:551–8.
53. Goodpaster BH, Delany JP, Otto AD, et al. Effects of diet and physical activity interventions on weight loss and cardiometabolic risk factors in severely obese adults: a randomized trial. JAMA 2010;304:1795–802.
54. Shah K, Stufflebam A, Hilton TN, et al. Diet and exercise interventions reduce intrahepatic fat content and improve insulin sensitivity in obese older adults. Obesity (Silver Spring) 2009;17:2162–8.
55. Garber CE, Blissmer B, Deschenes MR, et al. Quantity and quality of exercise for developing and maintaining cardiorespiratory, musculoskeletal, and neuromotor fitness in apparently healthy adults: guidance for prescribing exercise. Med Sci Sports Exerc 2011;43:1334–59.
56. Keating SE, Hackett DA, George J, et al. Exercise and nonalcoholic fatty liver disease: a systematic review and meta-analysis. J Hepatol 2012;57:157–66.
57. McCall GE, Byrnes WC, Fleck SJ, et al. Acute and chronic hormonal responses to resistance training designed to promote muscle hypertrophy. Can J Appl Physiol 1999;24:96–107.
58. Wu T, Gao X, Chen M, et al. Long-term effectiveness of diet-plus-exercise interventions vs diet-only interventions for weight loss: a meta-analysis. Obes Rev 2009;10:313–23.
59. Redman LM, Huffman KM, Landerman LR, et al. Effect of caloric restriction with and without exercise on metabolic intermediates in non-obese men and women. J Clin Endocrinol Metab 2011;96:E312–21.
60. Tieland M, van de Rest O, Dirks ML. Protein supplementation improves physical performance in frail elderly people: a randomized, double-blind, placebo-controlled trial. J Am Med Dir Assoc 2012;13:720–6.

61. Phillips SM. Protein requirements and supplementation in strength sports. Nutrition 2004;20:689–95.
62. Birerdinc A, Stepanova M, Pawloski L, et al. Caffeine is protective in patients with non-alcoholic fatty liver disease. Aliment Pharmacol Ther 2012;1:76–82.
63. Ristow M, Zarse K, Oberbach A, et al. Antioxidants prevent health-promoting effects of physical exercise in humans. Proc Natl Acad Sci U S A 2009;106:8665–70.
64. Fenkel JM, Navarro VJ. Herbal and dietary supplement induced liver injury. Gastroenterol Hepatol 2011;10:695–6.
65. Hagger M, Chatzisarantis N. The social psychology of exercise and sport. New York, NY: Open University Press; 2005.
66. Roberts GC. Advances in motivation in sport and exercise. Champaign (IL): Human Kinetics; 2001.
67. Haber D. Health promotion and aging: practical applications for health professionals. J Gerontol Soc Work 2013;56(6):569–71.
68. Kahn EB, Ramsey LT, Brownson RC, et al. The effectiveness of interventions to increase physical activity. A systematic review. Am J Prev Med 2002;22(Suppl 4):73–107.
69. Shinitzky HE, Kub J. The art of motivating behavior change: the use of motivational interviewing to promote health. Public Health Nurs 2001;18:178–85.
70. Cullen KW, Baranowski T, Smith SP. Using goal setting as a strategy for dietary behavior change. J Am Diet Assoc 2001;101:562–6.
71. Roitman JL, La Fontaine T. The exercise professional's guide to optimizing health: strategies for preventing and reducing chronic disease. Baltimore, MD: Lippincott Williams & Wilkins; 2011.
72. Haber D, Rhodes D. Health contract with sedentary older adults. Gerontologist 2004;44:827–35.
73. Ogden J, Karim L, Choudry A, et al. Understanding successful behaviour change: the role of intentions, attitudes to the target and motivations and the example of diet. Health Educ Res 2007;22:397–405.
74. Flora SR. The power of reinforcement. Albany, NY: SUNY Press; 2004.
75. Mondadori C, Waser PG, Huston JP. Time-dependent effects of post-trial reinforcement, punishment or ECS on passive avoidance learning. Physiol Behav 1977;18:1103–9.
76. Addy CL, Wilson DK, Kirtland KA, et al. Associations of perceived social and physical environmental supports with physical activity and walking behavior. Am J Public Health 2004;94:440–3.
77. Towers A, Flett R, Seebeck R. Assessing potential barriers to exercise adoption in middle-aged men: over-stressed, under-controlled, or just too unwell? Internet J Ment Health 2005;4:13–27.
78. Steptoe A, Wardle J, Pollard T, et al. Stress, social support and health-related behavior: a study of smoking, alcohol consumption and physical exercise. J Psychosom Res 1996;41:171–80.
79. Rogers LQ, Vicari S, Courneya KS. Lessons learned in the trenches. Cancer Nurs 2010;33:E10–7.
80. Melton B. Strategies to increase exercise adherence in older adults. Human Kinetics 2008. Available at: http://www.humankinetics.com/excerpts/excerpts/strategies-to-increase-exercise-adherence-in-older-adults. Accessed July 23, 2013.

Surgical Management of Obesity in Patients with Morbid Obesity and Nonalcoholic Fatty Liver Disease

John B. Dixon, PhD, MBBS, FRACGP, FRCP Edin[a,b],*

KEYWORDS

- Metabolic • Weight loss • Surgery • Diabetes • Hypertension • Gastric
- Malabsorption • Mortality

KEY POINTS

- Weight loss following conventional nonmalabsorptive bariatric-metabolic procedures reduces steatosis and lobular inflammation, but does not have a consistent effect on liver fibrosis.
- Rapid weight loss, especially with malabsorptive procedures, may produce a transient or prolonged increase in liver disease.
- The place for bariatric-metabolic surgery in patients with compensated cirrhosis is not established, but is contraindicated in decompensated cirrhosis.
- Long-term population studies are needed to establish the effect of bariatric-metabolic surgery on major liver morbidity and mortality, within the context of the effects of broader morbidity and mortality changes.

INTRODUCTION

Severe obesity with its associated comorbidities, including nonalcoholic fatty liver disease (NAFLD), can be considered as a chronic, relapsing disease and therefore needs a chronic disease approach to management. Chronic disease management requires a

Funding Sources: NHMRC, Allergan Inc.

Conflict of Interest: Professor Dixon is a consultant for Allergan Inc, and Metagenics (Bariatric Advantage); is on the Medical Advisory Board for Optifast, Nestle Australia, and has received speakers' fees from iNova Pharmaceuticals (Duromine). His research group has received research funding from Allergan Inc, Medtronics (formerly ARDIAN Inc), Abbott (formerly Solvay) Pharmaceuticals, and Servier.

[a] Clinical Obesity Research, Baker IDI Heart & Diabetes Institute, PO Box 6492, St Kilda Road Central, Melbourne, Victoria 8008, Australia; [b] Primary Care Research Unit, Monash University, Melbourne, Australia

* Baker IDI Heart & Diabetes Institute, Monash University, PO Box 6492, St Kilda Road Central, Melbourne, Victoria 8008, Australia.

E-mail address: john.dixon@bakeridi.edu.au

range of effective therapeutic options so that treatment can be stepped up or altered in relation to the severity of the individual's condition and response to the current therapy.[1] This management model also centers on the patient being well informed and critically engaged in the self-care aspects of the disease and having understanding of the options available for the management of the disease. There are many options for managing obesity-related comorbidity such as type 2 diabetes, hypertension, depression, and sleep apnea effectively, but there are limited options for managing the obesity effectively.

Weight loss is difficult because body weight and body fat are regulated by a range of highly efficient homeostatic mechanisms that have a bias toward preventing weight loss rather than weight gain.[2] Mechanisms that defend against weight (fat) loss include reduced energy expenditure through loss of lean body mass, energy adaptation with reduced thyroid activity, reduced sympathetic nervous activity, and improved muscle efficiency.[3] In contrast, intake is also influenced: weight loss generates feelings of hunger, changes the perceptions of food intake, increases the attractiveness and taste of food, reduces cognitive restraint, and increases the hedonic response to food.[4] As a result of these physiologic effects, lifestyle-behavioral interventions generate only modest long-term weight loss and maintaining weight loss is difficult. Drug therapy for weight loss has been limited and, with some drugs withdrawn from the market because of safety issues, a cautious approach has been taken to the regulatory approval and introduction of new medications. However, 2 new medications, lorcaserin[5] and an extended-release combination of phentermine and topiramate,[6] have recently been approved by the US Food and Drug Administration (FDA). In general, drug therapy has led to a useful 3% to 8% weight loss compared with placebo.[7–9] However, bariatric surgery is the most effective therapy available, with the most commonly used procedures generating sustained weight loss of 20% to 30% of body weight.[10]

LAPAROSCOPIC BARIATRIC-METABOLIC SURGERY

Bariatric surgery was revolutionized with the introduction of laparoscopic surgery in the early to mid-1990s and all currently used standard procedures (Roux-en-Y gastric bypass [RYGB], laparoscopic adjustable gastric band [LAGB], sleeve gastrectomy [SG], and biliopancreatic diversion with or without a duodenal switch [BPD+/−DS]) are performed laparoscopically (**Fig. 1**). Overall, there was a rapid increase in the use of bariatric surgery globally between 1995 and 2008, but this has been followed by a plateau effect at an annual global level of 340,000 procedures, which is considered to be a low (<1%) annual uptake among those eligible for surgery.[11,12] Procedure choice varies internationally and trends change with time in a manner resembling other fashions.[12] At present, RYGB, SG, and LAGB are the dominant three in all global regions, but the proportions vary and BPD+/−DS, which is the only procedure that is associated with significant malabsorption of macronutrients, makes up less than 3% of all procedures.

Indications

The indication for bariatric surgery follows a similar pattern internationally, with the more recent guidelines and position statements considering type 2 diabetes as a specific entity (**Table 1**).[13,14] The recognition that bariatric surgery has a role in managing obesity-related metabolic conditions, especially type 2 diabetes, has led to the inclusion of metabolic in national bariatric surgery societies' names, and the combined term bariatric-metabolic (BM) to describe the surgical specialty and the range of procedures used.

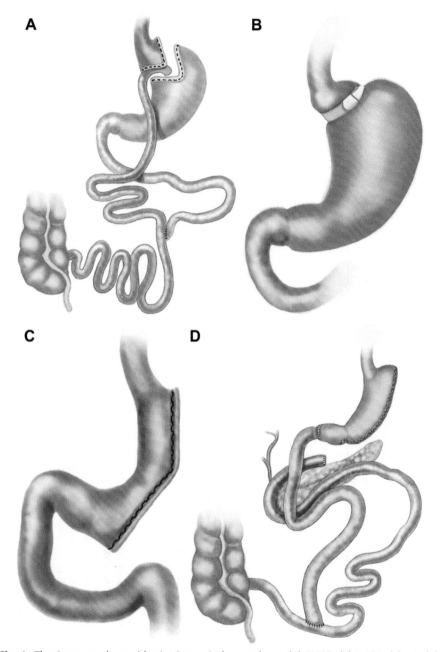

Fig. 1. The 4 commonly used bariatric surgical procedures. (*A*) RYGB, (*B*) LAGB, (*C*) SG, (*D*) BPD+DS.

NAFLD is considered an obesity-related comorbidity, with hepatic metabolites and steatosis playing a pivotal role in the development of hepatic insulin resistance,[15] and energy restriction generating a rapid improvement in hepatic insulin sensitivity.[16] NAFLD, and in particular nonalcoholic steatohepatitis (NASH), is critically linked to

Table 1
National and international guidelines for eligibility for bariatric-metabolic (BM) surgery in adults

	NIH (United States, 1991)[a]	NICE (United Kingdom, 2006)	European (2007)	SIGN (Scotland, 2010)	IDF (2011)	NHMRC (Australia, 2013)
Recommended BMI	NA	>50	NA	NA	>40, or >35 if diabetes and other comorbidities not controlled by optimal medical therapy	NA
Eligible BMI based on BMI only	>40	>40	>40	NA	>35	>40
Eligible BMI based on BMI and comorbid conditions	35–40 with 1 serious weight loss–responsive comorbidity	35–40 with 1 serious weight loss–responsive comorbidity	35–40 with 1 serious weight loss responsive comorbidity	>35 with 1 serious weight loss–responsive comorbidity	>30 if diabetes and other comorbidities not controlled by optimal medical therapy	35–40 with comorbidity that may improve with weight loss
Comment	US Medicare National Coverage Determinations 2004 removed "serious" for BMI 35–40	NA	Weight loss before surgery does not change eligibility	NA	—	Surgery can also be considered in: BMI>30 with poorly controlled diabetes and at increased cardiovascular risk

Abbreviations: BMI, body mass index; IDF, International Diabetes Federation; NA, not available; NHMRC, National Health and Medical Research Council; NICE, National Institutes for Health and Clinical Excellence; NIH, National Institutes of Health; SIGN, Scottish Intercollegiate Guidelines Network.

[a] Outdated, but of historical interest.

Data from Refs. [13,14,66-69]

central obesity, insulin resistance, dyslipidemia, hypertension, and the full array of perturbations and consequences of the metabolic syndrome.

Mechanism of Action

How BM surgery is able to alter energy balance and deliver sustained weight loss remains poorly understood, but the old concepts of restriction and malabsorption are naive and not the mechanisms for the most commonly used procedures, including RYGB, LAGB, and SG. None of the procedures significantly delay the absorption of oral intake, and the prolonged satisfaction of a small meal is not related to delayed absorption.[17] None of these procedures is accompanied by any significant malabsorption of macronutrients.[18] The answers lie in how the gastrointestinal (GI) tract communicates with the brain and alters the energy balance set-point, which is then defended at a lower level. Several putative mechanisms involving gut hormones, GI mechanical receptors, and neural afferent pathways are starting to provide insights.[10,19]

Procedure Choice

Choice of procedure depends on many factors including local expertise and experience in the different BM surgical procedures and their aftercare, and the complexity and reversibility of a procedure. In addition, the patient's age, general health, and co-morbidity can all influence the risk/benefit ratio for any given procedure. Once the range of risks and benefits, the importance of compliance, and the effects on eating choices and behaviors are fully described to the patient, personal preference is vital. The commonly used procedures have a range of different outcome characteristics as shown in **Table 2**. Complications are usually procedure dependent, and revisional surgery to correct abnormalities or convert to alternative procedures, is common and carries additional risk. All procedures have been gradually refined to improved safety and reduce the need for surgical revisions.

In addition to the conventional surgical procedures, many novel GI surgical procedures and GI devices are being explored for their efficacy, safety, and applicability. The FDA currently approves none of the devices, but several intragastric balloons and a duodenal endoluminal liner are available outside the United States. These are placed endoscopically and need to be removed after 6 or 12 months, depending on the device.

THE ESTABLISHED BENEFITS BM SURGERY

BM surgery presents an array of impressive outcome measures when performed for the conventional indication of a body mass index (BMI) greater than 35 kg/m². Several large case-control studies show a reduction in mortality,[20] notably deaths related to cardiovascular disease, diabetes, and cancer[21,22]; randomized controlled trials show improvement or remission of type 2 diabetes,[23–26] reduced cardiovascular risk, and improved health-related quality of life[27]; and longitudinal series show major improvements in all obesity-related metabolic, mechanical, and psychological comorbidity.[10,28] The effect on NAFLD is discussed separately. Many health economic analyses report that surgery is cost-effective and many studies show that surgery produces a return on investment, especially in patients with diabetes.[29–31]

BM SURGERY IN PATIENTS WITH NAFLD

Most patients presenting for BM surgery have NAFLD, with most (approximately 70%) having nonalcoholic fatty liver; 25% nonalcoholic steatohepatitis (NASH); and, of those

Table 2
The characteristics of the currently used conventional BM surgical procedures

	RYGB	LAGB	BPD+/−DS	SG
Mean weight loss (%)	25–35	20–30	30–40 (with duodenal switch)	20–30
Excess weight loss at 3–5 y[a] (%)	60 (75 with banded RYGB)	54	75	45–60 (limited reports at ≥5 y)
Pattern of weight loss	Rapid; maximal at 1–2 y Weight regain in 3–5 y	Gradual; usually maximal at 2–3 y	Very rapid and extensive; maximal at 1–2 y	Rapid; maximal at 1–2 y[b]
30-d postoperative mortality (%)	0.3–0.5	0.05–0.1	0.75–1.0	0.4[b]
Major 30-d morbidity (%)	Laparoscopic 4.8 Open 7.8	1	NR	NR
Morbidity at 1 y (%)	16	4	34	10
Long-term data available (≥10 y)	Yes	Yes	Yes	No
Evidence of reduced mortality	Yes	Yes	No	No
Nutritional concerns	Moderate (deficiencies in thiamine, iron, B12, folate, calcium, vitamin D, copper, zinc)	Low (deficiencies in thiamine, iron, B12, folate)	High (deficiencies in thiamine, iron, B12, folate, calcium, vitamin D, copper, zinc, fat-soluble vitamins)	High thiamine Moderate (deficiencies in iron, B12, folate, calcium, vitamin D, copper, zinc)
Follow-up requirements	Lifelong (assessment and nutritional support)	Lifelong (high in the first 12 mo)	Lifelong (assessment and nutritional support)	Lifelong (assessment and nutritional support)
Key complications	Abdominal pain, staple line leak, stomal ulcer, intestinal obstruction, internal hernia, gallstones, nutritional deficiency, weight regain	Gastric pouch dilatation, erosion of band into the stomach, leaks to the LAGB system, weight regain	As for RYGB and malabsorption, hypoalbuminemia, excessive fat malabsorption, progressive liver damage, renal calculi	Staple line leak and bleeding, chronic fistula, GERD, dilatation of the gastric remnant, nutritional deficiency, weight regain

Abbreviations: GERD, gastroesophageal reflux disease; NR, not reported.
[a] Excess weight defined as the weight of an individual in excess of their weight at BMI 25 kg/m^2.
[b] Thirty-day postoperative mortality for SG is based on fewer than 1000 cases.
Data from Refs.[20,70–78]

with NASH, half have advanced fibrosis and 1% to 2% have cirrhosis.[32] In our unselected series, less than 5% had a normal liver biopsy. Given this overwhelming association, the interaction between BM surgery and NAFLD should have been well understood, but this is not the case. To date there are no published randomized controlled trials specifically examining NAFLD, and data are restricted to longitudinal series in which the ability to obtain a follow-up liver biopsy was opportunistic and usually at the time of cholecystectomy, revisional BM surgery, or ventral hernia repair.[33] Some studies have targeted those with more advanced disease for a follow-up biopsy and 1 large series has performed planned biopsies at 1 and 5 years after surgery.[34,35]

A formal Cochrane Review of BM surgery as a treatment of NASH did not identify any randomized controlled trials or quasirandomized clinical trials, but did examine 21 cohort studies, and although there were consistent improvements in steatosis and inflammatory scores, 4 studies did report some deterioration in fibrosis.[36] The investigators concluded that evidence was generally positive, but, given that data were subject to bias and the potential risk of increased fibrosis, there was insufficient evidence to allow any firm conclusions regarding BM surgery as a treatment of NASH. Randomized controlled trials were recommended.[36]

The recently released practice guidelines for the management of NAFLD by the American Association for the Study of Liver Diseases, American College of Gastroenterology, and the American Gastroenterological Association, evaluating the same data, provide the following recommendations regarding BM surgery in patients with NAFLD[33]:

1 Foregut surgery is not contraindicated in otherwise eligible obese individuals with NAFLD and NASH (but without established cirrhosis).
2 The type, safety, and efficacy of foregut bariatric surgery in otherwise eligible individuals with established cirrhosis caused by NAFLD are not established.
3 It is premature to consider foregut bariatric surgery as an established option specifically to treat NASH.

There are 2 major studies of mortality and cause of death in patients following BM surgery that have compared them with matched community controls. The US study by Adams and colleagues[37] examined the long-term mortality and cause of death, using the National Death Index, in a cohort of 7925 patients having BM surgery and 7925 matched controls from US drivers' licenses followed for the same period of time. Adjusted all-cause mortality was reduced by 40% in the surgical group, with cardiovascular, diabetes, and cancer deaths reduced by 56%, 92%, and 60%, respectively.[22] Liver disease would have been grouped with other disease if the reduction in the surgical group was 40%. Nondisease causes of death were higher in the surgical group, and suicide, poisonings, and accidents contributed to this increase. There has been no signal to indicate an increase in liver related mortality following gastric bypass surgery in the large Utah case controlled mortality study (Ted Adams – personal communication).[22] The mortality reduction in the surgical group of the large, longitudinal, case-control Swedish Obese Subjects (SOS) study was similarly associated with reduced cardiovascular and cancer deaths, but no signal of increased liver mortality was evident.[21] The prospective SOS study has examined transaminase levels at 2 and 10 years after recruitment and reports lower alanine aminotransferase (ALT) and aspartate aminotransferase (AST) levels, lower incidence and prevalence of increased ALT and ALT levels, and a lower prevalence of ALT/AST of less than 1 in the surgical versus usual care group at both time points.[38]

It is also important to consider that the most common causes of death in patients with NAFLD are ischemic heart disease and cancer,[37,39] and that type 2 diabetes is a risk factor for NAFLD-related hepatic mortality. It is likely that BM surgery is an effective therapy for NAFLD, and, because almost all patients proceeding to surgery have NAFLD, with the severity usually unknown, it is important to identify those at greater risk of hepatic morbidity and mortality following surgery. The constant call for randomized controlled trials in bariatric surgery may seem logical, but the logistics are difficult; ethical implications considerable; and, for NAFLD, hard morbidity and mortality end points for liver and other diseases including cardiovascular, diabetes, and cancer, are necessary to assess the balance of risk and benefit for patients. However, examining liver histology as the primary outcome measure has several limitations because (1) it is likely to represent a single observation following surgery and may not reflect a continuing change; (2) it does not necessarily provide information about hard long-term liver-related morbidity and mortality; (3) it does not necessarily put into context liver morbidity and mortality with all-cause morbidity and mortality; and (4) the standard of diagnosis, and the reliability of histologic features of a biopsy from a single region, can be discordant with second biopsy from another region in the same patient at the same time.[40,41] National death registries, bariatric surgical registries, and linked comprehensive health data sets may combine to answer the critical question regarding BM surgery and long-term hepatic morbidity and mortality.

Studies Examining Paired Liver Biopsies

There are a range of studies that report the effect of weight loss following BM surgery on the histologic features of NAFLD. The studies are heterogeneous in size; patient selection criteria; time between biopsies; and, most notably, in how individual histologic features were scored. They are listed in **Table 3** in chronologic order so that the reader can reflect on the rigor and nature of histologic reporting systems of the time. All studies of BM surgery report that patients had lost considerable weight and the weight loss follows the pattern and extent detailed in **Table 2**.

There are some consistent findings from the studies of paired liver biopsies:

- All but 1 study, of a more recent version of jejunoileal bypass (JIB),[42] reported reductions in steatosis and the reductions were usually substantial.
- With the same exception,[42] there are consistent reports of improved lobular inflammation. However, reports of portal inflammation, when examined specifically, suggest minimal change.[34]
- The pattern of change in fibrosis is less clear, with most reports showing improvement, but some a modest increase in fibrosis. As for inflammation, several studies have noted a reduction in lobular fibrosis, but not in portal fibrosis.[34,43–45]

The largest prospective study followed 381 patients receiving BPD, LAGB, or gastric bypass, and planned a full clinical assessment and repeat biopsies at 1 and 5 years after surgery.[35] Suitable biopsies were obtained from 362, 267, and 211 participants at baseline, 1 year, and 5 years respectively. This study reported major reductions in steatosis and ballooning degeneration; no change in inflammation; and a small increase in fibrosis score at both 1 and 5 years compared with the baseline biopsies. Improvements in steatosis and ballooning degeneration were associated with changes in insulin sensitivity.[35,46] At baseline, 27% of the patients had probable or definite NASH and at 5-year the proportion had reduced to 14% ($P<.001$). Changes in fibrosis were small and at 5 years more than 95% of patients had a fibrosis score of less than or equal to 1. Perhaps the most important finding from this study was the stability of all aspects of liver histology between 1 and 5 years following surgery, suggesting that both the improvements in steatosis and ballooning degeneration and the increase in fibrosis occurred during the phase of rapid weight loss and there was no signal of progressive disease over the next 4 years.[35]

Table 3
Twenty-four studies that have examined liver histology in individuals before and following BM surgery

Study	Sample Size	Surgery Type	Mean Follow-up Time	Change in Steatosis	Change in Inflammation	Change in Fibrosis	Comments
Ranlov and Hardt,[79] 1990	15	RYGB or gastroplasty	12 mo	↓	NR	NR	Improved liver enzymes
Silverman et al,[43] 1995	91	RYGB	18.4 mo	↓	↓/0	↓	Improved lobular but no change in portal fibrosis
Luyckx et al,[80] 1998	69	Gastroplasty or adjustable gastric banding (LAGB)	Not declared	↓	↓	0	—
Dixon et al,[34] 2004	36	LAGB	25.6 ± 10 mo	↓	↓	↓	Significant improvement in all liver panel enzymes; Portal inflammation and fibrosis unchanged
Kral et al,[54] 2004	104	BPD	74 ± 27 mo	↓	NR	↑	Increase in fibrosis overall was small, but individual changes could be major (good and bad)
Clark et al,[81] 2005	16	RYGB	10 ± 4 mo	↓	↓	↓	Improvement in lobular and portal fibrosis; Improvement in ALT and AST
Keshishian et al,[55] 2005	78	BPD–DS	36 mo	↓	↓	NR	NASH grade improved. No significant reduction in liver function tests
Mattar et al,[82] 2005	70	RYGB, LAGB or SG	15 ± 9 mo	↓	↓	↓	—
Mottin et al,[83] 2005	90	RYGB	12 mo	↓	NR	NR	—
Stratopoulos et al,[84] 2005	216	Vertical banded gastroplasty	18 ± 9.6 mo	↓	↓	↓	Improvement in ALT and AST

(continued on next page)

Table 3
(continued)

Study	Sample Size	Surgery Type	Mean Follow-up Time	Change in Steatosis	Change in Inflammation	Change in Fibrosis	Comments
Meinhardt et al,[42] 2006	30	End-to-side jejunoileal bypass	70 ± 42.8 mo	0	0	0	After excellent weight loss there was no change in histology scores. ALT and AST levels tended higher
Barker et al,[85] 2006	19	RYGB	21.4 mo	↓	↓	↓	Improvement in portal and lobular fibrosis. No change in liver enzymes
Csendes et al,[86] 2006	16	RYGB with resection of bypassed stomach	22 mo	NR	NR	NR	Steatosis, inflammation, and fibrosis not reported independently; normalization of histology reported and showed significant normalization/improvement (12/16)
de Almeida et al,[87] 2006	16	RYGB	23.5 ± 8.4 mo	NR	↓	NR	Reductions in hepatocellular ballooning and lobular inflammation
Dixon et al,[88] 2006	60	LAGB	29.5 ± 16 mo	↓	↓	↓	Improvements in inflammation and fibrosis with lowering in GGT
Klein et al,[89] 2006	7	RYGB	12 mo	↓	NR	NR	—
Furuya et al,[90] 2007	18	RYGB	24 mo	↓	NR	↓	GGT was the only enzyme to decrease significantly

Liu et al,[44] 2007	39	RYGB	18 mo	↓	NR	↓	No improvement in portal fibrosis. ALT improved
Mathurin et al,[35,46] 2006; 2009	185	BPD, LAGB, RYGB	12 mo and 60 mo	↓	0	↑	Results did not differ between 1-y and 5-y follow-up; Reduced ALT and GGT
Bell et al,[91] 2010	20	RYGB, LAGB, SG	15 mo	↓	↓	↓	—
Weiner et al,[92] 2010	116	LAGB, RYGB, BPD–DS	18 mo	↓	↓	↓	—
Tai et al,[93] 2012	21	RYGB	12 mo	↓	↓	↓	Low levels of baseline fibrosis in this series; Reduced ALT and GGT
Moretto et al,[94] 2012	78	RYGB	Not stated	NR	NR	↓	Changes lobular fibrosis was modest and variable. There was no overall improvement in portal fibrosis
Vargas et al,[45] 2012	26	Banded RYGB	16 mo	↓	↓	↓	—

Abbreviations: 0, unchanged; GGT, Gamma-glutamyl transpeptidase; NR, not reported.
Data from Refs.[34,35,42–46,54,55,79–94]

Procedure-specific Concerns

BM surgical procedures currently in use vary in the degree and nature of disruption to the GI tract from the least disruptive LAGB, through to SG, RYGB, and the malabsorptive BPD+/−DS. It is therefore important to consider the potential for hepatotoxicity effects of GI interventions beyond their beneficial effects in insulin sensitivity and weight loss. The early experience with JIB should not be forgotten.

From a historical perspective, the first BM surgical procedure, JIB, had a serious hepatotoxic effect. Early series reported that most JIB-related deaths were caused by liver failure,[47] and a large proportion of patients having the procedure developed histologic evidence of progressive liver disease on serial biopsy.[48,49] Rapid weight loss, protein-calorie malnutrition, global malabsorption, and endotoxins from an isolated segment of gut setting up immune and metabolic changes have all been implicated in the development of progressive liver disease.[47,50] This procedure has now been abandoned and there has been a major trend away from any procedures that generate major malabsorption, blind loops, and risk of protein malnutrition.

Hepatic failure has been reported following BPD, the form of BM surgery that is associated with significant malabsorption of macronutrients.[51,52] Nicola Scopinaro, the surgeon who developed the procedure, and his team in Genoa had not experienced this issue, but tracked transaminase levels following surgery in 90 consecutive patients and found an increase in mean AST levels 2 months after surgery with a subsequent decrease by 12 months. The extent of the increase was associated with higher preoperative BMI and fasting glucose, and the extent of weight loss.[53] Kral and colleagues[54] described changes in liver histology following BPD/BPD−DS. Paired operative and opportunistic postoperative biopsies were available in 104 patients. Steatosis scores reduced and the reduction was associated with the weight loss; however, the effect on fibrosis and inflammatory scores was mixed and overall unchanged. There were 3 cases of incident cirrhosis and a fibrosis score increase was found in those with a postoperative decrease in serum albumin and with excessive diarrhea. In those with established cirrhosis at baseline (n = 11) there was a remarkable mean reduction in fibrosis and necroinflammatory changes. There was no lowering of hepatic transaminase levels following the BPD procedure.[55] Findings suggest that rapid early weight loss, low albumin levels, malnutrition, excessive malabsorption, blind loop bacterial overgrowth, and endotoxemia may be associated with either transient or long-term hepatotoxic state.

The rate of weight loss has been of concern when assessing the use of very low calorie diets because of transient enzyme increases, portal inflammation and fibrosis, and a high risk for gallstone development.[56,57] Weight loss greater than 1.6 kg per week increased the risk for portal fibrosis.[58] These observations may explain the early fibrosis changes reported at 12 months following surgery but no subsequent change in an additional 4 years.[35] Rate of weight loss may be a consideration in patients with more advanced NAFLD because any early hepatotoxic changes may be attenuated by a slower rate of loss (rates are detailed in **Table 2**).

BM Surgery in Patients with Cirrhosis

Data from a US nationwide sample indicate that early postoperative mortality is increased in patients with cirrhosis following BM surgery.[59] Compared with patients without cirrhosis, patients with compensated cirrhosis and decompensated cirrhosis had a mortality-adjusted odds ratio of 2.17 (1.03–4.55) and 21.2 (5.39–82.9) respectively. This study also found a lower mortality in centers performing more than 100 procedures a year. The investigators concluded that BM surgery should only be considered if cirrhosis was well compensated, there was no evidence of portal hypertension, and the surgery is performed in a high-volume center.[59] Several retrospective series confirm the relative safety of laparoscopic surgery and laparoscopic BM surgery in those with compensated cirrhosis.[60–62] Patients with cirrhosis electing to have surgery have high frequencies of type 2 diabetes, hypertension, and dyslipidemia.[60] Long-term outcomes in patients with cirrhosis have not been well reported, but some remarkable case studies of improvements in liver histology have been reported.[54]

BM Surgery Complements Established Therapy

BM surgery is used to treat severe complex obesity. It is used in conjunction with lifestyle interventions[63] and conventional medical therapies,[33] but is not intended to replace them. Effective models of chronic disease management involve the scaling up of therapy as needed, but not replacing general lifestyle advice or removing effective therapy for specific comorbidity. There is opportunity to reduce, or even stop, medications following BM surgery, but only when the condition is in remission and will be carefully monitored in the future.[64,65] Severely obese individuals with the more advanced forms of NAFLD have a broad range of obesity-related and obesity-responsive comorbidity and therefore BM surgery is indicated for the patient's global health state, rather than NAFLD specifically.[60] In this context, the statements within the 2012 US guidelines are cautious, but not restrictive, and the clinician should focus patient selection on NAFLD contraindications rather than considering NAFLD a specific stand-alone indication of surgery.[33] The position of patients with compensated cirrhosis is a gray area in which a cautious balance of risk versus benefit for the patient needs to be carefully evaluated. This need for balance provides an ethical dilemma when cirrhosis is first diagnosed laparoscopically at the time of a BM procedure.

FUTURE DIRECTION

There are some important gaps in current knowledge that reduce the clinical usefulness of the most commonly used BM procedures as a therapy for the spectrum of NAFLD. Uncertainty about any alteration to the long-term natural history of NAFLD and lingering doubts about surgery exacerbating NAFLD remain. Large case-control studies have not reported any signal of increased liver major morbidity or mortality following the commonly used procedures. Studies need to focus on several fundamental questions and the study design may be challenging:

- Do current procedures broadly alter, favorably or unfavorably, the short-term and long-term risk of cirrhosis, liver failure, hepatocellular carcinoma, or liver-related mortality?
- Is BM surgery an effective therapy or contraindicated for a patient with NAFLD-related compensated cirrhosis?
- How can clinicians reliably track patients with NAFLD without the need for a liver biopsy?

Of all therapies for NAFLD, BM surgery seems to have the optimal credentials for attenuating putative mechanisms associated with disease progression, but clinicians lack the confidence to deliver therapy to those who may benefit most.

REFERENCES

1. Wagner EH. Chronic disease management: what will it take to improve care for chronic illness? Eff Clin Pract 1998;1(1):2–4.

2. Schwartz MW, Woods SC, Seeley RJ, et al. Is the energy homeostasis system inherently biased toward weight gain? Diabetes 2003;52(2):232–8.
3. Rosenbaum M, Goldsmith R, Bloomfield D, et al. Low-dose leptin reverses skeletal muscle, autonomic, and neuroendocrine adaptations to maintenance of reduced weight. J Clin Invest 2005;115(12):3579–86.
4. Rosenbaum M, Kissileff HR, Mayer LE, et al. Energy intake in weight-reduced humans. Brain Res 2010;1350:95–102.
5. Chan EW, He Y, Chui CS, et al. Efficacy and safety of lorcaserin in obese adults: a meta-analysis of 1-year randomized controlled trials (RCTs) and narrative review on short-term RCTs. Obes Rev 2013;14(5):383–92.
6. Cameron F, Whiteside G, McKeage K. Phentermine and topiramate extended release (Qsymia): first global approval. Drugs 2012;72(15):2033–42.
7. Padwal R, Li SK, Lau DC. Long-term pharmacotherapy for overweight and obesity: a systematic review and meta-analysis of randomized controlled trials. Int J Obes Relat Metab Disord 2003;27(12):1437–46.
8. Gadde KM, Allison DB, Ryan DH, et al. Effects of low-dose, controlled-release, phentermine plus topiramate combination on weight and associated comorbidities in overweight and obese adults (CONQUER): a randomised, placebo-controlled, phase 3 trial. Lancet 2011;377(9774):1341–52.
9. Smith SR, Weissman NJ, Anderson CM, et al. Multicenter, placebo-controlled trial of lorcaserin for weight management. N Engl J Med 2010;363(3):245–56.
10. Dixon JB, Straznicky NE, Lambert EA, et al. Surgical approaches to the treatment of obesity. Nat Rev Gastroenterol Hepatol 2011;8:429–37.
11. Buchwald H, Oien DM. Metabolic/bariatric surgery worldwide 2008. Obes Surg 2009;19(12):1605–11.
12. Buchwald H, Oien DM. Metabolic/bariatric surgery worldwide 2011. Obes Surg 2013;23(4):427–36.
13. NHMRC. National Health and Medical Research Council: clinical practice guidelines for the management of overweight and obesity in adults, adolescents and children in Australia. Melbourne (Australia): National Health and Medical Research Council; 2013.
14. Dixon JB, Zimmet P, Alberti KG, et al. Bariatric surgery: an IDF statement for obese type 2 diabetes. Diabet Med 2011;28(6):628–42.
15. Magkos F, Su X, Bradley D, et al. Intrahepatic diacylglycerol content is associated with hepatic insulin resistance in obese subjects. Gastroenterology 2012;142:1444–6.e2.
16. Lim EL, Hollingsworth KG, Aribisala BS, et al. Reversal of type 2 diabetes: normalisation of beta cell function in association with decreased pancreas and liver triacylglycerol. Diabetologia 2011;54(10):2506–14.
17. Dixon JB, Straznicky NE, Lambert EA, et al. Laparoscopic adjustable gastric banding and other devices for the management of obesity. Circulation 2012;126(6):774–85.
18. Odstrcil EA, Martinez JG, Santa Ana CA, et al. The contribution of malabsorption to the reduction in net energy absorption after long-limb Roux-en-Y gastric bypass. Am J Clin Nutr 2010;92(4):704–13.
19. Ionut V, Burch M, Youdim A, et al. Gastrointestinal hormones and bariatric surgery induced weight loss. Obesity (Silver Spring) 2013;21:1093–103.
20. Pontiroli AE, Morabito A. Long-term prevention of mortality in morbid obesity through bariatric surgery. a systematic review and meta-analysis of trials performed with gastric banding and gastric bypass. Ann Surg 2011;253(3):484–7.

21. Sjostrom L, Narbro K, Sjostrom CD, et al. Effects of bariatric surgery on mortality in Swedish obese subjects. N Engl J Med 2007;357(8):741–52.
22. Adams TD, Gress RE, Smith SC, et al. Long-term mortality after gastric bypass surgery. N Engl J Med 2007;357(8):753–61.
23. Mingrone G, Panunzi S, De Gaetano A, et al. Bariatric surgery versus conventional medical therapy for type 2 diabetes. N Engl J Med 2012;366:1577–85.
24. Schauer PR, Kashyap SR, Wolski K, et al. Bariatric surgery versus intensive medical therapy in obese patients with diabetes. N Engl J Med 2012;366:1567–76.
25. Dixon JB, O'Brien PE, Playfair J, et al. Adjustable gastric banding and conventional therapy for type 2 diabetes: a randomized controlled trial. JAMA 2008; 299(3):316–23.
26. Ikramuddin S, Korner J, Lee WJ, et al. Roux-en-Y gastric bypass vs intensive medical management for the control of type 2 diabetes, hypertension, and hyperlipidemia: the Diabetes Surgery Study randomized clinical trial. JAMA 2013;309(21):2240–9.
27. O'Brien PE, Dixon JB, Laurie C, et al. Treatment of mild to moderate obesity with laparoscopic adjustable gastric banding or an intensive medical program: a randomized trial. Ann Intern Med 2006;144(9):625–33.
28. Sjöström L. Review of the key results from the Swedish Obese Subjects (SOS) trial: a prospective controlled intervention study of bariatric surgery. J Intern Med 2013;273:219–34.
29. Picot J, Jones J, Colquitt JL, et al. The clinical effectiveness and cost-effectiveness of bariatric (weight loss) surgery for obesity: a systematic review and economic evaluation. Health Technol Assess 2009;13(41):1–190, 215–357, iii–iv.
30. Finkelstein EA, Allaire BT, Burgess SM, et al. Financial implications of coverage for laparoscopic adjustable gastric banding. Surg Obes Relat Dis 2011;7(3): 295–303.
31. Keating CL, Dixon JB, Moodie ML, et al. Cost-effectiveness of surgically induced weight loss for the management of type 2 diabetes: modeled lifetime analysis. Diabetes Care 2009;32(4):567–74.
32. Dixon JB, Bhathal PS, O'Brien PE. Nonalcoholic fatty liver disease: predictors of nonalcoholic steatohepatitis and liver fibrosis in the severely obese. Gastroenterology 2001;121(1):91–100.
33. Chalasani N, Younossi Z, Lavine JE, et al. The diagnosis and management of non-alcoholic fatty liver disease: practice Guideline by the American Association for the Study of Liver Diseases, American College of Gastroenterology, and the American Gastroenterological Association. Hepatology 2012;55(6): 2005–23.
34. Dixon JB, Bhathal PS, Hughes NR, et al. Nonalcoholic fatty liver disease: improvement in liver histological analysis with weight loss. Hepatology 2004; 39(6):1647–54.
35. Mathurin P, Hollebecque A, Arnalsteen L, et al. Prospective study of the long-term effects of bariatric surgery on liver injury in patients without advanced disease. Gastroenterology 2009;137(2):532–40.
36. Chavez-Tapia NC, Tellez-Avila FI, Barrientos-Gutierrez T, et al. Bariatric surgery for non-alcoholic steatohepatitis in obese patients. Cochrane Database Syst Rev 2010;(1):CD007340.
37. Adams LA, Lymp JF, St Sauver J, et al. The natural history of nonalcoholic fatty liver disease: a population-based cohort study. Gastroenterology 2005;129(1): 113–21.

38. Burza MA, Romeo S, Kotronen A, et al. Long-term effect of bariatric surgery on liver enzymes in the Swedish Obese Subjects (SOS) Study. PLoS One 2013; 8(3):e60495.
39. Treeprasertsuk S, Bjornsson E, Enders F, et al. NAFLD fibrosis score: a prognostic predictor for mortality and liver complications among NAFLD patients. World J Gastroenterol 2013;19(8):1219–29.
40. Arun J, Jhala N, Lazenby AJ, et al. Influence of liver biopsy heterogeneity and diagnosis of nonalcoholic steatohepatitis in subjects undergoing gastric bypass. Obes Surg 2007;17(2):155–61.
41. Ratziu V, Charlotte F, Heurtier A, et al. Sampling variability of liver biopsy in nonalcoholic fatty liver disease. Gastroenterology 2005;128(7):1898–906.
42. Meinhardt NG, Souto KE, Ulbrich-Kulczynski JM, et al. Hepatic outcomes after jejunoileal bypass: is there a publication bias? Obes Surg 2006;16(9): 1171–8.
43. Silverman EM, Sapala JA, Appelman HD. Regression of hepatic steatosis in morbidly obese persons after gastric bypass. Am J Clin Pathol 1995;104(1):23–31.
44. Liu X, Lazenby AJ, Clements RH, et al. Resolution of nonalcoholic steatohepatits after gastric bypass surgery. Obes Surg 2007;17(4):486–92.
45. Vargas V, Allende H, Lecube A, et al. Surgically induced weight loss by gastric bypass improves non alcoholic fatty liver disease in morbid obese patients. World J Hepatol 2012;4(12):382–8.
46. Mathurin P, Gonzalez F, Kerdraon O, et al. The evolution of severe steatosis after bariatric surgery is related to insulin resistance. Gastroenterology 2006;130(6): 1617–24.
47. DeWind LT, Payne JH. Intestinal bypass surgery for morbid obesity. Long-term results. JAMA 1976;236(20):2298–301.
48. Rucker RD Jr, Horstmann J, Schneider PD, et al. Comparisons between jejunoileal and gastric bypass operations for morbid obesity. Surgery 1982;92(2): 241–9.
49. Hocking MP, Davis GL, Franzini DA, et al. Long-term consequences after jejunoileal bypass for morbid obesity. Dig Dis Sci 1998;43(11):2493–9.
50. O'Leary JP. Hepatic complications of jejunoileal bypass. Semin Liver Dis 1983; 3(3):203–15.
51. Antal SC. Prevention and reversal of liver damage following biliopancreatic diversion for obesity. Obes Surg 1994;4(3):285–90.
52. Castillo J, Fabrega E, Escalante CF, et al. Liver transplantation in a case of steatohepatitis and subacute hepatic failure after biliopancreatic diversion for morbid obesity. Obes Surg 2001;11(5):640–2.
53. Papadia F, Marinari GM, Camerini G, et al. Short-term liver function after biliopancreatic diversion. Obes Surg 2003;13(5):752–5.
54. Kral JG, Thung SN, Biron S, et al. Effects of surgical treatment of the metabolic syndrome on liver fibrosis and cirrhosis. Surgery 2004;135(1):48–58.
55. Keshishian A, Zahriya K, Willes EB. Duodenal switch has no detrimental effects on hepatic function and improves hepatic steatohepatitis after 6 months. Obes Surg 2005;15(10):1418–23.
56. Andersen T, Larsen U. Dietary outcome in obese patients treated with a gastroplasty program. Am J Clin Nutr 1989;50(6):1328–40.
57. Andersen T. Liver and gallbladder disease before and after very-low-calorie diets. Am J Clin Nutr 1992;56(1 Suppl):235S–9S.
58. Andersen T, Gluud C, Franzmann MB, et al. Hepatic effects of dietary weight loss in morbidly obese subjects. J Hepatol 1991;12(2):224–9.

59. Mosko JD, Nguyen GC. Increased perioperative mortality following bariatric surgery among patients with cirrhosis. Clin Gastroenterol Hepatol 2011;9(10):897–901.
60. Shimizu H, Phuong V, Maia M, et al. Bariatric surgery in patients with liver cirrhosis. Surg Obes Relat Dis 2013;9(1):1–6.
61. Cobb WS, Heniford BT, Burns JM, et al. Cirrhosis is not a contraindication to laparoscopic surgery. Surg Endosc 2005;19(3):418–23.
62. Dallal RM, Mattar SG, Lord JL, et al. Results of laparoscopic gastric bypass in patients with cirrhosis. Obes Surg 2004;14(1):47–53.
63. Peng L, Wang J, Li F. Weight reduction for non-alcoholic fatty liver disease. Cochrane Database Syst Rev 2011;(6):CD003619.
64. Serrot FJ, Dorman RB, Miller CJ, et al. Comparative effectiveness of bariatric surgery and nonsurgical therapy in adults with type 2 diabetes mellitus and body mass index <35 kg/m(2). Surgery 2011;150(4):684–91.
65. Arterburn DE, Bogart A, Sherwood NE, et al. A multisite study of long-term remission and relapse of type 2 diabetes mellitus following gastric bypass. Obes Surg 2013;23:93–102.
66. NIH. Gastrointestinal surgery for severe obesity: National Institutes of Health Consensus Development Conference Statement. Am J Clin Nutr 1992;55(2 Suppl):615S–9S.
67. NICE. Obesity: guidance on the prevention, identification, assessment and management of overweight and obesity in adults and children. London: National Institute for Health and Clinical Excellence; 2006.
68. Fried M, Hainer V, Basdevant A, et al. Inter-disciplinary European guidelines on surgery of severe obesity. Int J Obes (Lond) 2007;31(4):569–77.
69. Logue J, Thompson L, Romanes F, et al. Management of obesity: summary of SIGN guideline. BMJ 2010;340:c154.
70. Brethauer SA, Hammel JP, Schauer PR. Systematic review of sleeve gastrectomy as staging and primary bariatric procedure. Surg Obes Relat Dis 2009; 5(4):469–75.
71. O'Brien PE, McPhail T, Chaston TB, et al. Systematic review of medium-term weight loss after bariatric operations. Obes Surg 2006;16(8):1032–40.
72. Fischer L, Hildebrandt C, Bruckner T, et al. Excessive weight loss after sleeve gastrectomy: a systematic review. Obes Surg 2012;22(5):721–31.
73. Chapman A, Kiroff G, Game P, et al. Laparoscopic adjustable gastric banding in the treatment of obesity: a systematic review. Surgery 2004;135:326–51.
74. Buchwald H, Estok R, Fahrbach K, et al. Trends in mortality in bariatric surgery: a systematic review and meta-analysis. Surgery 2007;142(4):621–32.
75. Flum DR, Belle SH, King WC, et al. Perioperative safety in the longitudinal assessment of bariatric surgery. N Engl J Med 2009;361(5):445–54.
76. DeMaria EJ, Pate V, Warthen M, et al. Baseline data from American Society for Metabolic and Bariatric Surgery-designated Bariatric Surgery Centers of Excellence using the Bariatric Outcomes Longitudinal Database. Surg Obes Relat Dis 2010;6(4):347–55.
77. O'Brien PE, Macdonald L, Anderson M, et al. Long-term outcomes after bariatric surgery: fifteen-year follow-up of adjustable gastric banding and a systematic review of the bariatric surgical literature. Ann Surg 2013;257(1):87–94.
78. Mechanick JI, Youdim A, Jones DB, et al. Clinical practice guidelines for the perioperative nutritional, metabolic, and nonsurgical support of the bariatric surgery patient–2013 update: cosponsored by American Association of Clinical Endocrinologists, The Obesity Society, and American Society for Metabolic & Bariatric Surgery. Obesity (Silver Spring) 2013;21(Suppl 1):S1–27.

79. Ranlov I, Hardt F. Regression of liver steatosis following gastroplasty or gastric bypass for morbid obesity. Digestion 1990;47(4):208–14.
80. Luyckx FH, Desaive C, Thiry A, et al. Liver abnormalities in severely obese subjects: effect of drastic weight loss after gastroplasty. Int J Obes Relat Metab Disord 1998;22(3):222–6.
81. Clark JM, Alkhuraishi AR, Solga SF, et al. Roux-en-Y gastric bypass improves liver histology in patients with non-alcoholic fatty liver disease. Obes Res 2005;13(7):1180–6.
82. Mattar SG, Velcu LM, Rabinovitz M, et al. Surgically-induced weight loss significantly improves nonalcoholic fatty liver disease and the metabolic syndrome. Ann Surg 2005;242(4):610–7 [discussion: 618–20].
83. Mottin CC, Moretto M, Padoin AV, et al. Histological behavior of hepatic steatosis in morbidly obese patients after weight loss induced by bariatric surgery. Obes Surg 2005;15(6):788–93.
84. Stratopoulos C, Papakonstantinou A, Terzis I, et al. Changes in liver histology accompanying massive weight loss after gastroplasty for morbid obesity. Obes Surg 2005;15(8):1154–60.
85. Barker KB, Palekar NA, Bowers SP, et al. Non-alcoholic steatohepatitis: effect of Roux-en-Y gastric bypass surgery. Am J Gastroenterol 2006;101(2):368–73.
86. Csendes A, Smok G, Burgos AM. Histological findings in the liver before and after gastric bypass. Obes Surg 2006;16(5):607–11.
87. de Almeida SR, Rocha PR, Sanches MD, et al. Roux-en-Y gastric bypass improves the nonalcoholic steatohepatitis (NASH) of morbid obesity. Obes Surg 2006;16(3):270–8.
88. Dixon JB, Bhathal PS, O'Brien PE. Weight loss and non-alcoholic fatty liver disease: falls in gamma-glutamyl transferase concentrations are associated with histologic improvement. Obes Surg 2006;16(10):1278–86.
89. Klein S, Mittendorfer B, Eagon JC, et al. Gastric bypass surgery improves metabolic and hepatic abnormalities associated with nonalcoholic fatty liver disease. Gastroenterology 2006;130(6):1564–72.
90. Furuya CK Jr, de Oliveira CP, de Mello ES, et al. Effects of bariatric surgery on nonalcoholic fatty liver disease: preliminary findings after 2 years. J Gastroenterol Hepatol 2007;22(4):510–4.
91. Bell LN, Temm CJ, Saxena R, et al. Bariatric surgery-induced weight loss reduces hepatic lipid peroxidation levels and affects hepatic cytochrome P-450 protein content. Ann Surg 2010;251(6):1041–8.
92. Weiner RA. Surgical treatment of non-alcoholic steatohepatitis and non-alcoholic fatty liver disease. Dig Dis 2010;28(1):274–9.
93. Tai CM, Huang CK, Hwang JC, et al. Improvement of nonalcoholic fatty liver disease after bariatric surgery in morbidly obese Chinese patients. Obes Surg 2012;22(7):1016–21.
94. Moretto M, Kupski C, da Silva VD, et al. Effect of bariatric surgery on liver fibrosis. Obes Surg 2012;22(7):1044–9.

The Impact of Obesity and Metabolic Syndrome on Chronic Hepatitis C

Nicolas Goossens, MD, MSc[a], Francesco Negro, MD[a,b],*

KEYWORDS

- Liver • Hypertension • Steatosis • Fibrosis • Insulin resistance • Diabetes

KEY POINTS

- The interplay between the metabolic syndrome and hepatitis C virus (HCV) infection is complex and multilayered.
- HCV alters glucose metabolism and can lead to insulin resistance (IR) or overt diabetes in susceptible individuals, whereas in the case of IR and/or diabetes, the clinical outcome of HCV-infected individuals worsen.
- The strong relationship between HCV, especially genotype 3 HCV, and steatosis is also clear; however, its clinical consequences, if any, need further study.
- Insulin sensitizers seem to be a logical target to try and improve IR, however clinical trials in the context of antiviral treatment did not document a clear benefit in virologic outcomes.
- The optimal management of HCV-infected individuals with the metabolic syndrome should focus on lifestyle interventions, treatment of diabetes, and aggressive management of cofactors.

INTRODUCTION

Approximately 2.35% of the world's population, or 185 million people, are infected with the hepatitis C virus (HCV).[1] HCV is a major cause of chronic liver disease, culminating in cirrhosis, hepatocellular carcinoma (HCC), and increased mortality from both hepatic and extrahepatic disease.[2] On the other hand, the metabolic syndrome is a

The authors' quoted work is supported by Swiss National Science Foundation grant numbers 314730-130498 and 314730-146991 and by the Foundation for Liver and Gut Studies, Geneva, Switzerland.

Conflicts of Interest: F. Negro is advising Roche, MSD, Gilead, Janssen Novartis, and Boehringer Ingelheim and has received unrestricted research grants from Roche, Novartis, and Gilead. N. Goossens has nothing to disclose.

[a] Division of Gastroenterology and Hepatology, Geneva University Hospital, 4 rue Gabrielle-Perret-Gentil, 1211 Geneva 4, Switzerland; [b] Division of Clinical Pathology, Geneva University Hospital, 4 rue Gabrielle-Perret-Gentil, 1211 Geneva 4, Switzerland

* Corresponding author. Division of Clinical Pathology, Geneva University Hospital, 4 rue Gabrielle-Perret-Gentil, 1211 Geneva 4, Switzerland.

E-mail address: Francesco.Negro@hcuge.ch

global health burden associated with increased cardiovascular disease and diabetes.[3,4] Its prevalence varies from 23.7% of adults in the United States in one cross-sectional survey and 9.8% to 17.8% of Chinese adults in another study.[5,6]

In view of their high prevalence, there is bound to be significant interaction between these 2 conditions. However, it is becoming clear that their relationship is complex. First, HCV is associated with insulin resistance (IR), a fundamental characteristic of the metabolic syndrome.[7,8] Second, the metabolic syndrome and especially IR and/or diabetes play a role on the progression of HCV and on clinically relevant endpoints such as liver-related mortality[9] or the development of HCC.[10,11] Third, HCV has a very peculiar relationship with lipid metabolism: HCV virions circulate bound to lipoproteins, lipids modulate the HCV life cycle, and HCV is associated, in a distinct subgroup of patients, with severe steatosis.[12]

In this review therefore the relationship between the metabolic syndrome and HCV infection, its clinical impact, and potential management strategies are discussed.

DEFINITIONS

The metabolic syndrome is a cluster of risk factors for cardiovascular disease and type 2 diabetes mellitus. Its definition has gradually evolved from the initial definition by the World Health Organization[13] to the latest harmonized definition from the International Diabetes Federation Task Force on Epidemiology and Prevention, the National Heart, Lung, and Blood Institute, the American Heart Association, the World Heart Federation, the International Atherosclerosis Society, and the International Association for the Study of Obesity.[14] Essentially, to qualify for metabolic syndrome, a patient should have 3 or more abnormal findings of the 5 criteria, namely, raised blood pressure, dyslipidemia (elevated triglycerides or low high-density lipoprotein cholesterol [HDL-C]), elevated waist circumference, and raised fasting glucose (**Table 1**). Defining thresholds for abdominal obesity is difficult due to a lack of clear clinical thresholds and ethnic differences, but in common practice the thresholds defined by the International Diabetes Federation are used (ie, more than 94 cm waist circumference for men and more than 80 cm for women).[14]

Table 1
Criteria for the clinical diagnosis of the metabolic syndrome

Clinical Parameter	Threshold
Abdominal obesity	Population-specific. In general ≥94 cm waist circumference in men, ≥80 cm in women
Dyslipidemia	
Low HDL-C	<40 mg/dL (1.0 mmol/L) in men <50 mg/dL (1.3 mmol/L) in women or Treated for low HDL-C
Raised triglycerides	≥150 mg/dL (1.7 mmol/L) or Treated for raised triglycerides
Raised blood pressure	Systolic ≥130 mm Hg and/or Diastolic ≥85 mm Hg or Treated for hypertension
Impaired fasting glucose	≥100 mg/dL (5.6 mmol/L) or Treated for diabetes

Three or more positive criteria qualify a patient for the metabolic syndrome.
Abbreviation: HDL-C, high-density lipoprotein cholesterol.

Over the years, an international expert committee has been assessing and adapting guidelines to diagnose diabetes by measuring blood glucose (in the fasting state or after a glucose challenge, see **Table 2**).[15] Due to recent, improved standardization of glycated hemoglobin (HbA$_{1c}$), this biochemical test has been implemented in the diagnosis of diabetes. Importantly, the expert committee recognized a group of patients with higher than normal glucose levels, without reaching the criteria for diabetes, due to either high fasting glucose levels (impaired fasting glucose) or raised glucose levels after an oral glucose challenge (impaired glucose tolerance) (see **Table 2**).[15] These patients, sometimes referred to as having "prediabetes," have a higher risk of developing diabetes as well as cardiovascular disease and often have other components of the metabolic syndrome as mentioned above.[4,16]

Finally, IR is defined as a condition in which higher than normal insulin concentrations are needed to achieve normal metabolic responses or, alternatively, normal insulin concentrations are unable to achieve normal metabolic responses.[17] IR is often measured using the homeostasis model assessment of IR, or HOMA-IR, although its in vivo gold-standard measurement is the hyperinsulinemic-euglycemic clamp.[18]

HCV AND IR

Evidence from clinical, epidemiologic, and experimental fields concurs to suggest that there is a link between HCV infection and IR, an important feature of the metabolic syndrome.[7,8] Population-based cross-sectional studies have found an increased proportion of diabetics in HCV-positive patients compared with HCV-negative controls.[19–21] This association was verified in longitudinal, prospective studies comparing the incidence of diabetes in HCV-positive and HCV-negative individuals. In one trial of 1084 adults, HCV-positive patients at high risk of developing diabetes (based on body mass index and age) were 11 times more likely to develop diabetes than HCV-negative individuals, although this effect was not found in patients at low risk of developing diabetes.[22] Similar results were found in a Taiwanese cohort with a

Table 2
Definition of diabetes and prediabetic states according to the American Diabetes Association guidelines

Test	Normal	Prediabetes		Diabetes
		IFG	IGT	
Fasting plasma glucose	<100 mg/dL (5.6 mmol/L)	100 mg/dL (5.6 mmol/L) to 125 mg/dL (6.9 mmol/L)	—	≥126 mg/dL (7.0 mmol/L)
2 h values of plasma glucose in the 75 g OGTT	<140 mg/dL (7.8 mmol/L)	—	140 mg/dL (7.8 mmol/L) to 199 mg/dL (11.0 mmol/L)	≥200 mg/dL (11.1 mmol/L)
HbA$_{1c}$	<5.7%	5.7%–6.4%		≥6.5%

In patients without classic symptoms of hyperglycemia, the diagnostic test must be repeated to confirm the diagnosis of diabetes, but in patients with classic symptoms, a random plasma glucose of ≥200 mg/dL (11.1 mmol/L) is sufficient to diagnose diabetes. Note that there is not 100% concordance between the different tests (fasting glucose, 2 h post oral glucose load and HbA$_{1c}$), and it is not yet clear how to characterise patients clinically with differing glycemic statuses according to these tests.

Abbreviations: HbA$_{1c}$, glycosylated hemoglobin; IFG, impaired fasting glucose; IGT, impaired glucose tolerance; OGTT, oral glucose tolerance test.

hazard ratio of 1.7 of developing diabetes for HCV-positive patients; alternatively, a recent study from Southern Italy with a follow-up of 20 years of 2472 subjects only found such an association in HCV-infected patients with elevated alanine transaminase levels.[23,24] To define the epidemiologic interaction between IR and HCV further, a systematic review pooled all studies analyzing the risk of diabetes in patients with HCV.[25] In this review, combining 34 studies and a total of more than 300,000 patients, the pooled estimate of type 2 diabetes in HCV patients was an adjusted odds ratio of approximately 1.68 (95% confidence interval [CI] 1.15–2.20), significant in both prospective and retrospective meta-analyses.[25] Therefore, there is a clear epidemiologic association between HCV and the development of diabetes.

The mechanism by which HCV infection alters glucose metabolism seems to be related to an increase in IR rather than a change in β-cell function.[7] In a study of 260 HCV-positive subjects, IR, as measured by HOMA-IR, was increased as compared with healthy matched controls, even in subjects with minimal fibrosis.[26] This increase was confirmed in other studies, where IR was more frequent in HCV patients than in matched HCV-negative patients with or without chronic HBV, also suggesting a role of HCV on glucose metabolism.[27,28] However, not all studies have reproduced this finding[29] and further longitudinal, prospective studies are warranted to clarify this point of debate.

If HCV plays a role in glucose metabolism, then its eradication should improve IR. Two independent studies show that sustained viral response (SVR) is associated with a reduction in the risk of type 2 diabetes development in patients with HCV[30,31]; however, other studies did not show a significant difference in IR after SVR.[32,33] A recent large study, presented in abstract form, including 20,486 veterans treated for HCV noted a reduced incidence of diabetes (hazard ratio 0.76, 95% CI 0.70–0.82) in patients achieving SVR.[34] Therefore, overall data tend to show a reduction of the incidence of diabetes, and possibly IR, in HCV-positive patients achieving SVR.

Taken together, this data suggest that HCV affects glucose metabolism at early stages of the natural course of the disease by inducing IR. HCV seems to increase the progression from IR to overt diabetes in susceptible patients and curing HCV seems to improve IR and decrease the risk of diabetes. Below, the effect of IR on the natural history of HCV infection is discussed.

HCV AND STEATOSIS

Although steatosis is not a component of the metabolic syndrome definition per se, these 2 conditions interact closely and potentiate each other's effect.[35,36] Steatosis occurs in up to 80% of hepatitis C patients and was used in the preserology era as a diagnostic tool to identify non-A, non-B hepatitis patients.[37,38] Even when controlling for other factors known to induce a fatty liver, the prevalence of steatosis is still double that seen in chronic hepatitis B patients, suggesting a role for viral factors in the development of steatosis.[39,40]

The major piece of evidence arguing in favor of HCV-induced fatty liver is the strong association with genotype 3, where steatosis is more frequent and severe and its severity correlates with HCV replication, in both serum and liver,[41,42] whereas in non-3 genotypes, steatosis seems to correlate with traditional metabolic factors associated with a fatty liver.[43] Furthermore, in genotype 3, steatosis disappears after successful antiviral therapy in patients, while in most patients with other genotypes it is largely unaffected even in case of SVR.[42,44,45]

Therefore, there is a strong epidemiologic link between steatosis and HCV, although the clinical consequences of this link have yet to be completely unraveled.

HCV AND OTHER COMPONENTS OF THE METABOLIC SYNDROME

Although there is a close relationship between IR and HCV infection, the other components of the metabolic syndrome are not as clearly associated with HCV. The metabolic syndrome is characterized by hypertriglyceridemia and low HDL-C concentrations, whereas the lipid profile in patients with HCV, especially genotype 3, is characterized by low levels of total cholesterol and triglycerides.[12] On the other hand, recent data show an association between HCV infection and hypertension (odds ratio of 2.06) in a cohort of 19,741 participants of whom 0.88% were HCV-positive.[46] This data must be confirmed in further longitudinal studies.

HCV AND THE METABOLIC SYNDROME: DOES IT MATTER?

Although there seems to be a clear association between HCV and the metabolic syndrome, especially IR, what is the clinical consequence of this interaction and how does it affect patients? The clinical impact of this association and its relevance on patient-relevant outcomes such as mortality, incidence of HCC, and influence on HCV cure rates, are discussed.

In a large NHANES III population-based study, an association was demonstrated between IR or type 2 diabetes and all-cause mortality in chronic HBV-infected patients, nonalcoholic fatty liver disease, and alcoholic liver disease but not in patients with HCV. However, diabetes and IR were independent predictors of liver-related mortality in HCV in the same study,[9] suggesting that IR and diabetes act together with HCV infection to increase liver-related mortality, possibly by favoring progression of liver fibrosis and increasing incidence of HCC (see below).

Due to the close link between HCV, type 2 diabetes, and other metabolic factors, one of the first legitimate questions is whether the interaction of all these factors is reflected in an increased cardiovascular morbidity and mortality in patients with HCV. A large retrospective cohort study showed an increase in cardiovascular mortality among HCV-positive blood donors (hazard ratio 2.21, 95% CI: 1.41, 3.46) and another study showed larger carotid intima-media thickness (IMT), an index of early atherosclerosis, in HCV-positive patients when compared with controls.[47,48] A further, more recent, study demonstrated an association between HCV infection and congestive heart failure subtype of cardiovascular diseases but not ischemic heart disease and stroke.[46] In another prospective cohort, the REVEAL study based in Taiwan, anti-HCV seropositivity was associated, in multivariable analysis, with multiple extrahepatic complications, including mortality from circulatory diseases (adjusted hazard ratio 1.50, 95% CI 1.10–2.33).[2] In this study, showing that HCV-infected patients had a higher mortality from hepatic and extrahepatic disease, HCV was associated with mortality from circulatory disease only if HCV patients had detectable HCV RNA levels, suggesting that patients with undetectable HCV RNA levels return to their baseline cardiovascular risk.[2] Other studies, however, did not confirm this association; for example, a large German cross-sectional study failed to find an association between HCV positivity and IMT or other cardiovascular endpoints.[49] In a more recent Egyptian cross-sectional study, IMT and number of patients with carotid plaques did not seem increased in patients with HCV compared with healthy controls, although there was an association after complete adjustment for other cardiovascular risk factors.[50] A weakness of many of these studies is a lack of liver biopsies to exclude superimposed NAFLD. Whether the weak association between cardiovascular diseases and HCV infection may be related to the favorable lipid profile in HCV-infected individuals, namely low LDL cholesterol, is open to debate.[12]

A series of recent studies and meta-analyses confirmed that the risk of several types of malignancies, including HCC, is increased in the setting of type 2 diabetes.[51] In population-based data of 19,349 diabetic patients and 77,396 controls in Taiwan, Lai and colleagues[52] found that diabetes was associated with a doubled incidence of HCC and that HCV increased that risk with a hazard ratio of 5.61. A systematic review pooled 13 case-control studies and cohort studies and showed a significant association between diabetes and HCC in both cases.[53] A recent retrospective study of 4302 Japanese HCV-positive patients treated with interferon found that type 2 diabetes was associated with a 1.73-fold increase in the risk of development of HCC or other malignancies, but this risk decreased when HbA1c levels were maintained less than 7.0%, suggesting a role for improved glycemic control as a strategy to decrease HCC occurrence.[54] Other factors associated with HCC development in this study were advanced fibrosis, lack of SVR, male sex, age of $\geq$50 years, and alcohol abuse.[54] Another meta-analysis showed that HCC is increased by 17% in overweight subjects and by 89% in obese individuals, but the combined risk factors of diabetes, obesity, and HBV or HCV infection increased the risk more than 100 times in one follow-up study of 23,820 Taiwan residents,[10,11] which underlines the importance of the synergistic links between features of the metabolic syndrome and viral factors in the pathogenesis of HCC. Interestingly, pathologic data studying HCV-positive liver explants and retrospective clinical data of HCV-positive individuals suggest that steatosis is also associated with increased HCC incidence.[55,56] Unfortunately, the relative contribution of viral versus metabolic steatosis was not assessed in these studies and must be further studied.

IR also seems to accelerate fibrosis progression rates in patients with HCV. For instance, in 260 HCV-infected patients HOMA-IR was an independent predictor for the degree of fibrosis (P<.001) and the rate of fibrosis progression ($P = .03$).[26] However, a matter of debate is whether hepatic steatosis or IR mediates the increased fibrosis progression rate, although IR seems to be the best predictor for advanced fibrosis.[57]

IR also seems to affect the rate of virologic response to anti-HCV interferon-based therapy. In a systematic review of 14 studies, SVR was less frequent in patients with IR (as assessed with baseline HOMA-IR) with a mean difference of -13.0% (95% CI: -22.6% to -3.4%, $P = .008$).[58] Speculative pathogenic mechanisms include increased viral replication, impairment of interferon-α, and insulin signaling or increased liver fibrosis.[8] Interestingly, similarly to what is reported for liver steatosis, it seems to be host-induced IR (rather than IR caused by HCV) that affects the response to viral therapy, although this remains speculative and must be confirmed in further research.[59,60] In the meantime, it remains to be seen whether IR will continue to predict treatment response in the era of newer direct-acting antivirals. Recent data in genotype 1-infected patients show that virologic response was not affected by IR in treatment-naïve or experienced HCV patients treated with telaprevir-based therapy.[61,62]

Of all the factors in the metabolic syndrome, IR and type 2 diabetes seem to have the greatest importance in the clinical consequence of the metabolic syndrome on HCV infection. Fibrosis progression rate is increased and liver-related mortality is higher. HCC incidence is also increased and these patients seem to respond less well to interferon-based therapy. As discussed above, curing HCV may be associated with reduced incidence of diabetes and possibly an improved cardiovascular risk profile.[2,30] Therefore, although longer term studies are warranted, achieving SVR in these patients could lead to reduced morbidity and mortality linked to cardiovascular disease and diabetes.

SUMMARY

The interplay between the metabolic syndrome and HCV infection is complex and multilayered. HCV alters glucose metabolism and can lead to IR or overt diabetes in susceptible individuals, whereas in the case of IR and/or diabetes the clinical outcome of HCV-infected individuals worsen. The relationship between genotype 3 HCV and steatosis is also clear; however, its clinical consequences, if any, need further studies.

Insulin sensitizers seem to be a logical target to try and improve IR especially in the setting of antiviral therapy for HCV. Unfortunately, results involving pioglitazone and metformin are discouraging without a clear improvement in virologic outcomes.[60,63–65]

Therefore, for the time being, the optimal management of HCV-infected individuals with the metabolic syndrome should focus on lifestyle interventions, treatment of diabetes, and aggressive management of cofactors.

REFERENCES

1. Mohd Hanafiah K, Groeger J, Flaxman AD, et al. Global epidemiology of hepatitis C virus infection: new estimates of age-specific antibody to HCV seroprevalence. Hepatology 2013;57(4):1333–42.
2. Lee MH, Yang HI, Lu SN, et al. Chronic hepatitis C virus infection increases mortality from hepatic and extrahepatic diseases: a community-based long-term prospective study. J Infect Dis 2012;206:469–77.
3. Ford ES. Risks for all-cause mortality, cardiovascular disease, and diabetes associated with the metabolic syndrome: a summary of the evidence. Diabetes Care 2005;28(7):1769–78.
4. Ford ES, Zhao G, Li C. Pre-diabetes and the risk for cardiovascular disease: a systematic review of the evidence. J Am Coll Cardiol 2010;55(13):1310–7.
5. Ford ES, Giles WH, Dietz WH. Prevalence of the metabolic syndrome among US adults: findings from the third National Health and Nutrition Examination Survey. JAMA 2002;287(3):356–9.
6. Gu D, Reynolds K, Wu X, et al. Prevalence of the metabolic syndrome and overweight among adults in China. Lancet 2005;365(9468):1398–405.
7. Kaddai V, Negro F. Current understanding of insulin resistance in hepatitis C. Expert Rev Gastroenterol Hepatol 2011;5(4):503–16.
8. Bugianesi E, Salamone F, Negro F. The interaction of metabolic factors with HCV infection: does it matter? J Hepatol 2012;56(Suppl 1):S56–65.
9. Stepanova M, Rafiq N, Younossi ZM. Components of metabolic syndrome are independent predictors of mortality in patients with chronic liver disease: a population-based study. Gut 2010;59(10):1410–5.
10. Chen CL, Yang HI, Yang WS, et al. Metabolic factors and risk of hepatocellular carcinoma by chronic hepatitis B/C infection: a follow-up study in Taiwan. Gastroenterology 2008;135(1):111–21.
11. Larsson SC, Wolk A. Overweight, obesity and risk of liver cancer: a meta-analysis of cohort studies. Br J Cancer 2007;97(7):1005–8.
12. Negro F. Abnormalities of lipid metabolism in hepatitis C virus infection. Gut 2010;59(9):1279–87.
13. Alberti KG, Zimmet PZ. Definition, diagnosis and classification of diabetes mellitus and its complications. Part 1: diagnosis and classification of diabetes mellitus provisional report of a WHO consultation. Diabet Med 1998;15(7):539–53.
14. Alberti KG, Eckel RH, Grundy SM, et al. Harmonizing the metabolic syndrome: a joint interim statement of the International Diabetes Federation Task Force on Epidemiology and Prevention; National Heart, Lung, and Blood Institute;

American Heart Association; World Heart Federation; International Atherosclerosis Society; and International Association for the Study of Obesity. Circulation 2009;120(16):1640–5.

15. American Diabetes Association. Diagnosis and classification of diabetes mellitus. Diabetes Care 2013;36(Suppl 1):S67–74.
16. Tabak AG, Herder C, Rathmann W, et al. Prediabetes: a high-risk state for diabetes development. Lancet 2012;379(9833):2279–90.
17. Bugianesi E, McCullough AJ, Marchesini G. Insulin resistance: a metabolic pathway to chronic liver disease. Hepatology 2005;42(5):987–1000.
18. Matthews DR, Hosker JP, Rudenski AS, et al. Homeostasis model assessment: insulin resistance and beta-cell function from fasting plasma glucose and insulin concentrations in man. Diabetologia 1985;28(7):412–9.
19. Allison ME, Wreghitt T, Palmer CR, et al. Evidence for a link between hepatitis C virus infection and diabetes mellitus in a cirrhotic population. J Hepatol 1994; 21(6):1135–9.
20. Negro F, Alaei M. Hepatitis C virus and type 2 diabetes. World J Gastroenterol 2009;15(13):1537–47.
21. Mehta SH, Brancati FL, Sulkowski MS, et al. Prevalence of type 2 diabetes mellitus among persons with hepatitis C virus infection in the United States. Ann Intern Med 2000;133(8):592–9.
22. Mehta SH, Brancati FL, Strathdee SA, et al. Hepatitis C virus infection and incident type 2 diabetes. Hepatology 2003;38(1):50–6.
23. Wang CS, Wang ST, Yao WJ, et al. Hepatitis C virus infection and the development of type 2 diabetes in a community-based longitudinal study. Am J Epidemiol 2007;166(2):196–203.
24. Montenegro L, De Michina A, Misciagna G, et al. Virus C hepatitis and type 2 diabetes: a cohort study in southern Italy. Am J Gastroenterol 2013;108(7):1108–11.
25. White DL, Ratziu V, El-Serag HB. Hepatitis C infection and risk of diabetes: a systematic review and meta-analysis. J Hepatol 2008;49(5):831–44.
26. Hui JM, Sud A, Farrell GC, et al. Insulin resistance is associated with chronic hepatitis C virus infection and fibrosis progression [corrected]. Gastroenterology 2003;125(6):1695–704.
27. Dai CY, Yeh ML, Huang CF, et al. Chronic hepatitis C infection is associated with insulin resistance and lipid profiles. J Gastroenterol Hepatol 2013. [Epub ahead of print].
28. Moucari R, Asselah T, Cazals-Hatem D, et al. Insulin resistance in chronic hepatitis C: association with genotypes 1 and 4, serum HCV RNA level, and liver fibrosis. Gastroenterology 2008;134(2):416–23.
29. Tanaka N, Nagaya T, Komatsu M, et al. Insulin resistance and hepatitis C virus: a case-control study of non-obese, non-alcoholic and non-steatotic hepatitis virus carriers with persistently normal serum aminotransferase. Liver Int 2008;28(8): 1104–11.
30. Arase Y, Suzuki F, Suzuki Y, et al. Sustained virological response reduces incidence of onset of type 2 diabetes in chronic hepatitis C. Hepatology 2009; 49(3):739–44.
31. Romero-Gomez M, Fernandez-Rodriguez CM, Andrade RJ, et al. Effect of sustained virological response to treatment on the incidence of abnormal glucose values in chronic hepatitis C. J Hepatol 2008;48(5):721–7.
32. Brandman D, Bacchetti P, Ayala CE, et al. Impact of insulin resistance on HCV treatment response and impact of HCV treatment on insulin sensitivity using direct measurements of insulin action. Diabetes Care 2012;35(5):1090–4.

33. Giordanino C, Bugianesi E, Smedile A, et al. Incidence of type 2 diabetes mellitus and glucose abnormalities in patients with chronic hepatitis C infection by response to treatment: results of a cohort study. Am J Gastroenterol 2008; 103(10):2481–7.
34. Hyder SM, Krishnan S, Promrat K. #608 Sustained virological response prevents the development of new type 2 diabetes in patients with chronic hepatitis C. Gastroenterology 2013;144(5):S951.
35. Marchesini G, Brizi M, Bianchi G, et al. Nonalcoholic fatty liver disease: a feature of the metabolic syndrome. Diabetes 2001;50(8):1844–50.
36. Marchesini G, Bugianesi E, Forlani G, et al. Nonalcoholic fatty liver, steatohepatitis, and the metabolic syndrome. Hepatology 2003;37(4):917–23.
37. Dienes HP, Popper H, Arnold W, et al. Histologic observations in human hepatitis non-A, non-B. Hepatology 1982;2(5):562–71.
38. Wiese M, Haupt R. Histomorphologic picture of chronic non-A, non-B hepatitis. Dtsch Z Verdau Stoffwechselkr 1985;45(3):101–10 [in German].
39. Czaja AJ, Carpenter HA, Santrach PJ, et al. Host- and disease-specific factors affecting steatosis in chronic hepatitis C. J Hepatol 1998;29(2):198–206.
40. Peng D, Han Y, Ding H, et al. Hepatic steatosis in chronic hepatitis B patients is associated with metabolic factors more than viral factors. J Gastroenterol Hepatol 2008;23(7 Pt 1):1082–8.
41. Fartoux L, Poujol-Robert A, Guechot J, et al. Insulin resistance is a cause of steatosis and fibrosis progression in chronic hepatitis C. Gut 2005;54(7):1003–8.
42. Rubbia-Brandt L, Quadri R, Abid K, et al. Hepatocyte steatosis is a cytopathic effect of hepatitis C virus genotype 3. J Hepatol 2000;33(1):106–15.
43. Adinolfi LE, Gambardella M, Andreana A, et al. Steatosis accelerates the progression of liver damage of chronic hepatitis C patients and correlates with specific HCV genotype and visceral obesity. Hepatology 2001;33(6):1358–64.
44. Kumar D, Farrell GC, Fung C, et al. Hepatitis C virus genotype 3 is cytopathic to hepatocytes: reversal of hepatic steatosis after sustained therapeutic response. Hepatology 2002;36(5):1266–72.
45. Poynard T, Ratziu V, McHutchison J, et al. Effect of treatment with peginterferon or interferon alfa-2b and ribavirin on steatosis in patients infected with hepatitis C. Hepatology 2003;38(1):75–85.
46. Younossi ZM, Stepanova M, Nader F, et al. Associations of chronic hepatitis C with metabolic and cardiac outcomes. Aliment Pharmacol Ther 2013;37(6):647–52.
47. Guiltinan AM, Kaidarova Z, Custer B, et al. Increased all-cause, liver, and cardiac mortality among hepatitis C virus-seropositive blood donors. Am J Epidemiol 2008;167(6):743–50.
48. Targher G, Bertolini L, Padovani R, et al. Differences and similarities in early atherosclerosis between patients with non-alcoholic steatohepatitis and chronic hepatitis B and C. J Hepatol 2007;46(6):1126–32.
49. Volzke H, Schwahn C, Wolff B, et al. Hepatitis B and C virus infection and the risk of atherosclerosis in a general population. Atherosclerosis 2004;174(1):99–103.
50. Mostafa A, Mohamed MK, Saeed M, et al. Hepatitis C infection and clearance: impact on atherosclerosis and cardiometabolic risk factors. Gut 2010;59(28):1135–40.
51. Vigneri P, Frasca F, Sciacca L, et al. Diabetes and cancer. Endocr Relat Cancer 2009;16(4):1103–23.
52. Lai SW, Chen PC, Liao KF, et al. Risk of hepatocellular carcinoma in diabetic patients and risk reduction associated with anti-diabetic therapy: a population-based cohort study. Am J Gastroenterol 2012;107(1):46–52.

53. El-Serag HB, Hampel H, Javadi F. The association between diabetes and hepatocellular carcinoma: a systematic review of epidemiologic evidence. Clin Gastroenterol Hepatol 2006;4(3):369–80.

54. Arase Y, Kobayashi M, Suzuki F, et al. Effect of type 2 diabetes on risk for malignancies includes hepatocellular carcinoma in chronic hepatitis C. Hepatology 2013;57(3):964–73.

55. Ohata K, Hamasaki K, Toriyama K, et al. Hepatic steatosis is a risk factor for hepatocellular carcinoma in patients with chronic hepatitis C virus infection. Cancer 2003;97(12):3036–43.

56. Pekow JR, Bhan AK, Zheng H, et al. Hepatic steatosis is associated with increased frequency of hepatocellular carcinoma in patients with hepatitis C-related cirrhosis. Cancer 2007;109(12):2490–6.

57. Bugianesi E, Marchesini G, Gentilcore E, et al. Fibrosis in genotype 3 chronic hepatitis C and nonalcoholic fatty liver disease: role of insulin resistance and hepatic steatosis. Hepatology 2006;44(6):1648–55.

58. Deltenre P, Louvet A, Lemoine M, et al. Impact of insulin resistance on sustained response in HCV patients treated with pegylated interferon and ribavirin: a meta-analysis. J Hepatol 2011;55(6):1187–94.

59. Fattovich G, Covolo L, Pasino M, et al. The homeostasis model assessment of the insulin resistance score is not predictive of a sustained virological response in chronic hepatitis C patients. Liver Int 2011;31(1):66–74.

60. Negro F. Steatosis and insulin resistance in response to treatment of chronic hepatitis C. J Viral Hepat 2012;19(Suppl 1):42–7.

61. Serfaty L, Forns X, Goeser T, et al. Insulin resistance and response to telaprevir plus peginterferon alpha and ribavirin in treatment-naive patients infected with HCV genotype 1. Gut 2012;61(10):1473–80.

62. Younossi Z, Negro F, Serfaty L, et al. The homeostasis model assessment of insulin resistance does not seem to predict response to telaprevir in chronic hepatitis C in the REALIZE trial. Hepatology 2013, in press.

63. Overbeck K, Genne D, Golay A, et al. Pioglitazone in chronic hepatitis C not responding to pegylated interferon-alpha and ribavirin. J Hepatol 2008;49(2):295–8.

64. Harrison SA, Hamzeh FM, Han J, et al. Chronic hepatitis C genotype 1 patients with insulin resistance treated with pioglitazone. Hepatology 2012;56:464–73.

65. Romero-Gomez M, Diago M, Andrade RJ, et al. Treatment of insulin resistance with metformin in naive genotype 1 chronic hepatitis C patients receiving peginterferon alfa-2a plus ribavirin. Hepatology 2009;50(6):1702–8.

The Impact of Obesity and Metabolic Syndrome on Alcoholic Liver Disease

Dian J. Chiang, MD, MPH[a], Arthur J. McCullough, MD[b],*

KEYWORDS

- Obesity • Diabetes • Insulin resistance • Metabolic syndrome
- Alcoholic liver disease

KEY POINTS

- Obesity and metabolic syndrome are common in alcoholic liver disease (ALD) patients and increase the risk of liver-related mortality.
- Obesity is an independent risk factor for steatosis, acute alcoholic hepatitis, and cirrhosis in ALD.
- Obesity and alcohol synergistically enhance hepatic carcinogenesis.
- Diabetes is an independent risk factor for hepatic carcinogenesis in alcoholics and increases mortality in both cirrhosis and precirrhosis patients.

EPIDEMIOLOGY OF ALD

ALD is a major health burden in the United States. Approximately 18 million people abuse alcohol and 10 million people suffer from ALD.[1,2] ALD includes a spectrum of liver pathology from alcoholic fatty liver and alcoholic steatohepatitis (AH) to liver fibrosis and cirrhosis.[3] In the general population, the prevalence and mortality from ALD closely follows per capita ethanol consumption and increases as the per capita alcohol consumption increases.[4] ALD remains a major cause of liver failure and contributes to more than 20,000 deaths annually in the United States.[2]

This work was supported in part by grant from ABMRF/The Foundation for Alcohol Research to D.J. Chiang and AA021893 grant from the National Institute of Alcohol Abuse and Alcoholism to A.J. McCullough.
The authors have nothing to disclose.
[a] Department of Gastroenterology and Hepatology, Digestive Disease Institute, Cleveland Clinic, A51, 9500 Euclid Avenue, Cleveland, OH 44195, USA; [b] Department of Gastroenterology and Hepatology, Digestive Disease Institute, Cleveland Clinic, A31, 9500 Euclid Avenue, Cleveland, OH 44195, USA
* Corresponding author.
E-mail address: mcculla@ccf.org

SPECTRUM OF ALD

Studies of the incidence and prevalence of different stages of ALD prior to the development of cirrhosis in the general population are difficult to conduct because patients with compensated liver disease usually do not seek medical attention.[5] Up to 90% of alcoholics have fatty liver, which usually resolves within 2 weeks if alcohol consumption is discontinued.[6] Although patients with pure alcoholic fatty liver are mostly asymptomatic, they have a 10% risk of progressing to cirrhosis and an 18% risk of cirrhosis or fibrosis over a median time period of 10.5 years. In those who drink more than 40 units of alcohol per week, the risk dramatically increases, with a 30% risk of cirrhosis and a 37% risk of cirrhosis or fibrosis[7,8]; 10% to 35% of all alcoholics have changes on liver biopsy consistent with alcoholic hepatitis.[8] The amount of alcohol intake that puts an individual at risk for alcoholic hepatitis is unknown, but a majority of patients have a history of heavy alcohol use (more than 100 g/d) for 2 or more decades.[9] Once alcoholic hepatitis has developed, the risk of cirrhosis is increased compared with simple steatosis. In one study, over a 5-year period, cirrhosis developed in 16% of patients with steatohepatitis and in 7% of patients with simple steatosis.[10] A subset of patients with ALD develops severe AH, which often presents acutely against a background of chronic liver disease and has a substantially worse short-term prognosis.[11] The progression to cirrhosis is a leading cause of morbidity and mortality in ALD.[2] Hepatic decompensation is common among patients with alcoholic cirrhosis. The risk of complications, including the development of ascites, variceal bleeding, or hepatic encephalopathy, is approximately 25% after 1 year and 50% after 5 years.[12] Once hepatic decompensation develops, the expected 5-year transplant-free survival rate is 60% for those who stop drinking alcohol and 30% for those who continue to drink alcohol.[13] Only 10% to 15% of alcoholics, however, develop cirrhosis. Although the amount and patterns of alcohol consumption are important, they do not fully account for the differences in cirrhosis incidence rates.[3] Several studies have been performed to investigate risk factors (gender, genetics, diet, type of alcohol, pattern of drinking, and hepatitis C virus infection) in the progression of ALD.[14] Given the rising prevalence of obesity and metabolic syndrome, this review focuses on current understanding of the potential impact of obesity and metabolic syndrome in the progression of ALD.

OBESITY ON THE PROGRESSION OF ALD

The World Health Organization and the National Center for Health Statistics define overweight as a body mass index (BMI) greater than 25 kg/m^2 and less than or equal to 29.9 kg/m^2 and obesity as a BMI greater than 30 kg/m^2.[15] Alcohol and obesity synergistically increase the risk of liver injury as measured by elevated serum alanine aminotransferase and aspartate aminotransferase levels.[16] A study of 1604 alcoholic patients revealed that overweight (as determined by BMI$\geq$25 kg/m^2 in women and $\geq$27 kg/m^2 in men) is a risk factor for the progression of alcoholic liver disease.[9] Being overweight for at least 10 years is independently correlated with the presence of steatosis, acute alcoholic hepatitis, and cirrhosis. These results show that the presence of excess weight for at least 10 years is a risk factor for progression of ALD.[9] Another study of asymptomatic alcoholic patients revealed that higher body weight is a risk factor for more severe histologic liver damage.[17]

Whether the exacerbation of ALD in overweight patients is a result of additive injury from nonalcoholic steatohepatitis (NASH), which is a hepatic manifestation of metabolic syndrome, or the metabolic derangement in obesity that exacerbates ethanol-induced liver injury remains a subject of further investigation. Ethanol feeding results in more pronounced hepatic steatosis and liver injury in genetically obese mice (ob/ob) compared with control lean wild-type mice.[18] Furthermore, ethanol feeding augments the impairment of hepatic sirtuin 1–AMP-activated protein kinase signaling in the ob/ob mice, which is associated with altered hepatic lipid metabolism pathways.[18] Emerging evidence also suggests that adipose tissue has a critical regulatory function in metabolism and immunity through adipose tissue–derived bioactive substances, including tumor necrosis factor α, interleukin 6, monocyte/macrophage chemoattractant protein 1, and adipokines, which may regulate insulin resistance and tissue inflammation.[19] Also, chronic ethanol exposure results in inflammation in adipose tissue in mice[20] and alcohol intake can alter adipokine expression in adipose tissue and adipokine plasma levels.[21] The direct effects of alcohol on the metabolic and innate immune activity of adipose tissue likely contribute to ethanol-induced liver injury.

OBESITY AND METABOLIC SYNDROME ON THE MORTALITY OF ALD

Obesity, in particular abdominal obesity, is associated with insulin resistance on peripheral glucose and fatty acid utilization, which leads to type 2 diabetes mellitus.[22] Insulin resistance, the associated hyperinsulinemia and hyperglycemia, and adipokines may lead to increased risk for cardiovascular disease (CVD) due to vascular endothelial dysfunction, abnormal lipid profile, hypertension, and vascular inflammation.[22] The co-occurrence of metabolic risk factors for type 2 diabetes mellitus and CVD (abdominal obesity, hyperglycemia, dyslipidemia, and hypertension) suggests the existence of metabolic syndrome.[23] Obesity and metabolic syndrome are among the most important public health problems in the United States given the rising prevalence and comorbidities.[24] The prevalence of the metabolic syndrome, as defined by the 2001 Adult Treatment Panel III criteria, was evaluated in the third National Health and Nutrition Examination Survey (NHANES III, 1988–1994).[25] The overall prevalence of metabolic syndrome is 22% in this population.[25] The prevalence rates of obesity and metabolic syndrome in ALD patients in the NHANES III cohort are 44.5% and 32.4%, respectively (**Table 1**).[26] Furthermore, obesity and metabolic syndrome are associated with increased liver-related mortality in ALD patients (see **Table 1**).[26] There is no increased overall mortality risk with either obesity or metabolic syndrome in this cohort. Type 2 diabetes mellitus and insulin resistance, however, are both associated with increased overall mortality in ALD patients (see **Table 1**).[26] The findings from this

Table 1
Prevalence and adjusted hazard ratio for overall and liver-related mortality of obesity and metabolic syndrome in ALD patients in NHANES III

	Prevalence (%)	Overall Mortality (aHRs and 95% CIs)	Liver-related Mortality (aHRs and 95% CIs)
Obesity	44.56 ± 5.9	1.58 (0.57–4.40)	16.22[a] (1.91–137.68)
Metabolic syndrome	32.46 ± 5.2	2.37 (0.50–11.18)	2.06[a] (1.21–3.31)
Type 2 diabetes mellitus	7.46 ± 2.4	3.00[a] (1.06–8.54)	3.60 (0.96–13.52)
Insulin resistance	33.76 ± 5.1	3.21[a] (1.56–6.58)	2.43 (0.28–21.38)
Hypercholesterolemia	64.56 ± 6.0	0.79 (0.25–2.53)	0.04 (0.01–0.24)
Hypertension	36.56 ± 5.7	1.76 (0.46–6.70)	1.77 (0.40–7.72)

[a] P value for the adjusted hazard ratio (aHR) is ≤.05.
Data from Stepanova M, Rafiq N, Younossi ZM. Components of metabolic syndrome are independent predictors of mortality in patients with chronic liver disease: a population-based study. Gut 2010;59(10):1410–5.

large population-based study suggest a detrimental effect of concomitant obesity and components of metabolic syndrome in patients with ALD.

Data from two Scottish prospective cohorts also reveal that obesity and alcohol consumption are strongly associated with liver disease mortality in analyses adjusted for other confounders (P = .001 and P<.0001, respectively).[27] Drinkers of 15 or more units per week have adjusted relative rates for liver disease mortality of 3.16 (95% CI, 1.28–7.8) for underweight/normal weight men, 7.01 (95% CI, 3.02–16.3) for overweight men, and 18.9 (95% CI, 6.84–52.4) for obese men. The relative excess risk due to interaction between BMI and alcohol consumption is 5.58 (95% CI, 1.09–10.1) with a synergy index of 2.89 (95% CI, 1.29–6.47), suggesting obesity and alcohol consumption synergistically increase mortality in this population.[27]

OBESITY AND ALCOHOL ON HEPATIC CARCINOGENESIS

Hepatocellular carcinoma (HCC) is one of the complications of ALD and cirrhosis. Several epidemiologic studies have suggested that both alcoholic and nonalcoholic fatty liver disease are associated with increased risk of HCC.[28–30] Given the enhanced liver injury and fibrosis from concomitant alcohol consumption and obesity,[16] it is plausible that alcohol and obesity may enhance hepatic carcinogenesis. In a population-based study of 23,712 Taiwanese residents from January 1, 1991, to December 31, 2004, there was an association between alcohol use (defined as those who consume alcohol at least 4 days per week for at least a year) and obesity (BMI$\geq$30 kg/m^2) with the risk of HCC incidence in an unadjusted analysis (hazard ratio 7.19; 95% CI, 3.69–14.00; P<.01) and a multivariable-adjusted analyses (hazard ratio 3.82; 95% CI, 1.94–7.52; P<.01).[31] The data suggest a multiplicative interaction between alcohol use and obesity and that obesity and alcohol synergistically increase the risk of HCC incidence.[31] In addition, alcohol consumption is associated with increased risk of HCC in a cohort of patients with NASH cirrhosis from a tertiary referral center in the United States.[32]

DIABETES ON THE PROGRESSION OF ALD

Concomitant diabetes mellitus in alcoholics includes a wide spectrum of causes, including insulin insufficiency due to alcoholic pancreatitis,[33] hyperinsulinemia and insulin resistance associated with liver cirrhosis,[34] and type 2 diabetes mellitus associated with the metabolic syndrome. The presence of diabetes is a significant risk factor for mortality in a Japanese cohort of alcoholic patients, in both cirrhosis and noncirrhosis groups.[35] Furthermore, diabetes is an independent risk factor for hepatic carcinogenesis in patients with alcoholic cirrhosis.[36] Autonomic nerve dysfunction occurs in both alcoholics and diabetics. It is generally reversible in alcoholics if they abstain[37] but is irreversible in diabetics.[38]

CLINICAL MANAGEMENT AND FUTURE DIRECTION

The cornerstone of clinical management of ALD is alcohol cessation.[14] Because obesity and metabolic syndrome may exacerbate progression of ALD, it is critical for physicians to counsel patients with concomitant metabolic syndrome on their increased risk of ALD progression. Treatment options for patients with concomitant obesity, metabolic syndrome, and advanced ALD remain limited. Therefore, detection of early-stage disease and prevention of progression are critical in addressing this issue. Both obesity and alcohol use are modifiable risk factors; lifestyle interventions should be undertaken to reduce the risks of disease progression. Early referral to alcohol rehabilitation program should be considered in these patients prior to the development of cirrhosis or severe AH to avoid disease progression. Treatment of components of metabolic syndrome also may improve the outcomes in these patients. Prospective studies are instrumental to demonstrate the clinical efficacy of such intervention. Further understanding of the mechanistic link of synergism among alcohol, obesity, and metabolic syndrome in the progression of ALD may provide novel targets of intervention in this high-risk population.

SUMMARY

The intersection of the obesity epidemic and ALD poses a challenging health care issue with significant morbidity and mortality. Obesity and metabolic syndrome exacerbate progression of ALD and increase mortality and HCC incidence. Furthermore, alcohol may modulate the metabolic and innate immune activity of adipose tissue and thus contribute to ethanol-induced liver injury. Recognition of these increased risks is crucial in patient counseling and disease management. Detection of early stage of liver injury in asymptomatic patients may offer the opportunity to prevent disease progression. Lifestyle modifications, including alcohol cessation and weight loss, should be pursued along with the management of components of metabolic syndrome.

REFERENCES

1. Mandayam S, Jamal MM, Morgan TR. Epidemiology of alcoholic liver disease. Semin Liver Dis 2004;24(3):217–32.
2. Peery AF, Dellon ES, Lund J, et al. Burden of gastrointestinal disease in the United States: 2012 update. Gastroenterology 2012;143(5):1179–87.e1–3.
3. Mann RE, Smart RG, Govoni R. The epidemiology of alcoholic liver disease. Alcohol Res Health 2003;27(3):209–19.
4. Corrao G, Ferrari P, Zambon A, et al. Are the recent trends in liver cirrhosis mortality affected by the changes in alcohol consumption? Analysis of latency period in European countries. J Stud Alcohol 1997;58(5):486–94.
5. Kim WR, Brown RS Jr, Terrault NA, et al. Burden of liver disease in the United States: summary of a workshop. Hepatology 2002;36(1):227–42.
6. Diehl AM. Alcoholic liver disease: natural history. Liver Transpl Surg 1997;3(3): 206–11.
7. Sorensen TI, Orholm M, Bentsen KD, et al. Prospective evaluation of alcohol abuse and alcoholic liver injury in men as predictors of development of cirrhosis. Lancet 1984;2(8397):241–4.
8. Teli MR, Day CP, Burt AD, et al. Determinants of progression to cirrhosis or fibrosis in pure alcoholic fatty liver. Lancet 1995;346(8981):987–90.
9. Naveau S, Giraud V, Borotto E, et al. Excess weight risk factor for alcoholic liver disease. Hepatology 1997;25(1):108–11.
10. Deleuran T, Gronbaek H, Vilstrup H, et al. Cirrhosis and mortality risks of biopsy-verified alcoholic pure steatosis and steatohepatitis: a nationwide registry-based study. Aliment Pharmacol Ther 2012;35(11):1336–42.
11. Orrego H, Blake JE, Blendis LM, et al. Prognosis of alcoholic cirrhosis in the presence and absence of alcoholic hepatitis. Gastroenterology 1987;92(1):208–14.
12. Jepsen P, Ott P, Andersen PK, et al. Clinical course of alcoholic liver cirrhosis: a Danish population-based cohort study. Hepatology 2010;51(5):1675–82.

13. Morgan MY. The prognosis and outcome of alcoholic liver disease. Alcohol Alcohol Suppl 1994;2:335–43.
14. O'Shea RS, Dasarathy S, McCullough AJ, Practice Guideline Committee of the American Association for the Study of Liver Diseases, Practice Parameters Committee of the American College of Gastroenterology. Alcoholic liver disease. Hepatology 2010;51(1):307–28.
15. Clinical guidelines on the identification, evaluation, and treatment of overweight and obesity in adults–the evidence report. National Institutes of Health. Obes Res 1998;6(Suppl 2):51S–209S.
16. Loomba R, Bettencourt R, Barrett-Connor E. Synergistic association between alcohol intake and body mass index with serum alanine and aspartate aminotransferase levels in older adults: the Rancho Bernardo Study. Aliment Pharmacol Ther 2009;30(11–12):1137–49.
17. Iturriaga H, Bunout D, Hirsch S, et al. Overweight as a risk factor or a predictive sign of histological liver damage in alcoholics. Am J Clin Nutr 1988;47(2): 235–8.
18. Everitt H, Hu M, Ajmo JM, et al. Ethanol administration exacerbates the abnormalities in hepatic lipid oxidation in genetically obese mice. Am J Physiol Gastrointest Liver Physiol 2013;304(1):G38–47.
19. Tilg H, Moschen AR. Adipocytokines: mediators linking adipose tissue, inflammation and immunity. Nature reviews. Immunology 2006;6(10):772–83.
20. Sebastian BM, Roychowdhury S, Tang H, et al. Identification of a cytochrome P4502E1/Bid/C1q-dependent axis mediating inflammation in adipose tissue after chronic ethanol feeding to mice. J Biol Chem 2011;286(41):35989–97.
21. Pravdova E, Fickova M. Alcohol intake modulates hormonal activity of adipose tissue. Endocr Regul 2006;40(3):91–104.
22. Reaven GM. Banting lecture 1988. Role of insulin resistance in human disease. Diabetes 1988;37(12):1595–607.
23. Eckel RH, Grundy SM, Zimmet PZ. The metabolic syndrome. Lancet 2005; 365(9468):1415–28.
24. Ogden CL, Flegal KM, Carroll MD, et al. Prevalence and trends in overweight among US children and adolescents, 1999–2000. JAMA 2002;288(14): 1728–32.
25. Ford ES, Giles WH, Dietz WH. Prevalence of the metabolic syndrome among US adults: findings from the third National Health and Nutrition Examination Survey. JAMA 2002;287(3):356–9.
26. Stepanova M, Rafiq N, Younossi ZM. Components of metabolic syndrome are independent predictors of mortality in patients with chronic liver disease: a population-based study. Gut 2010;59(10):1410–5.
27. Hart CL, Morrison DS, Batty GD, et al. Effect of body mass index and alcohol consumption on liver disease: analysis of data from two prospective cohort studies. BMJ 2010;340:c1240.
28. Franceschi S, Montella M, Polesel J, et al. Hepatitis viruses, alcohol, and tobacco in the etiology of hepatocellular carcinoma in Italy. Cancer Epidemiol Biomarkers Prev 2006;15(4):683–9.
29. Hassan MM, Hwang LY, Hatten CJ, et al. Risk factors for hepatocellular carcinoma: synergism of alcohol with viral hepatitis and diabetes mellitus. Hepatology 2002;36(5):1206–13.
30. Marrero JA, Fontana RJ, Su GL, et al. NAFLD may be a common underlying liver disease in patients with hepatocellular carcinoma in the United States. Hepatology 2002;36(6):1349–54.

31. Loomba R, Yang HI, Su J, et al. Synergism between obesity and alcohol in increasing the risk of hepatocellular carcinoma: a prospective cohort study. Am J Epidemiol 2013;177(4):333–42.
32. Ascha MS, Hanouneh IA, Lopez R, et al. The incidence and risk factors of hepatocellular carcinoma in patients with nonalcoholic steatohepatitis. Hepatology 2010;51(6):1972–8.
33. Bank S. Chronic pancreatitis: clinical features and medical management. Am J Gastroenterol 1986;81(3):153–67.
34. Iversen J, Vilstrup H, Tygstrup N. Kinetics of glucose metabolism in relation to insulin concentrations in patients with alcoholic cirrhosis and in healthy persons. Gastroenterology 1984;87(5):1138–43.
35. Yokoyama A, Matsushita S, Ishii H, et al. The impact of diabetes mellitus on the prognosis of alcoholics. Alcohol Alcohol 1994;29(2):181–6.
36. Torisu Y, Ikeda K, Kobayashi M, et al. Diabetes mellitus increases the risk of hepatocarcinogenesis in patients with alcoholic cirrhosis: a preliminary report. Hepatol Res 2007;37(7):517–23.
37. Yokoyama A, Takagi T, Ishii H, et al. Impaired autonomic nervous system in alcoholics assessed by heart rate variation. Alcohol Clin Exp Res 1991;15(5):761–5.
38. Ewing DJ, Campbell IW, Clarke BF. The natural history of diabetic autonomic neuropathy. Q J Med 1980;49(193):95–108.

The Impact of Obesity and Metabolic Syndrome on Chronic Hepatitis B and Drug-Induced Liver Disease

Raluca Pais, MD, PhD[a], Elena Rusu, MD, PhD[b], Vlad Ratziu, MD, PhD[a,*]

KEYWORDS

- Fatty liver • Steatosis • Metabolic syndrome • Chronic hepatitis B
- Drug-induced liver injury • Fibrosis • Cirrhosis • Hepatocellular carcinoma

KEY POINTS

- In chronic hepatitis B, steatosis is not more frequent than in the general population, a notable difference with the high prevalence seen in chronic hepatitis C.
- Both steatosis and insulin resistance (IR) are related to host metabolic risk factors and therefore occur mainly through epidemiologic association; viral factors (viral genotype, viral load, and hepatitis B e antigen status) do affect liver fat content or IR levels.
- Experimental data suggest that at the molecular level, the HBx protein might induce liver fat accumulation, but human studies do not show evidence for a viral-induced mechanism.
- A wealth of experimental data suggest that the steatotic liver is more susceptible to liver injury and that intrinsic abnormalities associated with excessive hepatic fat deposition in animal models should promote hepatotoxicity in patients with nonalcoholic or metabolic fatty liver disease.
- Diabetes and possibly obesity could favor methotrexate-induced liver fibrosis in patients treated for psoriasis.

CHRONIC HEPATITIS B

Because overweight and diabetes, the 2 main predisposing conditions for nonalcoholic or metabolic fatty liver disease (NAFLD), are increasingly prevalent worldwide,

The study was partially supported by grant PN-II-ID-PCE-2011-3-0917, no. 297/2011 of the Romanian Ministry of Education represented by UEFISDCI.

Financial Disclosures: V. Ratziu declares associations with the following companies: Astellas, Abbott, Axcan, Enterome, Galmed, Genfit, Gilead, Intercept, Phenex, Roche-Genentech.

[a] Department of Hepatogastroenterology, Université Pierre et Marie Curie, Assistance Publique Hôpitaux de Paris, Hôpital Pitié-Salpêtrière, Inserm UMR_S 938, Paris 75013, France; [b] Institutul Clinic Fundeni, Bucharest, Romania
* Corresponding author.
E-mail address: vlad.ratziu@upmc.fr

chronic hepatitis B (CHB) can frequently coexist with NAFLD. Type 2 diabetes and obesity are risk factors for fibrosis progression, cirrhosis, and related complications in the general population,[1,2] in patients with chronic hepatitis C,[3] and in patients with alcoholic liver disease.[4,5] In the following sections, the evidence linking these conditions to the severity of liver disease in patients with CHB is reviewed.

PREVALENCE AND DETERMINANTS OF STEATOSIS IN PATIENTS WITH CHB

The prevalence of steatosis in CHB ranges widely from 14% to 71%, with a median of 31% (**Fig. 1, Table 1**). This prevalence is close to that in the general population, as assessed by ultrasonography in Asian and Western surveys (20%–30%).[6,7] The prevalence is higher in European series[8–14] (46%) than in those from the Asia-Pacific region[15–24] (24%), which might be explained by differences in alcohol consumption (higher in some European studies) or in body mass index (BMI, calculated as weight in kilograms divided by the square of height in meters). When only studies including patients without alcohol consumption are considered, the prevalence decreases to 26%.[25] Although most patients have mild steatosis, only a few (22%), have marked steatosis (ie, >30% of hepatocytes showing fat droplets). In chronic hepatitis C, the prevalence of steatosis (any degree of fat infiltration) was 69%, ranging from 62% to 76%.[25] Thus, the prevalence of steatosis in CHB (1) seems to be similar to that in the general population and (2) is most probably around 2-fold lower than in chronic hepatitis C virus (HCV) infection.

Steatosis in patients with CHB virus (HBV) infection is correlated exclusively with metabolic risk factors (BMI, diabetes, triglyceride levels) and no direct association has been identified with viral factors.[25] The same holds true for steatohepatitis when strictly defined, histologically.[26] This finding suggests that steatosis is caused by chance association with metabolic abnormalities predisposing to NAFLD rather than a direct role of the virus, as is the case with genotype 3 HCV. Data from the National Health and Nutrition Examination Survey III[27] have confirmed that HBV carriers do not have a higher level of insulin resistance (IR) (measured by Homeostatic Model Assessment levels), or higher prevalence of diabetes or obesity than the general population, and therefore steatosis is probably not specifically related to the presence of HBV. This finding was supported by Chinese magnetic resonance spectroscopy studies showing that HBV carriers younger than 60 years had a lower content of liver fat compared with non-HBV carriers, even after adjustment for alcohol consumption, demographic and metabolic factors, or dietary intake.[28] Further reinforcing the lack of an association between HBV and steatosis is the evidence that viral genotype, viral load or hepatitis B e antigen (HBeAg) status do not affect hepatic fat in the same Chinese series.[5,28]

Concerning the precise subtype of NAFLD, only 1 study with detailed histology is available. Of 163 US-based patients with HBV, half of whom were overweight or obese, the proportion of NAFLD was 19%.[26] On rigorous histologic criteria, two-thirds of these patients had steatohepatitis (13% of the total cohort).[26] This is a lower prevalence than would be expected from a non–HBV-infected population with the same level of increased body weight. Why HBV carriers would have a lower than expected prevalence of metabolic syndrome is unclear. It has been hypothesized that HBV might interfere with lipid metabolism and result in lower triglyceride and cholesterol levels.[28] It is also unknown whether the current, lower levels of metabolic syndrome, overweight, and IR in HBV carriers, especially in Asia, will still hold true with the future expansion of the prevalence of obesity and diabetes worldwide. Data from Wong and colleagues[20] show that the prevalence of metabolic syndrome clearly increases with age: patients with HBV older than 60 years have a 3-fold higher

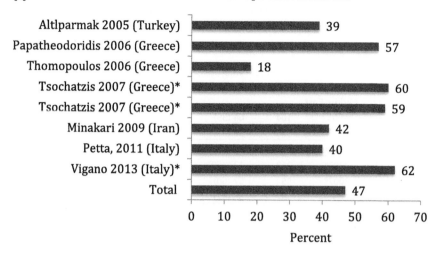

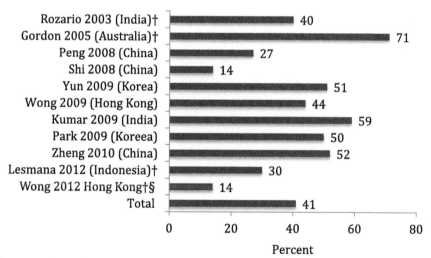

Fig. 1. Studies evaluating the prevalence of steatosis in patients with CHB in Europe and the Middle East (*A*) and Asia-Pacific region (*B*). *Patients consuming alcohol not excluded; †patients drinking alcohol not excluded; §general population. (*Data from* Refs.[8–19,21–24,28,33,35])

prevalence of metabolic syndrome than those aged 21 to 40 years. It is therefore highly probable that in both the West and the East, the trends of obesity epidemics will considerably affect the association between steatosis and HBV infection.

MOLECULAR MECHANISMS AND FACTORS ASSOCIATED WITH STEATOSIS IN PATIENTS WITH CHB

In stark contrast with clinical data, there is some experimental evidence that HBV can induce hepatic steatosis, mainly through the HBV *X* (HBx) protein. Both the livers of

Table 1
Prevalence and distribution of hepatic steatosis in patients with CHB and chronic hepatitis C (CHC)

	Patients with CHB			Patients with CHC	
Reference	Patients (N)	Steatosis >5% (n, %)	Marked Steatosis >30% (n, %)	Patients (N)	Steatosis (n, %)
Europe and the Middle East					
Altlparmak et al,[9] 2005	164	64 (39)	19 (12)	—	—
Papatheodoridis et al,[8] 2006	174	99 (57)	38 (22)	260	180 (69)
Thomopoulos et al,[10] 2006	233	42 (18)	11 (5)	—	—
Tsochatzis et al,[11] 2007[a]	213	127 (59)	46 (22)	163	117 (72)
Tsochatzis et al,[12] 2007[a]	95	57 (60)	13 (14)	176	117 (66)
Minakari et al,[13] 2009	132	56 (42)	20 (15)	—	—
Petta et al,[14] 2011	170	68 (40)	NR	170	80 (47)
Vigano et al,[35] 2013[a]	235	146 (62)	24 (10)	—	—
Total	1416	659 (46)	171 (12)	769	494 (64)
Asia-Pacific Region					
Rozario & Ramakrishna,[15] 2003[a]	82	33 (40)	NR	45	28 (62)
Gordon et al,[16] 2005[a]	17	12 (71)	3 (18)	74	53 (72)
Peng et al,[17] 2008	153	41 (27)	10 (6)	—	—
Shi et al,[18] 2008	1915	260 (14)	25 (1)	—	—
Yun et al,[19] 2009	86	44 (51)	2 (2)	—	—
Wong et al,[33] 2009	266	116 (44)	21 (8)	—	—
Kumar et al,[21] 2009	69	41 (59)	7 (10)	—	—
Park et al,[22] 2009	80	40 (50)	NR	—	—
Zheng et al,[23] 2010	204	106 (52)	83 (40)	—	—
Lesmana et al,[24] 2012[a]	174	52 (30)	14 (8)	—	—
Wong et al,[28] 2012[a,b]	91	13 (14)	NR	—	—
Total	3137	758 (24)	165 (5)	119	81 (68)
Overall total	4553	1417 (31)	336 (7)	888	575 (65)

Abbreviation: NR, not reported.
[a] Patients drinking alcohol not excluded.
[b] General population.
Data from Refs.[8–19,21–24,28,33,35]

transgenic mice expressing the HBx protein and hepatoma cell lines transfected with the HBx protein accumulate excessive amounts of cellular fat.[29] In these experimental models, the HBx protein induces expression of SREBP1c and of PPAR-γ, an action involving activation of the PI3K/AKT pathway and downregulation of PTEN expression.[29] HBx might also interact with the liver X receptor to induce SREBP1c activation.[30] This interaction results in increased expression of downstream genes involved in lipogenesis and accounting for fat accumulation.[29,31] The relevance of these findings to hepatitis B infection in humans is questionable, because no data point toward a virus-induced steatosis in HBV carriers.

IMPACT OF STEATOSIS AND METABOLIC COFACTORS ON THE SEVERITY OF LIVER INJURY AND DISEASE OUTCOMES

Diabetes and obesity are recognized risk factors for fibrosis progression and development of cirrhosis in the general population[1,2] and in patients with chronic liver diseases, such as chronic hepatitis C (CHC), NAFLD, and excessive alcohol consumption.[4,5,32] In the following sections, available data on the respective impact of steatosis, clinical metabolic risk factors, and IR on liver-related outcomes in HBV-infected patients are reviewed.

Role of Steatosis

In chronic HBV infection, steatosis is not correlated with either necroinflammatory activity or fibrosis stage.[9,10,13,17,18,23,33] Thus, metabolic steatosis by itself is not a predictor of histologic severity; whether the same holds true for steatohepatitis is unknown. The only study that specifically looked at superimposed nonalcoholic steatohepatitis in patients with HBV did not investigate associations with histologic severity.[26] However, there are some data suggesting that steatosis might be associated with reduced HBV viral load.[9,17,18,23] This theory is difficult to reconcile with experimental studies (see later discussion) showing that HBV might promote lipogenesis. Nonetheless, 1 study in HBV transgenic mice fed either a high-fat diet or a control diet has shown that animals fed the high-fat diet developed full-blown histologic lesions of steatohepatitis, despite a reduction in HBV DNA and hepatitis B surface antigen (HBsAg) levels.[34] Other clinical studies did not confirm this reduction of viral replication in patients with HBV with liver steatosis.[28]

Role of IR and Metabolic Factors

Large studies in Asian patients with HBV have confirmed that the metabolic syndrome is associated with higher fibrosis stages and a higher prevalence of cirrhosis.[20] This association is independent of other known fibrosis cofactors and has been confirmed when cirrhosis was diagnosed both by histology and by elastometry. The probability of cirrhosis increased with increasing number of components of the metabolic syndrome, with diabetes mellitus and hypertension showing a strong association.[20] BMI was an independent predictor of advanced fibrosis in European-based patients with HBV.[35] Other studies confirmed that overweight[36] or diabetes[27] are associated with an increased risk of cirrhosis and liver-related death in male HBsAg carriers.[36] Neither of these studies had data on insulin, and therefore IR, as a confounder, could not be assessed. A Taiwanese longitudinal study (a substudy of the REVEAL cohort) of 1142 patients with HBV with a median of 7.8 years of follow-up has shown that a high serum insulin at baseline is a strong and independent predictor of cirrhosis occurrence (detected by ultrasonography) at follow-up.[37] The risk for cirrhosis related to a BMI greater than 25 kg/m^2 or to diabetes mellitus was greatly attenuated and became statistically nonsignificant after adjustment for insulin.[37] Studies evaluating the factors associated with fibrosis severity are summarized in **Table 2**.

Obesity and diabetes are independent risk factors for hepatocellular carcinoma (HCC) in the general population.[38–40] There are numerous studies showing that overweight/obesity or diabetes significantly increase the risk of HCC in HBV carriers. In a Taiwanese community cohort of 23,567 patients followed prospectively for 14 years,[41] the association of obesity and diabetes increased at least 10-fold the risk of HCC in HBV carriers (relative risk of 21 in nonobese, nondiabetic HBV carriers vs 265 in obese, diabetic HBV carriers, after adjustment for common carcinogenic confounders). Diabetes alone significantly increased the risk of HCC in HBV carriers (2.4-fold).[41] A

Table 2
Factors associated with fibrosis severity

Reference	Patients (N)	Prevalence of Steatosis (N, %)	Prevalence of Advanced Fibrosis (N, %)	Factors Associated With Advanced Fibrosis in Multivariate Analysis
Papatheodoridis et al,[8] 2006	174	99 (57)	46 (26)[c]	Diabetes[a]
Thomopoulos et al,[10] 2006	233	42 (18)	37 (16)[c]	Necroinflammation
Peng et al,[17] 2008	153	41 (27)	30 (20)	Necroinflammation
Shi et al,[18] 2008	1915	260 (14)	NR	Age, necroinflammation
Yun et al,[19] 2009	86	44 (51)	16 (19)	Necroinflammation
Persico,[83] 2009	126	14 (13)	NR	Age
Wong et al,[33] 2009	266	116 (44)	68 (26)[c]	Male sex, BMI, metabolic syndrome
Park et al,[22] 2009	80	40 (50)	45 (56)	HBeAg[b], portal/periportal inflammation
Zheng et al,[23] 2010	204	106 (52)	70 (34)	BMI, cholesterol
Petta et al,[14] 2011	170	68 (40)	44 (26)	Age, steatosis, necroinflammation
Vigano et al,[35] 2013	235	146 (62)	94 (40)	Age, HBeAg status, BMI, alcohol

[a] If patients with cirrhosis were excluded, no associations were found between type 2 diabetes and fibrosis stages.
[b] Negative association between HBeAg status and fibrosis severity.
[c] Cirrhosis.
Data from Refs.[8,10,14,17–19,22,23,33,35,83]

smaller but prospective Taiwanese study with long follow-up[37] reported that type 2 diabetes is a determinant of HCC independent of hepatitis viral infection thus confirming the universal carcinogenic potential of diabetes on the liver (ie, irrespective of the level of endemicity for viral hepatitis). Again, as is the case for fibrosis, IR seems to hold the key to the deleterious effect of diabetes or obesity. These investigators[37] showed that a high fasting insulin level on admission is an independent predictor of incident HCC in male HBV carriers. The association between overweight and HCC disappeared after adjustment for insulin, thus suggesting a more direct role for hyperinsulinemia than for obesity or diabetes. Also, this association between insulin and incident HCC increased in strength with longer exposure (>8 years of follow-up),[37] which strengthens the biological plausibility of this statistical association. There are intrinsic methodological limits to the possibility of detecting an association between diabetes and HCC in HBV carriers: at least in Far-East Asia, HBV-related HCC has an earlier onset than type 2 diabetes (55 years old vs 57 years old) and HCV-related HCC (65 years old).[42]

IMPACT ON THERAPEUTIC OUTCOMES

The impact of steatosis, IR, or clinical metabolic risk factors on the response to antiviral therapy in patients with HBV was insufficiently studied. Given the potency of current analogue therapies for HBV, this impact is probably marginal. Two studies[43,44] failed to show any deleterious impact of steatosis on the response to pegylated interferon. Pivotal studies of pegylated interferon α-2a, entecavir, or tenofovir did not report reduced antiviral efficacy in patients with steatosis, overweight, or diabetes. A Chinese study claimed that the rates of HBV DNA clearance at 6, 12, and 24 months of treatment with entecavir were lower in patients with steatosis, high BMI, or high waist circumference.[45] In the absence of confirmation and of a strong pharmacologic rationale, the relevance of these findings is unclear. However, type 2 diabetes and obesity were significant negative predictors for the regression of cirrhosis in tenofovir-treated patients, despite similar HBV DNA control or HBsAg loss.[46]

SUMMARY

Despite some experimental data that show that the HBx protein can induce hepatic lipogenesis, clinical studies do not support the concept of viral-induced steatosis in CHB. Instead, HbsAg carriers diagnosed with steatosis usually have coexisting exposure to metabolic risk factors or alcohol consumption, as a result of the high prevalence of these conditions in the general population. Steatosis by itself is not associated with fibrosis or deleterious outcomes in CHB. In contrast, obesity, diabetes, and IR significantly increase the risk of advanced fibrosis, cirrhosis occurrence, and hepatocellular carcinoma in HBsAg carriers. These associations are often strongest for IR, suggesting that the latter is a major confounder for obesity and diabetes. In CHB, careful diagnosis of concurrent NAFLD and metabolic risk factors is therefore important for prognostic purposes. Future studies will need to address whether their correction benefits the long-term prognosis of HbsAg carriers.

DRUG-INDUCED LIVER DISEASE

Patients with NAFLD have numerous concurrent comorbidities (eg, diabetes, hypertension, dyslipidemia, hyperuricemia), which entail a large consumption of drugs, some of which have well-described liver toxicity. Overweight and obesity are the main risk factors of NAFLD, and it has been shown that obese individuals consume more drugs than those who are not obese.[47] The overall aging of the population and the relentless increase in the prevalence of obesity (and therefore NAFLD) are additional reasons why drug consumption in patients with NAFLD is increasing. Because of this high level of exposure of a sizable fraction of the general population, the question whether patients with NAFLD are at higher risk of drug-induced liver injury (DILI) than patients without NAFLD becomes highly relevant.

Over the past decade, it has become increasingly evident that an acute challenge in a steatotic liver results in extensive injury, more than results from the same challenge in a normal liver. In a landmark experiment, Diehl and colleagues[48] have shown that physiologic doses of lipopolysaccharide induce a higher increase in aminotransferase levels and higher levels of mortality in rodents with fatty liver than in those with normal liver. This vulnerability to necrosis was the result of the induction of proinflammatory cytokines and an increased susceptibility toward their actions but also a failure of compensatory regenerative mechanisms.[49] In a series of experiments, Feldstein and colleagues[50,51] have also shown that the steatotic liver is sensitized to apoptotic liver injury, a phenomenon that might be mediated by key regulators of lipid biosynthesis.[52] Others have shown that the steatotic liver is also more susceptible to bile acid–induced hepatotoxicity.[53] This higher susceptibility of the fatty liver to injury seems to occur irrespective of the experimental model of steatosis (genetic or dietary)[48,50,54] and irrespective of the noxious agent.[49,52,54] Preliminary human studies in patients with NAFLD have reported a dysfunctional replenishment of hepatic adenosine triphosphate stores after acute fructose challenge, which, arguably, could play a role in propagating liver injury.[55] Several studies have documented enhanced hepatic expression and activity of cytochrome P450 subtype 2E1 in the liver of obese patients or patients with NAFLD[56–58] (reviewed in Ref.[59]), which, given the central role of this cytochrome in drug biotransformation, suggests a higher risk of drug-induced liver disease in patients with steatosis (reviewed in Ref.[60]).

However exciting these experimental data, available data in humans do not offer much credence to an overall increased risk of DILI in obese, diabetic, or NAFLD populations. Traditionally, DILI is classified into 2 broad categories: idiosyncratic DILI, the most common form of DILI (acute liver failure excepted) and intrinsic DILI.[61,62] Idiosyncratic DILI is unpredictable and does not depend directly on the dose (although some dose dependency exists); intrinsic DILI is dose dependent, therefore predictable.

Idiosyncratic DILI

There is little clinical evidence that NAFLD increases the risk of idiosyncratic DILI. The 2 prospective, population-based studies of the incidence of DILI[63,64] do not mention BMI, diabetes, any concurrent metabolic comorbidity, or NAFLD as a predisposing factor of DILI. Although in the French study, this particular association might not have been studied or available for study, in the Icelandic DILI population the prevalence of obesity and diabetes was low (10% and 5%, respectively).[64] Large prospective registries of reported DILI do not mention either increased odds of hepatotoxicity in people with NAFLD or in those sharing metabolic risk factors of NAFLD.[65] Tarantino and colleagues[66] suggested that patients with NAFLD are at higher risk of DILI than patients with HCV. However, their study is based on few events (6 cases of DILI among 74 patients with NAFLD and 1 case among 174 patients with HCV) and questionable methodology.

Although NAFLD or components of the metabolic syndrome do not seem to increase the incidence of idiosyncratic DILI, a distinct question is whether they are associated with a more severe course of DILI. There is some evidence suggesting that this might be the case for diabetes mellitus. In a large series prospectively collected by the US DILI Network, Chalasani and colleagues[67] reported that among the first 300 collected cases, the proportion of diabetes was higher in the severe DILI cases (37% vs 25% in mild to moderate DILI), whereas there were no differences in BMI. Diabetes increased the risk of severe DILI by an odds ratio of 2.7, independent of age, alcohol, and the pattern of liver injury (cytolytic or cholestatic). This observation could not be confirmed by a Scandinavian series of severe DILI, because data on metabolic risk factors were not reported.[68] El Serag and Everson[69] noted that veterans with type 2 diabetes had a 40% higher risk of developing acute liver failure, even after excluding patients with chronic liver disease, viral hepatitis, or congestive heart failure. It is not clear how much of this excess risk of acute liver failure could be related to DILI. However, this observation suggests that diabetes, either directly or not, might increase the risk of severe liver injury in cases of acute liver injury, possibly iatrogenic in nature. This hypothesis still awaits confirmation. The Acute Liver Failure Study group investigated a series of 308 consecutive cases of acute liver failure admitted in referral centers, but no information on metabolic risk factors versus clinical outcome is available.[70]

Intrinsic DILI

Acetaminophen

NAFLD might increase the risk of acetaminophen hepatotoxicity. Nguyen and colleagues[71] studied 42,781 admissions for acetaminophen overdose reported over 8 years in the Nationwide Inpatient Sample, covering 20% of US hospitals. Only 7% of patients developed acute liver injury. Patients diagnosed with NAFLD had 7.5 higher odds of progressing to acute liver injury, independent of age, sex, or comorbidities.[71] This association was not driven by patients with cirrhosis. Although NAFLD increased the risk of acetaminophen-induced hepatitis, it did not increase the risk of severe liver failure (ie, acute liver injury with encephalopathy). However, the diagnosis of NAFLD was most certainly considerably underestimated in this series (as the 1.1% prevalence of HCV among patients with acetaminophen overdose vs only 0.1% prevalence of NAFLD suggests), because liver biopsy is usually not performed in patients with acetaminophen overdose. Nonetheless, this work based on hospitalization diagnosis codes is one of the few solid reports suggesting that NAFLD might increase the occurrence of acetaminophen-induced DILI. Experimental data have shown that obesity is associated with reduced glutathione levels,[72] a critical defense mechanism against hepatotoxic acetaminophen metabolites such as N-acetyl-P-benzoquinone imine (NAPQI). Also, CYP2E1 is responsible for NAPQI formation, and there are some data that hepatic CYP2E1 activity is enhanced in overweight individuals with NAFLD.[56,59] These experimental data might explain the clinical findings mentioned earlier.

Methotrexate
Methotrexate-induced hepatotoxicity consists of a chronic fibrogenic injury rather than an acute liver injury, typical of classic DILI. The potential for long-term liver fibrosis has been best described in patients receiving methotrexate for psoriasis, but in these patients the impact of NAFLD per se has not been studied. Because methotrexate can induce steatosis, the distinction between drug-induced and underlying, IR-induced steatosis is not a simple one. However, several studies have examined whether risk factors for NAFLD increase the risk of fibrosis in methotrexate-treated patients. Two studies clearly show that diabetes is associated with higher chances of developing liver fibrosis as well as advanced fibrosis.[73,74] One study[73] but not the other[74] found that overweight also contributes to fibrosis. Patients with both risk factors might develop advanced fibrosis at a higher rate and for a lower cumulative dose of methotrexate; fibrosis monitoring should be particularly stressed in these patients, preferably through noninvasive methods.[75,76]

Anesthetic drugs
It has been long recognized that halogenated anesthetic drugs such as halothane can induce acute hepatitis. The most severe form associates fever, rash, arthralgia, and eosinophilia and is believed to be caused by an immunoallergic mechanism, usually after repeated exposure. This particular form occurs frequently in obese individuals, although it is not well understood whether obesity specifically favors the hypersensitive reaction, because this has not been tested or reproduced in animal models.[77] In humans, the predominant mechanism of halothane biotransformation is oxidative, through cytochrome P4502E1. This situation results in a highly reactive intermediate metabolite, trifluoroacetyl chloride, which binds covalently to hepatocyte proteins and lipids and triggers an adaptive immune response. Obesity increases the activity of several P450 cytochromes, including CYP4502E1,[59] and this might account for a higher level of hepatotoxicity for halothane (and also for acetaminophen). Despite a lower rate of oxidative metabolism with isoflurane (0.2% compared with 30% with halothane), hepatotoxicity with isoflurane has still been described, including in an obese patient.[78] These events are too rare to infer any specific contribution of NAFLD, obesity, or diabetes in increasing the risk of isoflurane hepatitis. There is clearly cross-reactivity between halothane, isoflurane, and enflurane, to the extent that previous exposure to one of these drugs may increase the risk of hepatotoxicity for another compound.[79–82]

SUMMARY

Unsurprisingly for a disease process that is unpredictable, rare, and not dose related, intrinsic DILI does not seem to increase with NAFLD or associated metabolic risk factors. There is some clinical evidence that obese or diabetic patients with NAFLD might be at higher risk of hepatotoxicity from acetaminophen and at higher fibrotic risk from methotrexate. Because most registries of DILI did not specifically consider NAFLD or the metabolic syndrome as risk factors for hepatotoxicity, future studies will be critical for testing this association. Nonetheless, the contrast between the abundance of experimental data in favor of a heightened risk of hepatotoxicity in the fatty liver and the scarcity of human observations of DILI in patients with NAFLD point to a complex interplay between deleterious and protective mechanisms of cytotoxicity in human hepatic steatosis.

REFERENCES

1. Hart CL, Morrison DS, Batty GD, et al. Effect of body mass index and alcohol consumption on liver disease: analysis of data from two prospective cohort studies. BMJ 2010;340:c1240.
2. Liu B, Balkwill A, Reeves G, et al. Body mass index and risk of liver cirrhosis in middle aged UK women: prospective study. BMJ 2010;340:c912.
3. Younossi ZM, McCullough AJ. Metabolic syndrome, non-alcoholic fatty liver disease and hepatitis C virus: impact on disease progression and treatment response. Liver Int 2009;29(Suppl 2):3–12.
4. Naveau S, Giraud V, Borotto E, et al. Excess weight is a risk factor for alcoholic liver disease. Hepatology 1997;25:108–11.
5. Raynard B, Balian A, Fallik D, et al. Risk factors of fibrosis in alcohol-induced liver disease. Hepatology 2002;35:635–8.
6. Bellentani S, Saccoccio G, Masutti F, et al. Prevalence of and risk factors for hepatic steatosis in Northern Italy. Ann Intern Med 2000;132:112–7.
7. Fan JG, Farrell GC. Epidemiology of non-alcoholic fatty liver disease in China. J Hepatol 2009;50:204–10.
8. Papatheodoridis GV, Chrysanthos N, Savvas S, et al. Diabetes mellitus in chronic hepatitis B and C: prevalence and potential association with the extent of liver fibrosis. J Viral Hepat 2006;13:303–10.
9. Altlparmak E, Koklu S, Yalinkilic M, et al. Viral and host causes of fatty liver in chronic hepatitis B. World J Gastroenterol 2005;11:3056–9.
10. Thomopoulos KC, Arvaniti V, Tsamantas AC, et al. Prevalence of liver steatosis in patients with chronic hepatitis B: a study of associated factors and of relationship with fibrosis. Eur J Gastroenterol Hepatol 2006;18:233–7.
11. Tsochatzis E, Papatheodoridis GV, Manesis EK, et al. Hepatic steatosis in chronic hepatitis B develops due to host metabolic factors: a comparative approach with genotype 1 chronic hepatitis C. Dig Liver Dis 2007;39:936–42.
12. Tsochatzis E, Papatheodoridis GV, Manesis EK, et al. Metabolic syndrome is associated with severe fibrosis in chronic viral hepatitis and non-alcoholic steatohepatitis. Aliment Pharmacol Ther 2007;27:80–9.
13. Minakari M, Molaei M, Shalmani HM, et al. Liver steatosis in patients with chronic hepatitis B infection: host and viral risk factors. Eur J Gastroenterol Hepatol 2009;21:512–6.
14. Petta S, Cammà C, Marco VD, et al. Hepatic steatosis and insulin resistance are associated with severe fibrosis in patients with chronic hepatitis caused by HBV or HCV infection. Liver Int 2011;31:507–15.

15. Rozario R, Ramakrishna B. Histopathological study of chronic hepatitis B and C: a comparison of two scoring systems. J Hepatol 2003;38:223–9.
16. Gordon A, McLean CA, Pedersen JS, et al. Hepatic steatosis in chronic hepatitis B and C: predictors, distribution and effect on fibrosis. J Hepatol 2005;43: 38–44.
17. Peng D, Han Y, Ding H, et al. Hepatic steatosis in chronic hepatitis B patients is associated with metabolic factors more than viral factors. J Gastroenterol Hepatol 2008;23:1082–8.
18. Shi JP, Fan JG, Wu R, et al. Prevalence and risk factors of hepatic steatosis and its impact on liver injury in Chinese patients with chronic hepatitis B infection. J Gastroenterol Hepatol 2008;23:1419–25.
19. Yun JW, Cho YK, Park JH, et al. Hepatic steatosis and fibrosis in young men with treatment-naïve chronic hepatitis B. Liver Int 2009;29:878–83.
20. Wong GL, Wong VW, Choi PC, et al. Metabolic syndrome increases the risk of liver cirrhosis in chronic hepatitis B. Gut 2009;58:111–7.
21. Kumar M, Choudhury A, Manglik N, et al. Insulin resistance in chronic hepatitis B virus infection. Am J Gastroenterol 2009;104:76–82.
22. Park SH, Kim DJ, Lee HY. Insulin resistance is not associated with histologic severity in nondiabetic, noncirrhotic patients with chronic hepatitis B virus infection. Am J Gastroenterol 2009;104:1135–9.
23. Zheng RD, Xu CR, Jiang L, et al. Predictors of hepatic steatosis in HBeAg-negative chronic hepatitis B patients and their diagnostic values in hepatic fibrosis. Int J Med Sci 2010;7:272–7.
24. Lesmana LA, Lesmana CR, Pakasi LS, et al. Prevalence of hepatic steatosis in chronic hepatitis B patients and its association with disease severity. Acta Med Indones 2012;44:35–9.
25. Machado MV, Oliveira AG, Cortez-Pinto H. Hepatic steatosis in hepatitis B virus infected patients– meta-analysis of risk factors and comparison with hepatitis C infected patients. J Gastroenterol Hepatol 2011;26:1361–7.
26. Bondini S, Kallman J, Wheeler A, et al. Impact of non-alcoholic fatty liver disease on chronic hepatitis B. Liver Int 2007;27:607–11.
27. Stepanova M, Rafiq N, Younossi ZM. Components of metabolic syndrome are independent predictors of mortality in patients with chronic liver disease: a population-based study. Gut 2010;59:1410–5.
28. Wong VW, Wong GL, Chu WC, et al. Hepatitis B virus infection and fatty liver in the general population. J Hepatol 2012;56:533–40.
29. Kim KH, Shin HJ, Kim K, et al. Hepatitis B virus X protein induces hepatic steatosis via transcriptional activation of SREBP1 and PPARγ. Gastroenterology 2007;132:1955–67.
30. Na TY, Shin YK, Roh KJ, et al. Liver X receptor mediates hepatitis B virus X protein-induced lipogenesis in hepatitis B virus-associated hepatocellular carcinoma. Hepatology 2009;49:1122–31.
31. Kim K, Kim Kook H, Kim Hyeong H, et al. Hepatitis B virus X protein induces lipogenic transcription factor SREBP1 and fatty acid synthase through the activation of nuclear receptor LXRα. Biochem J 2008;416:219.
32. Bedossa P, Moucari R, Chelbi E, et al. Evidence for a role of nonalcoholic steatohepatitis in hepatitis C: a prospective study. Hepatology 2007;46: 380–7.
33. Wong VW, Wong GL, Yu J, et al. Interaction of adipokines and hepatitis B virus on histological liver injury in the Chinese. Am J Gastroenterol 2009; 105:132–8.

34. Zhang Z, Pan Q, Duan XY, et al. Fatty liver reduces hepatitis B virus replication in a genotype B hepatitis B virus transgenic mice model. J Gastroenterol Hepatol 2012;27:1858–64.
35. Vigano M, Valenti L, Lampertico P, et al. Patatin-like phospholipase domain-containing 3 I148M affects liver steatosis in patients with chronic hepatitis B. Hepatology 2013;58(4):1245–52.
36. Yu MW, Shih WL, Lin CL, et al. Body-mass index and progression of hepatitis B: a population-based cohort study in men. J Clin Oncol 2008;26:5576–82.
37. Chao LT, Wu CF, Sung FY, et al. Insulin, glucose and hepatocellular carcinoma risk in male hepatitis B carriers: results from 17-year follow-up of a population-based cohort. Carcinogenesis 2011;32:876–81.
38. Chen Y, Wang X, Wang J, et al. Excess body weight and the risk of primary liver cancer: an updated meta-analysis of prospective studies. Eur J Cancer 2012; 48:2137–45.
39. Welzel TM, Graubard BI, Zeuzem S, et al. Metabolic syndrome increases the risk of primary liver cancer in the United States: a study in the SEER-Medicare database. Hepatology 2011;54:463–71.
40. El-Serag HB, Hampel H, Javadi F. The association between diabetes and hepatocellular carcinoma: a systematic review of epidemiologic evidence. Clin Gastroenterol Hepatol 2006;4:369–80.
41. Chen CL, Yang HI, Yang WS, et al. Metabolic factors and risk of hepatocellular carcinoma by chronic hepatitis B/C infection: a follow-up study in Taiwan. Gastroenterology 2008;135:111–21.
42. Wang CS, Yao WJ, Chang TT, et al. The impact of type 2 diabetes on the development of hepatocellular carcinoma in different viral hepatitis statuses. Cancer Epidemiol Biomarkers Prev 2009;18:2054–60.
43. Ateş F. Impact of liver steatosis on response to pegylated interferon therapy in patients with chronic hepatitis B. World J Gastroenterol 2011;17:4517.
44. Cindoruk M, Karakan T, Unal S. Hepatic steatosis has no impact on the outcome of treatment in patients with chronic hepatitis B infection. J Clin Gastroenterol 2007;41:513–7.
45. Jin X, Chen YP, Yang YD, et al. Association between hepatic steatosis and entecavir treatment failure in Chinese patients with chronic hepatitis B. PLoS One 2012;7:e34198.
46. Marcellin P, Gane E, Buti M, et al. Regression of cirrhosis during treatment with tenofovir disoproxil fumarate for chronic hepatitis B: a 5-year open-label follow-up study. Lancet 2013;381:468–75.
47. Stuart B, Lloyd J, Zhao L, et al. Obesity, disease burden, and prescription spending by community-dwelling Medicare beneficiaries. Curr Med Res Opin 2008;24:2377–87.
48. Yang SQ, Lin HZ, Lane MD, et al. Obesity increases sensitivity to endotoxin liver injury: implications for the pathogenesis of steatohepatitis. Proc Natl Acad Sci U S A 1997;94:2557–62.
49. Yang S, Lin H, Diehl AM. Fatty liver vulnerability to endotoxin-induced damage despite NF-kappaB induction and inhibited caspase 3 activation. Am J Physiol Gastrointest Liver Physiol 2001;281:G382–92.
50. Feldstein AE, Canbay A, Guicciardi ME, et al. Diet associated hepatic steatosis sensitizes to Fas mediated liver injury in mice. J Hepatol 2003;39:978–83.
51. Feldstein AE, Werneburg NW, Canbay A, et al. Free fatty acids promote hepatic lipotoxicity by stimulating TNF-alpha expression via a lysosomal pathway. Hepatology 2004;40:185–94.

52. Reinartz A, Ehling J, Leue A, et al. Lipid-induced up-regulation of human acyl-CoA synthetase 5 promotes hepatocellular apoptosis. Biochim Biophys Acta 2010;1801:1025–35.
53. Soden JS, Devereaux MW, Haas JE, et al. Subcutaneous vitamin E ameliorates liver injury in an in vivo model of steatocholestasis. Hepatology 2007;46:485–95.
54. Bjorkegren J, Beigneux A, Bergo MO, et al. Blocking the secretion of hepatic very low density lipoproteins renders the liver more susceptible to toxin-induced injury. J Biol Chem 2002;277:5476–83.
55. Cortez-Pinto H, Chatham J, Chacko VP, et al. Alterations in liver ATP homeostasis in human nonalcoholic steatohepatitis: a pilot study. JAMA 1999;282: 1659–64.
56. Chalasani N, Gorski JC, Asghar MS, et al. Hepatic cytochrome P450 2E1 activity in nondiabetic patients with nonalcoholic steatohepatitis. Hepatology 2003;37: 544–50.
57. Weltman MD, Farrell GC, Hall P, et al. Hepatic cytochrome P450 2E1 is increased in patients with nonalcoholic steatohepatitis. Hepatology 1998;27:128–33.
58. Niemela O, Parkkila S, Juvonen RO, et al. Cytochromes P450 2A6, 2E1, and 3A and production of protein-aldehyde adducts in the liver of patients with alcoholic and non-alcoholic liver diseases. J Hepatol 2000;33:893–901.
59. Aubert J, Begriche K, Knockaert L, et al. Increased expression of cytochrome P450 2E1 in nonalcoholic fatty liver disease: mechanisms and pathophysiological role. Clin Res Hepatol Gastroenterol 2011;35:630–7.
60. Fromenty B. Drug-induced liver injury in obesity. J Hepatol 2013;58:824–6.
61. Chalasani N, Björnsson E. Risk factors for idiosyncratic drug-induced liver injury. Gastroenterology 2010;138:2246–59.
62. Navarro VJ, Senior JR. Drug-related hepatotoxicity. N Engl J Med 2006;354: 731–9.
63. Sgro C. Incidence of drug-induced hepatic injuries: a French population-based study. Hepatology 2002;36:451–5.
64. Björnsson ES, Bergmann OM, Björnsson HK, et al. Incidence, presentation, and outcomes in patients with drug-induced liver injury in the general population of Iceland. Gastroenterology 2013;144:1419–25.e1–3.
65. Andrade RJ, Lucena MI, Fernandez MC, et al. Drug-induced liver injury: an analysis of 461 incidences submitted to the Spanish registry over a 10-year period. Gastroenterology 2005;129:512–21.
66. Tarantino G, Conca P, Basile V, et al. A prospective study of acute drug-induced liver injury in patients suffering from non-alcoholic fatty liver disease. Hepatol Res 2007;37:410–5.
67. Chalasani N, Fontana RJ, Bonkovsky HL, et al. Causes, clinical features, and outcomes from a prospective study of drug-induced liver injury in the United States. Gastroenterology 2008;135:1924–34, 1934.e1–4.
68. Bjornsson E, Olsson R. Outcome and prognostic markers in severe drug-induced liver disease. Hepatology 2005;42:481–9.
69. El-Serag HB, Everhart JE. Diabetes increases the risk of acute hepatic failure. Gastroenterology 2002;122:1822–8.
70. Ostapowicz G, Fontana RJ, Schiodt FV, et al. Results of a prospective study of acute liver failure at 17 tertiary care centers in the United States. Ann Intern Med 2002;137:947–54.
71. Nguyen GC, Sam J, Thuluvath PJ. Hepatitis C is a predictor of acute liver injury among hospitalizations for acetaminophen overdose in the United States: a nationwide analysis. Hepatology 2008;48:1336–41.

72. Begriche K, Massart J, Robin MA, et al. Mitochondrial adaptations and dysfunctions in nonalcoholic fatty liver disease. Hepatology 2013;58(4):1497–507.
73. Rosenberg P, Urwitz H, Johannesson A, et al. Psoriasis patients with diabetes type 2 are at high risk of developing liver fibrosis during methotrexate treatment. J Hepatol 2007;46:1111–8.
74. Malatjalian DA, Ross JB, Williams CN, et al. Methotrexate hepatotoxicity in psoriatics: report of 104 patients from Nova Scotia, with analysis of risks from obesity, diabetes and alcohol consumption during long term follow-up. Can J Gastroenterol 1996;10:369–75.
75. Laharie D, Seneschal J, Schaeverbeke T, et al. Assessment of liver fibrosis with transient elastography and FibroTest in patients treated with methotrexate for chronic inflammatory diseases: a case-control study. J Hepatol 2010;53: 1035–40.
76. Laharie D, Zerbib F, Adhoute X, et al. Diagnosis of liver fibrosis by transient elastography (FibroScan) and non-invasive methods in Crohn's disease patients treated with methotrexate. Aliment Pharmacol Ther 2006;23:1621–8.
77. Dugan CM, MacDonald AE, Roth RA, et al. A mouse model of severe halothane hepatitis based on human risk factors. J Pharmacol Exp Ther 2010;333:364–72.
78. Gunaratnam NT, Benson J, Gandolfi AJ, et al. Suspected isoflurane hepatitis in an obese patient with a history of halothane hepatitis. Anesthesiology 1995;83: 1361–4.
79. Christ DD, Satoh H, Kenna JG, et al. Potential metabolic basis for enflurane hepatitis and the apparent cross-sensitization between enflurane and halothane. Drug Metab Dispos 1988;16:135–40.
80. Hasan F. Isoflurane hepatotoxicity in a patient with a previous history of halothane-induced hepatitis. Hepatogastroenterology 1998;45:518–22.
81. Kusuma HR, Venkataramana NK, Rao SA, et al. Fulminant hepatic failure after repeated exposure to isoflurane. Indian J Anaesth 2011;55:290–2.
82. Turner GB, O'Rourke D, Scott GO, et al. Fatal hepatotoxicity after re-exposure to isoflurane: a case report and review of the literature. Eur J Gastroenterol Hepatol 2000;12:955–9.
83. Persico M. Clinical expression of insulin resistance in hepatitis C and B virus-related chronic hepatitis: differences and similarities. World J Gastroenterol 2009;15:462.

Nutrition in Cirrhosis and Chronic Liver Disease

Wassem Juakiem, MD[a], Dawn M. Torres, MD[b],
Stephen A. Harrison, MD[c],*

KEYWORDS

- Cirrhosis • Chronic liver disease • Nutrition • Assessment • Management

KEY POINTS

- Malnutrition is common in patients with cirrhosis and increases with disease severity.
- Deficiencies in vitamins and trace minerals such as vitamins A, D, B_{12}, folate, thiamine, and pyridoxine are common.
- Bacterial overgrowth is common in patients with cirrhosis and can result in increased bacterial translocation leading to infection and fat malabsorption.
- The European Society of Clinical Nutrition and Metabolism 2006 guidelines recommend the use of subjective global assessment, anthropometric parameters, or hand grip strength to evaluate nutritional status and detect the presence of malnutrition in patients with cirrhosis.

INTRODUCTION

Chronic liver disease was reported as the ninth leading cause of death in the United States between 1980 and 1989[1]; recent evidence indicates that liver-related mortality has been consistently underestimated in the last 2 decades.[2] This has traditionally been associated with viral and alcoholic liver diseases, but the obesity epidemic of the last 2 decades has led to an increase in the incidence of nonalcoholic fatty liver disease (NAFLD), and specifically its subtype nonalcoholic steatohepatitis (NASH), with its adherent risk for progression to cirrhosis. This creates an interesting dichotomy in the discussion of nutrition and chronic liver disease. NAFLD is associated

Disclaimer: The view(s) expressed herein are those of the author(s) and do not reflect the official policy or position of San Antonio Military Medical Center, the US Army Medical Department, the US Army Office of the Surgeon General, the Department of the Army, Department of Defense or the US Government.

[a] Department of Medicine, San Antonio Military Medical Center, 3851 Roger Brooke Dr, #3600 Fort Sam Houston, San Antonio, TX 78234, USA; [b] Division of Gastroenterology, Department of Medicine, Walter Reed National Military Medical Center, 8901 Wisconsin Avenue, Bethesda, MD 20889, USA; [c] Division of Gastroenterology and Hepatology, Department of Medicine, San Antonio Military Medical Center, 3851 Roger Brooke Dr, #3600 Fort Sam Houston, San Antonio, TX 78234, USA
* Corresponding author.
E-mail address: stephen.a.harrison.mil@mail.mil

with excessive caloric intake, metabolic syndrome, and insulin resistance. On the other hand, cirrhosis due to excessive alcohol consumption is typically a catabolic state, often with protein calorie and other nutrient malnutrition.[3]

The relationship between nutritional status and chronic liver disease is complicated; protein, carbohydrate and lipid metabolism are all affected by the liver. End-stage liver disease (ESLD) and its complications affect energy synthesis and metabolism, which in turn influence nutritional status. Poor nutritional status is linked to multiple medical and surgical complications and affects the outcome of chronic liver disease. Adequate and optimal nutrition regimens are now believed to be important, if not essential, to optimize outcomes including reductions in morbidity and mortality associated with ESLD. This review provides an overview of the common nutritional deficiencies associated with non-NAFLD cirrhosis as well as the nutrition supplementation and dietary strategies investigated to date to address this unmet need in cirrhosis management.

PREVALENCE

Malnutrition is common in patients with cirrhosis, particularly those with advanced disease; the malnutrition rate in patients with cirrhosis is 50% to 90%. In a study of 300 patients by Carvalho and Parise,[4] 75% of those with advanced liver disease displayed some degree of malnutrition. The same study also showed that malnutrition incidence increased with Child-Pugh class. Patients with Child-Pugh A had a 46% rate of malnutrition compared with 84% of patients with Child-Pugh B, and 95% with Child-Pugh C.

The prevalence of malnutrition among patients with cirrhosis is particularly concerning because of its association with mortality and inherent complications. In multiple studies, protein calorie malnutrition (PCM) has been described in 50% to 100% of patients with decompensated cirrhosis and at least 20% with compensated cirrhosis.[5–8] PCM is associated with an increased number of complications including ascites, variceal bleeding, increased surgical morbidity and mortality, reduced survival, and worsening hepatic function.[9] This was demonstrated in a large nationwide analysis of hospitalized patients with cirrhosis and portal hypertension; PCM was more frequently associated with ascites (65% vs 48%, $P<.0001$) and hepatorenal syndrome (5% vs 3%, $P<.0001$), longer hospitalization, and a 2-fold increase in in-hospital mortality compared with well-nourished patients.[10]

Another study focused on patients with Child-Pugh class A cirrhosis demonstrated that malnutrition, even in patients with well-compensated cirrhosis, affected prognosis. Among those that were malnourished, 20% had a 1-year mortality rate, whereas none of the patients who received proper nutrition died within a 1-year period.[11] Complications such as infections, hepatic encephalopathy (HE), ascites, and variceal bleeding were also significantly more common in malnourished patients compared with well-nourished patients (65% vs 11%; $P<.05$).

PATHOGENESIS

The pathogenesis of malnutrition in cirrhosis is multifactorial; protein, carbohydrate, and lipid metabolism are all affected by liver disease.[12] Contributing factors include inadequate dietary intake, impaired digestion and absorption, and altered metabolism.

POOR NUTRIENT INTAKE

Most patients with cirrhosis have low caloric intake, which contributes to the overall poor outcomes that are observed. Loss of appetite is a frequent complaint in these patients and is believed to be partially attributable to upregulation of multiple cytokines such as tumor necrosis factor α (TNF-α) and leptin.[13] TNF-α affects appetite and metabolism by acting on the central nervous system, altering the release and function of neurotransmitters.[14] Leptin, an appetite-regulating hormone that is secreted by adipose tissue, is increased 2-fold in patients with cirrhosis compared with healthy individuals and may contribute to anorexia.[15] Early satiety has been shown to occur with impaired gastric expansion capacity secondary to ascites and often results in inadequate nutrient intake.[16] Similarly, HE is often associated with poor oral intake as a result of altered consciousness. Irregular feeding was reported by 40% of patients with cirrhosis and 36% reported consuming only 1 meal per day.[12] Alcohol, independent of cirrhosis, can induce anorexia and the empty calories from alcohol often replace balanced nutrition.

IMPAIRED DIGESTION, ABSORPTION, AND METABOLISM

Portal hypertension likely contributes to impaired digestion and nutrient absorption in patients with cirrhosis. As cirrhosis progresses and portal hypertension worsens, nutrients bypass the liver without appropriate metabolic processing and the end result is impaired utilization of critical cellular constituents.[17] Cholestatic liver disease may also impair nutrient absorption, especially the fat-soluble vitamins such as A, D, E and K, because of reduced intraluminal bile salt concentration. Another issue commonly seen in patients with cirrhosis is bacterial overgrowth, which can result in mucosal and villous atrophy in the small intestine, further worsening absorption and utilization of nutrients.

There are multiple factors that lead to nutrient malabsorption, particularly of fat and protein, seen commonly in patients with cirrhosis. Bile acid is produced by the liver then stored in the gallbladder and is responsible for the formation of micelles and absorption of long chain fatty acids through the lymphatic system.[18] Intraluminal bile acid deficiency is common in patients with cirrhosis and leads to decreased capacity for bile production.[19]

Other factors that lead to reduced body protein are the inadequate synthesis of various proteins as well as the diminished storage capacity of the cirrhotic liver.[20] Furthermore, cirrhosis represents an accelerated state of starvation, and fuels other than glucose such as proteins and lipids are used.[21] It has been shown that, in patients with cirrhosis, an early switch to gluconeogenesis from amino acids originating from body proteins happens after an overnight fast. This process occurs via the mobilization of amino acids from the skeletal muscles so that the proper amount of glucose is provided due to the lack of sufficient amounts of hepatic glycogen reserves and impaired synthetic capacity of hepatic cells.[20] Comparatively, this condition is only observed in healthy individuals after a fasting period of approximately 3 days.

As previously mentioned, deficiencies in vitamins and trace minerals are often seen as a result of cholestasis as well as portal hypertensive enteropathy, which leads to impaired absorption of fat and fat-soluble vitamins. Deficiencies in vitamin A, vitamin D, vitamin B_{12}, folate, thiamine, and pyridoxine are common. Vitamin D malabsorption can lead to osteoporosis as the result of calcium loss.[20] In summary, a combination of poor oral intake and malabsorption as a result of an accelerated metabolic state all contribute to the malnutrition seen in cirrhosis (**Fig. 1**).

NUTRITIONAL ASSESSMENT

The goal of a nutritional assessment is to identify modifiable nutritional risk factors that influence morbidity and mortality. Nutritional assessment allows for a determination of the macronutrient (energy, protein, water) and micronutrient (electrolytes, minerals, vitamins, trace elements) state of a given individual. Although there is no gold standard

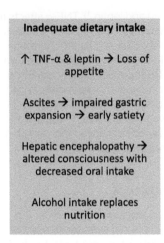 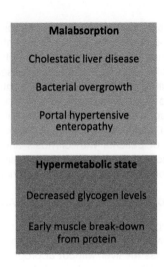

Fig. 1. Causes of malnutrition in cirrhosis.

for the assessment of nutritional status in patients with cirrhosis, and it is not practical to attempt detailed nutritional assessment in all patients, several approaches have been investigated with varying degrees of success. Most involve multiple stages, beginning with a complete history and physical examination and proceeding with more detailed testing if needed.

It is not unexpected that patients with compensated cirrhosis are more likely to be similar to a healthy population clinically and on laboratory investigations compared with those with decompensated cirrhosis. Thus, nutritional assessment is generally most warranted in patients with decompensated disease, although many of the standard nutritional assessment tools have limitations when applied to patients with decompensated cirrhosis because of the presence of salt and water retention and advanced hepatic synthetic dysfunction.

There are several key factors that should be evaluated in all patients with cirrhosis. Patients should be questioned about their usual weight and any recent weight loss. Severe weight loss is typically defined as unintentional weight loss of more than 10% over a 6-month period. Although these parameters are useful in patients with compensated cirrhosis, weight history is usually less accurate and can fluctuate as a result of salt and water retention and diuretic use in patients with more advanced cirrhosis.

Dietary intake can be assessed using 24-hour dietary recall whereby the patient recounts meals and snacks on a typical day. Although this process could be inaccurate, it does assist with overall appraisal of food intake. Alcohol intake should be quantified because it can account for a large proportion of caloric intake in some patients.

Gastrointestinal symptoms could also affect nutritional status. Duration and frequency of nausea, vomiting, diarrhea, anorexia, and steatorrhea should be assessed. Loose stool in a patient on lactulose may be difficult to distinguish from malabsorptive states. Symptoms that persist could pose a limitation in nutrient intake and thus outcomes in patients with cirrhosis.

The severity of the liver disease should be assessed and categorized using standard methods such as the Child-Pugh score or Model for End-Stage Liver Disease (MELD) score. The Child-Pugh classification includes factors predictive of disease severity including ascites and HE, as well as markers of liver function including bilirubin, albumin, and prothrombin time. Although the nutritional status has been well recognized as a factor affecting prognosis, it is not included in the Child-Pugh classification, which has also been criticized for its subjectivity in assessing HE and ascites leading to variable results among clinicians. The MELD score uses the less subjective laboratory parameters of internationalized normalized ratio, total bilirubin, and serum creatinine but it also omits nutritional status.

Although not included in the 2 most common methods of defining severity of cirrhosis, nutrition has been correlated with patient outcomes and thus it is important to accurately assess nutritional status using universal methods. The European Society of Clinical Nutrition and Metabolism (ESPEN) 2006 guidelines recommend the use of subjective global assessment (SGA), anthropometric parameters, or hand grip strength to evaluate nutritional status and detect the presence of malnutrition.[22]

The SGA is a questionnaire recommended by ESPEN as a bedside tool for assessing undernourished patients by collecting information on dietary intake, weight change, and gastrointestinal symptoms. The SGA also includes an evaluation of subcutaneous fat loss, muscle wasting, edema, and ascites.[23] A strength of the SGA is its reliability because it is not affected by fluid retention or ascites, and has been commonly used in patients with liver diseases because of its simplicity and cost-effectiveness.[24]

In addition to the SGA, the ESPEN guidelines also recommended the use of simple anthropometric parameters that are not affected by ascites and fluid retention when assessing malnutrition.[23] These parameters include midarm circumference, midarm muscle circumference, and triceps skin thickness. It is imperative that such measurements are performed by experienced clinicians to limit variability between observers. Malnutrition is diagnosed on values less than the fifth percentile in patients aged 18 to 74 years, or the 10th percentile in patients aged more than 74 years.[25]

Although these methods are accurate when performed correctly, a major limitation is the cumbersome and difficult nature of repeating these tests on a routine basis. Identifying a simpler method to evaluate for malnutrition has proved to be challenging and controversial. Albumin levels alone have been shown to be a poor nutritional marker due to the reduced levels in patients with advanced disease and albumin variability during periods of inflammation.[24] Similarly, multiple studies have reported that conventional methods such as determination of body mass by weight, or body composition with bioelectric impedance analysis, are not always accurate because of the prevalence of edema or ascites.[22] Campillo and colleagues[25] reported more encouraging results using body mass index (BMI); BMI was found to be a reliable parameter for the detection of malnutrition using BMI cutoff values depending on the severity of fluid retention. BMI values less than 22 kg/m^2 with no ascites versus 23 kg/m^2 with mild ascites and 25 kg/m^2 with tense ascites were considered to be malnourished with a positive predictive value of 92.7% and 93.6% in the study and validation populations, respectively.[26]

The handgrip strength test measures the strength of the hand and forearm muscles using a dynamometer and has been used as a simple method to detect malnutrition in patients with chronic liver disease. Alvares-da-Silva and Reverbal-da-Silveria[11] compared the handgrip test with the standard SGA and found handgrip to be a superior predictor of clinical complications such as uncontrolled ascites, HE, spontaneous bacterial peritonitis, and hepatorenal syndrome in a group of 50 patients with cirrhosis as well as 2 control groups with hypertension or general gastrointestinal disorders. At 1 year, 65% of those malnourished as defined by handgrip versus 37.5% who met the definition of malnourished by SGA experienced the clinical complications suggesting handgrip was a better prognostic indicator, although survival and rates of liver transplantation were not different between the 2 groups.

Other methods for analysis of body composition to measure nutritional status include bioelectrical impedance analysis, in vivo neutron activation analysis, isotope dilution, and dual-energy X-ray (DEXA) absorptometry. Although they provide relevant and accurate data, their widespread application has been limited to special centers because of the cost and technical complexity.[22,23]

In summary, the initial evaluation of a patient with cirrhosis should include a measure of their overall disease severity with either the Child-Pugh score or MELD (or both) as well as a clinical assessment of nutritional status. Although 1 approach has not proved to be universally efficacious, handgrip may be a reasonable option to consider. **Fig. 2** summarizes the commonly used nutritional assessment tools for all patients with cirrhosis as well as additional testing for those with more advanced stage disease.

NUTRITIONAL RECOMMENDATIONS

General guidelines have been developed for nutrition management in patients with chronic liver disease (**Table 1**). Current recommendations aim to provide sufficient energy intake for daily activities and account for the increased energy requirements associated with liver disease as well as to prevent further protein catabolism. Nutritional intervention is required in patients who are found to be malnourished. The ESPEN guidelines issued in 2006 provide recommendations that reflect the higher nutritional needs as well as the impaired absorption and altered metabolism seen in patients with cirrhosis or alcoholic hepatitis.[22]

Energy requirements are based on the severity of cirrhosis and their state of malnutrition. The energy intake recommendation in the ESPEN guidelines for patients with stable cirrhosis or alcoholic steatohepatitis is 35 to 40 kcal/kg/d (147–168 kJ/kg/d) versus the American Society of Parenteral and Enteral Nutrition (ASPEN) recommendations of 25 to 35 kcal/kg/d for patients without HE and 35 kcal/kg/d in patients with acute encephalopathy.[27] The ESPEN guidelines also recommend 1.2 to 1.5 g/kg/d protein intake and the use of supplementary enteral nutrition when patients cannot meet their caloric requirements. The use of nasogastric tube feeding has been recommended over percutaneous endoscopic gastrostomy tube placement, which has been associated with a higher risk of complications. A typical patient weighing 75 kg should intake 2625 to 3000 kcal/d with 90 to 120 g protein/d, which translates

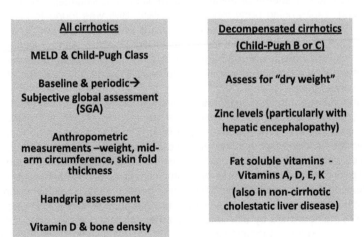

Fig. 2. Nutritional assessment in cirrhosis.

Table 1 Nutritional interventions in cirrhosis	
Overall Recommendations	**Specialized Recommendations**
25–35 kcal/kg/d, no HE 35 kcal/kg/d, HE 1.2–1.5 kcal/kg/d, protein	Ascites: low sodium (<2 g) daily
4–6 meals daily to prevent hypoglycemia	Hepatic encephalopathy: zinc replacement (if deficient); branched chain amino acid supplementation; avoid supplements with manganese; probiotics for minimal HE
Daily multivitamin	Alcoholic patients: thiamine and folate supplementation Vitamin D deficiency: 50,000 IU weekly for 12 wk, repeat level, and then daily 1000 IU replacement (with calcium) Vitamin A deficiency: 100,000–200,000 IU weekly for 12 wk

to approximately 360 to 480 kcal from protein. Whole protein formulas are generally recommended with more concentrated high-energy formulas in patients with ascites to reduce fluid overload. Total parenteral nutrition (TPN) should be limited to special situations where enteral nutrition is contraindicated. TPN has been associated with infectious complications and long-term use can actually worsen liver function.[28]

The prevalence of diabetes mellitus (DM) or some degree of insulin resistance (IR) is high in ESLD populations; approximately 40% to 50% of this population meet the criteria for DM.[29] Despite the high prevalence of DM, carbohydrate restriction has not been recommended for patients with cirrhosis because impaired glycogen synthesis and limited glycogen storage predisposes patients to episodes of hypoglycemia. When a reduction in liver function of ~80% is reached during cirrhosis progression, hypoglycemia may be seen with increasing frequency.[30] It is therefore recommended that patients consume multiple meals and snacks to reduce the risk of hypoglycemia with 4 to 6 meals containing food rich in carbohydrates accounting for 45% to 65% of caloric intake.[31]

Energy recommendations are based on the patient's dry weight, which is calculated based on ideal body weight in patients with ascites. Patients with edema and ascites are placed on sodium-restricted diets (<2 g/d) to combat the activation of the renin-angiotensin system that occurs with cirrhotic physiology and reduce fluid accumulation.[32,33] Sodium-restricted diets are difficult to sustain and diuretic therapy is often required.

Routine vitamin supplementation within recommended daily allowances has been considered to be a reasonable approach because vitamin deficiency is common in patients with cirrhosis with a particular emphasis on the fat-soluble vitamins (A, D, E, and K) as well as zinc and selenium. Vitamin levels may be checked if a deficiency is clinically suspected or routinely in all patients with cholestatic liver disease.[12] Vitamin A deficiency may be treated with 100,000 to 200,000 IU every 4 weeks as recommended to prevent night blindness and dry corneas.[29] Special attention should be paid to vitamin replacement, in particular parenteral thiamine administration, in alcoholic liver disease whenever Wernicke encephalopathy is suspected.

Zinc deficiency has been specifically associated with HE and low zinc levels are common in cirrhotic populations. Although zinc replacement is recommended when there is deficiency, many of the studies to date, including the largest randomized placebo controlled trial (RCT),[34] have failed to show improvements in cognitive function with zinc supplementation. On the other hand, total body manganese levels are often increased in patients with cirrhosis secondary to impaired biliary excretion as a result of portal-systemic shunting of blood leading to selective accumulation of manganese in specific areas of the brain.[35] The significance of this finding in relation to the development of HE is not clear, although it seems reasonable, and the recent recommendations from the International Society for Hepatic Encephalopathy and Nitrogen Metabolism Consensus statement recommended avoiding nutritional supplements with manganese.[36]

Osteoporosis has been commonly reported in cirrhosis; smoking, older age, heavy alcohol intake, or history of fractures increase the risk to the patient.[29] Vitamin D deficiency is common in cirrhosis from any cause and levels should be assessed as well as baseline bone density testing. Vitamin D deficiency is typically defined by a threshold of less than 20 ng/mL and insufficiency at a level of less than 30 ng/mL.[37] Supplementation with 1200 to 1500 mg of calcium and 400 to 800 IU of vitamin D daily is recommended in the presence of cirrhosis with additional interventions required for vitamin D deficiency or true osteoporosis. Typically, vitamin D levels may be repleted with 50,000 IU orally once weekly for 12 weeks in the setting of deficiency with repeat testing to confirm adequate replacement. Subsequent daily maintenance with 400 to 800 IU of vitamin D daily is typically adequate in the absence of a malabsorptive condition. In addition to its key role in bone homeostasis, vitamin D has essential immunomodulatory effects including steps essential in combating spontaneous bacterial peritonitis in cirrhosis where the active version of vitamin D is locally produced in response to infection.[38]

The use of branch-chain amino acids (BCAA) as directed therapy to improve outcomes in advanced cirrhosis warrants special discussion. Deficiency of the BCAAs (valine, leucine, isoleucine) relative to ammonia and aromatic amino acids (AAAs) has been well established in the setting of cirrhosis and there have been several studies suggesting positive effects on HE, protein levels, and overall liver function.[39–41] Theoretically this makes sense because BCAAs are essential for protein synthesis and turnover and may provide an alternate pathway of ammonia detoxification. AAAs are normally metabolized and detoxified by the liver; however, in chronic liver disease, AAAs accumulate as a result of dysfunctional hepatocytes with impaired capacity for deamination[42] as well as portal shunting and BCAA levels decrease because they are taken up by skeletal muscle cells as substrate for energy or ammonia degradation.[43] In theory, replacement of BCAAs stimulates the synthesis of glutamine from glutamate and ammonia in skeletal muscle.[44,45] A relative deficiency of BCAAs is also believed to lead to increased tryptophan uptake in the brain, which may also contribute to HE. BCAA supplementation would theoretically limit tryptophan uptake because the BCAAs compete for the same blood-brain barrier transporters.[46]

The ESPEN 2006 consensus guidelines support the use of BCAA supplements to improve clinical outcomes, largely based on the results of 3 studies investigating BCAAs in HE. Marchesini and colleagues[47] conducted a 1-year double-blinded RCT of 174 patients with advanced cirrhosis provided with BCAA (14 g/d) supplementation or 2 control groups with equicaloric amounts of lactoalbumin or maltodextrin. The primary end point was a combination of death and liver decompensation, defined by worsening HE, refractory ascites, or a Child-Pugh score of 12 or more. The BCAA arm had significantly lower rates of reaching this composite primary end point compared with the control group on lactoalbumin. Significant limitations of this study included a high dropout rate in the treatment arm because of inability to tolerate the taste of the BCAA formulation bringing into question whether or not this trial could truly be blinded. In terms of the overall conclusions from this study, it would suggest a modest albeit not striking benefit to BCAAs.

Subsequently, Muto and colleagues[48] performed a larger multicenter RCT of 646 patients who were given BCAAs (12 g/d) or a control group for 2 years. Although the study had a smaller number of dropouts because of better-tasting formulas, BCAAs did not improve important objective end points such as rates of variceal bleeding. There was an overall decreased rate of hepatic decompensation as defined by the development of refractory ascites or HE in the BCAA group and it was on this basis that these investigators recommended BCAA supplementation.

The most recent study conducted by Nakaya and colleagues[31] suggested that long-term use of BCAA mixtures was more beneficial than a late evening snack in improving serum albumin level, nitrogen balance, and respiratory quotient in 48 patients with cirrhosis. The study concluded that the catabolic state of the patients was improved and the prevalence of anorexia decreased although there was a high noncompliance rate secondary to poor taste of the BCAA and no change in overall quality of life based on a Short Form 36 questionnaire.

In summary, these studies generally support the use of BCAAs in advanced cirrhotic populations and are the basis for the ESPEN guidelines. However, the reality of poorly tolerated and expensive BCAA formulations has led to limited use of these agents in routine clinical practice.

Probiotics are live microorganisms believed to modulate gut microflora in a beneficial manner and have been investigated as potential therapy for a wide variety of gastroenterologic and other chronic medical conditions including cirrhosis.[36] Bacterial overgrowth is common in patients with cirrhosis and can result in increased bacterial translocation leading to infection and fat malabsorption. In 1 study, 33% of 24 patients with portal hypertension versus none in a control group of 33 patients demonstrated small bowel bacterial overgrowth.[49] This may be secondary to slower transit times in patients with more advanced liver disease. A recent study demonstrated 6.17-hour transit time versus 3.56 hours in patients with decompensated versus compensated cirrhosis.[50] Probiotics are live microorganisms and may be administered in tablet, capsule, power, or freeze-dried packets with the goal of reducing growth of pathogenic bacteria and improving mucosal integrity ultimately leading to less infection and reduced rates of HE. Lactulose has long been considered a prebiotic and established as useful in the treatment of HE.[51] Trials with probiotics have been mixed when used for HE prevention with some showing equivalent efficacy to lactulose,[52] but RCTs are lacking and recent reviews suggest their benefit may be limited to minimal HE.[53] Further study is needed before these agents can be recommended routinely for patients with cirrhosis with or without HE.

Nutritional intake in NAFLD populations is the focus of discussion elsewhere in this issue but NAFLD cirrhosis requires special mention. In broad terms, NAFLD is a disease of overnutrition associated with high carbohydrate and fat content in addition to a net excess caloric intake compared with total expended. Diabetes is especially common in patients with NASH and should be managed aggressively with early institution of insulin therapy if needed to maintain normal blood sugar levels along with small frequent meals to avoid hypoglycemia. The optimal NASH diet both early on and in the presence of cirrhosis has not been established although diet is believed to be an essential component of a multidisciplinary treatment regimen in precirrhotic NASH.

SUMMARY

Nutrition has not been a primary focus of many medical conditions despite its importance in the development and the severity of these diseases. This is certainly the case with nutrition and ESLD despite the well-established association of nutritional deficiencies and increases rates of complications and mortality in cirrhosis. It is important to assess nutritional status early in cirrhosis so that replacement and dietary modifications can be implemented. The optimal approaches are still under investigation but adequate caloric intake, particularly with protein, as well as nutrient replacement as needed are essential. Vitamin D and fat-soluble vitamin (A, D, E, K) levels should be checked with replacement if deficient. Thiamine and folate replacement are important in alcoholic cirrhotic populations and zinc levels should be checked in patients with cirrhosis with HE. Further study is required to better define whether specialized approaches such as probiotics and BCAAs can provide meaningful clinical benefit.

REFERENCES

1. Centers for Disease Control and Prevention (CDC). Death and hospitalizations from chronic liver disease and cirrhosis: Unites States 1980-1989. MMWR Morb Mortal Wkly Rep 1996;41:969–73.
2. Asrani SK, Larson JJ, Yawn B, et al. Underestimation of liver-related mortality in the United States. Gastroenterology 2013;145:375–82.
3. Rehm J, Samokhvalov AV, Shield KD. Global burden of alcoholic liver diseases. J Hepatol 2013;59(1):160–8.
4. Carvalho L, Parise ER. Evaluation of nutritional status of nonhospitalized patients with liver cirrhosis. Arq Gastroenterol 2006;43(4):269–74.
5. Simon D, Galambos JT. A randomized controlled study of peripheral parenteral nutrition in moderate and severe alcoholic hepatitis. J Hepatol 1988;7:200.
6. Mezey E, Potter JJ, Rennie-Tankersley L, et al. A randomized placebo controlled trial of vitamin E for alcoholic hepatitis. J Hepatol 2004;40:40.
7. Altamirano J, Higuera-de laTijera F, Duarte-Rojo A, et al. The amount of alcohol consumption negatively impacts short-term mortality in Mexican patients with alcoholic hepatitis. Am J Gastroenterol 2011;106:1472.
8. Liangpunsakul S. Clinical characteristics and mortality of hospitalized alcoholic hepatitis patients in the United States. J Clin Gastroenterol 2011;45:714.
9. Altamirano J, Fagundes C, Dominguez M, et al. Acute kidney injury is an early predictor of mortality for patients with alcoholic hepatitis. Clin Gastroenterol Hepatol 2012;10:65.
10. Sam J, Nguyen GC. Protein-calorie malnutrition as a prognostic indicator of mortality among patients hospitalized with cirrhosis and portal hypertension. Liver Int 2009;29:1396–402.
11. Alvares-da-Silva MR, Reverbel da Silveira T. Comparison between handgrip strength, subjective global assessment, and prognostic nutritional index in assessing malnutrition and predicting clinical outcome in cirrhotic outpatients. Nutrition 2005;21:113–7.
12. Cheung K, Lee SS, Raman M. Prevalence and mechanisms of malnutrition in patients with advanced liver disease, and nutrition management strategies. Clin Gastroenterol Hepatol 2012;10:117.
13. Plauth M, Schütz ET. Cachexia in liver cirrhosis. Int J Cardiol 2002;85:83–7.
14. Grsberg AJ, Scarlett JM, Marks DL. Hypothalamic mechanisms in cachexia. Physiol Behav 2010;100:478–89.
15. Kalaitzakis E, Bosaeus I, Ohman L, et al. Altered postprandial glucose, insulin, leptin, and ghrelin in liver cirrhosis: correlations with energy intake and resting energy expenditure. Am J Clin Nutr 2007;85:808–15.
16. Aqel BA, Scolapio JS, Dickson RC, et al. Contribution of ascites to impaired gastric function and nutritional intake in patients with cirrhosis and ascites. Clin Gastroenterol Hepatol 2005;3:1095–100.

17. Dudrick SJ, Kavic SM. Hepatobiliary nutrition: history and future. J Hepatobiliary Pancreat Surg 2002;9:459–68.
18. Badley BW, Murphy GM, Boucheir IA, et al. Diminished micellar phase lipid in patients with chronic non-alcoholic liver disease and steatorrhea. Gastroenterology 1970;58:781–9.
19. Vlahcevic ZR, Buhac I, Farrar JT, et al. Bile acid metabolism in patients with cirrhosis. I. Kinetic aspects of cholic acid metabolism. Gastroenterology 1971; 60(4):491.
20. Tsiaousi ET, Hatzitolios AI, Trygonis SK, et al. Malnutrition in end of stage liver disease: recommendation and nutritional support. J Gastroenterol Hepatol 2008;23:527–33.
21. Charlton M. Alcoholic liver disease: energy and protein metabolism in alcoholic liver disease. Clin Liver Dis 1998;2:781.
22. Plauth M, Cabré E, Rggio O, et al. ESPEN guidelines on enteral nutrition: liver disease. Clin Nutr 2006;25:285–94.
23. Gunsar F, Raimondo ML, Jones S, et al. Nutrition status and prognosis in cirrhotic patients. Aliment Pharmacol Ther 2006;24:563–72.
24. Mathan LK, Escott-Stump S. Krauses's food nutrition and diet therapy. Philadelphia: WB Saunders; 2000.
25. Campillo B, Richardet JP, Bories PN. Enteral nutrition in severely malnourished and anorectic cirrhotic patients in clinical practice. Gastroenterol Clin Biol 2005; 29:645–51.
26. Campillo B, Richardet JP, Bories PN. Validation of body mass index for the diagnosis of malnutrition in patients with liver cirrhosis. Gastroenterol Clin Biol 2006; 30(10):1137–43.
27. Delich PC, Siepler JK, Parker P. Liver disease. In: Gottschlich MM, editor. The A.S.P.E.N. nutrition support core curriculum: a case based approach-the adult patient. Silver Spring (MD): American Society for Parenteral and Enteral Nutrition; 2007. p. 540–57.
28. Plauth M, Cabre E, Campillo B, et al. ESPEN guidelines on parenteral nutrition: hepatology. Clin Nutr 2009;28:436–44.
29. Gundling F, Teich N, Strebel HM, et al. Ernahrung beileberzirrhose. Med Klin 2007;102:435–44.
30. Matos C, Porayko MK, Francisco-Ziller N, et al. Nutrition and chronic liver disease. J Clin Gastroenterol 2002;35:391–7.
31. Nakaya Y, Okita K, Suzuki K, et al. BCAA-enriched snack improves nutritional state of cirrhosis. Nutrition 2007;23:113–20.
32. Moore KP, Aithal GP. Guidelines on the management of ascites in cirrhosis. Gut 2006;55:1–12.
33. Salerno F, Guevara M, Bernardi M, et al. Refractory ascites: pathogenesis, definition and therapy of a severe complication in patients with cirrhosis. Liver Int 2010;30:937–47.
34. Bresci G, Paris G, Banti S. Management of hepatic encephalopathy with oral zinc supplementation: a long-term treatment. Eur J Med 1993;2:414–6.
35. Inoue E, Hori S, Narumi Y, et al. Portal-systemic encephalopathy; presence of basal ganglia lesions with high signal intensity on MR images. Radiology 1991;179:551–5.
36. Amodio P, Bemeur C, Butterworth R, et al. The nutritional management of hepatic encephalopathy in patients with cirrhosis: international society for hepatic encephalopathy and nitrogen metabolism consensus. Hepatology 2013;58: 325–36.

37. Weisman Y. Vitamin D deficiency and insufficiency. Isr Med Assoc J 2013;15: 377–8.
38. Zhang C, Zhao L, Ma L, et al. Vitamin D status and expression of vitamin D receptor and LL-37 in patients with spontaneous bacterial peritonitis. Dig Dis Sci 2012;57(1):182–8.
39. Rossi Fanelli F, Cangiano C, Capocaccia L, et al. Use of branched chain amino acids for treating hepatic encephalopathy: clinical experience. Gut 1986;27: 111–5.
40. Holecek M, Simek J, Palicka V, et al. Effect of glucose and branched chain amino acids (BCAA) infusion on onset of liver regeneration and plasma amino acid pattern in a partially hepatectomized rat. J Hepatol 1991;13:14–20.
41. Alexander WF, Spindel E, Harty RF, et al. The usefulness of branched chain amino acids in patients with acute or chronic hepatic encephalopathy. Am J Gastroenterol 1989;84:91–6.
42. Lam V, Poon RT. Role of branched chain amino acids in management of cirrhosis and hepatocellular carcinoma. Hepatol Res 2008;38(Suppl 1):107–15.
43. Holecek M. Three targets of branched-chain amino acid supplementation in the treatment of liver disease. Nutrition 2010;26:482–90.
44. Holecek M. Branched-chain amino acids and ammonia metabolism in liver disease: therapeutic implications. Nutrition 2013;29(10):1186–91.
45. Chadalavada R, Sappati Biyyani RS, Maxwell J, et al. Nutrition in hepatic encephalopathy. Nutr Clin Pract 2010;25:257–64.
46. James JH, Ziparo V, Jeppsson B, et al. Hyperammonaemia, plasma aminoacid inbalance, and blood-brain aminoacid transport: a unified theory of portal-systemic encephalopathy. Lancet 1979;2:772–5.
47. Marchesini G, Bianchi G, Merli M, et al. Nutritional supplementation with branched-chain amino acids in advanced cirrhosis: double blind randomized trial. Gastroenterology 2003;124:1792–801.
48. Muto Y, Sato S, Watanabe A, et al. Effects of oral branched chain amino acid granules on event-free survival in patients with liver cirrhosis. Clin Gastroenterol Hepatol 2005;3:705–13.
49. Gunnarsdottir SA, Sadik R, Shev S, et al. Small intestinal motility disturbances and bacterial overgrowth in patients with liver cirrhosis and portal hypertension. Am J Gastroenterol 2003;98(6):1362–70.
50. Chandler Roland B, Garcia-Tsao G, Ciarleglio MM, et al. Decompensated cirrhotics have slower intestinal transit times as compared with compensated cirrhotics and healthy controls. J Clin Gastroenterol 2013 [Epub head of print].
51. Shukla S, Shukla A, Mehboog S, et al. Meta-analysis: the effects of gut flora modulation using prebiotics, probiotics and synbiotics on minimal hepatic encephalopathy. Aliment Pharmacol Ther 2011;33:662–71.
52. Agrawal A, Sharma BC, Sharma P, et al. Secondary prophylaxis of hepatic encephalopathy in cirrhosis: an open-label, randomized controlled trial of lactulose, probiotics, and no therapy. Am J Gastroenterol 2012;107:1043–50.
53. McGee RG, Bakens A, Wiley K, et al. Probiotics for patients with hepatic encephalopathy. Cochrane Database Syst Rev 2011;(11):CD008716.

Obesity and Liver Cancer

Ester Vanni, MD, PhD, Elisabetta Bugianesi, MD, PhD*

KEYWORDS

- Obesity • Hepatocellular carcinoma • Nonalcoholic fatty liver disease
- Carcinogenesis

KEY POINTS

- Obesity has become an alarming threat to health worldwide, because of its pandemic spread and increasing prevalence among children.
- Hepatocellular carcinoma (HCC) is the cancer most strongly enhanced by obesity, mainly through the increased risk for nonalcoholic fatty liver disease (NAFLD).
- The lower rates of HCC incidence compared with virus or alcohol-related etiology are outweighed by the much larger spread of NAFLD, thus foreseeing the future trends of HCC in the general population.
- The diagnosis of nonalcoholic steatohepatitis–related HCC is often made at the first referral, when the tumor is at a more advanced stage.
- HCC may also develop in noncirrhotic livers with NAFLD.
- The mechanisms of obesity-induced hepatocarcinogenesis are under active investigation to identify new targets for therapeutic interventions.

INTRODUCTION

Obesity and cancer represent 2 of the most important public health challenges of the twenty-first century. The prevalence of obesity has reached epidemic proportions, with a steep increase over the last decades (**Fig. 1**). In 2005 approximately 1.6 billion people worldwide were overweight and 400 million adults were obese; according to World Health Organization estimates, by 2015 these figures will have doubled.[1] One of the most worrisome aspects of this pandemic spread of obesity is the constant increase among children and adolescents; in 2006, one-third of children aged 2 to 19 years had a body mass index (BMI) above the 85th percentile, with 16% above the 95th percentile.[2] Overweight in early childhood increases the likelihood of being obese in later childhood,[3] and in up to one-half of cases leads to obesity and its complications in adulthood.[4]

Obesity is an established risk factor for cancers in several sites. In a well-known study from the American Cancer Society, death rates from all cancers in the heaviest

Division of Gastroenterology and Hepatology, Department of Medical Sciences, University of Torino, Corso Dogliotti 14, I-10126 Torino, Italy
* Corresponding author.
E-mail address: elisabetta.bugianesi@unito.it

Clin Liver Dis 18 (2014) 191–203
http://dx.doi.org/10.1016/j.cld.2013.09.001
1089-3261/14/$ – see front matter © 2014 Elsevier Inc. All rights reserved.

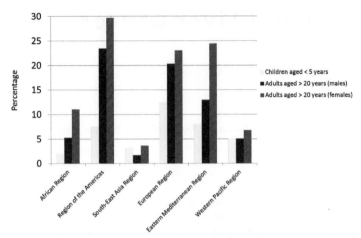

Fig. 1. Global burden of increased body mass index (>25 kg/m²) in children and of obesity in adults. (*Data from* World Health Organization. World Health Statistics Report 2013.)

members of the cohort (BMI ≥35 kg/m²) were 52% higher in men and 62% higher in women when compared with lean subjects. Based on the relative risks observed in this study and on the current patterns of overweight and obesity, the proportion of all cancer deaths in United States adults older than 50 years that is attributable to overweight/obesity may be as high as 14% in men and 20% in women.[5] An important and still controversial point is the relative importance of fat distribution. Visceral fat (VF), evaluated as waist circumference or by computed tomography (CT), can be more important than general adiposity for cancer induction, although the threshold for the increased risk is still unclear.[6] Regarding obesity, VF is also associated with worse clinical outcomes, such as recurrence of the primary cancer, shorter disease-free survival, reduced overall survival, and reduced responsiveness to chemotherapy.[6]

Sites of cancer whose risk is increased by obesity include endometrium, breast, kidney, and bone marrow. Regarding the gastrointestinal tract, obesity increases the risk of colorectal, esophageal, pancreatic, and, above all, primary liver cancer (**Fig. 2**).[7]

OBESITY AND HEPATOCELLULAR CARCINOMA

Liver cancer is the fifth most common cancer in men (7.9% of the total), the seventh most common in women (6.5% of the total), and the third most common cause of death from cancer worldwide.[8] Hepatocellular carcinoma (HCC) accounts for 70% to 85% of the total burden of liver cancer. Most cases of HCC (70%–90%) develop against a background of advanced chronic liver disease, related mainly to hepatitis B virus (HBV), hepatitis C virus (HCV), and alcohol abuse.[8] Whereas in eastern Asia and sub-Saharan Africa the dominant risk factor is HBV, in the developed countries time trends in the incidence of HCC paralleled the timing of HCV spread, but in approximately 15% to 50% of HCC cases the etiology is unrelated to viruses or alcohol. Lately, a strong association between HCC and the metabolic syndrome (MS) has become evident.[9] The definition of the MS is constantly updated, but basically refers to a cluster of interrelated risk factors, including visceral obesity, atherogenic dyslipidemia, arterial hypertension, and hyperglycemia/type 2 diabetes, which exponentially increase the risk of developing cardiovascular diseases.[10] Among the components of the MS, both obesity and type 2 diabetes are independent risk factors

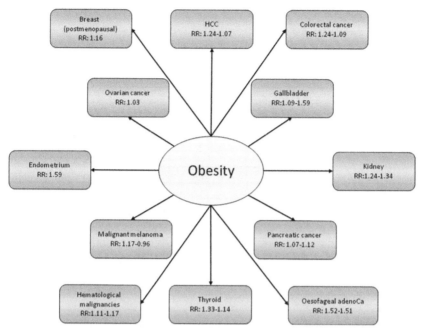

Fig. 2. The risk ratio (RR) of obesity-related cancers in men and women per 5 kg/m² increase in body mass index. (*Adapted from* Renehan AG, Tyson M, Egger M, et al. Body-mass index and incidence of cancer: a systematic review and meta-analysis of prospective observational studies. Lancet 2008;371:569–78; with permission.)

for HCC.[5,11] Large-scale epidemiologic studies have associated the increasing prevalence of overweight/obesity with a higher risk of HCC and a worse clinical outcome **(Table 1)**. In a large mortality study, the risk of dying from liver cancer was 4.5 times higher in obese than in lean people.[5] Several meta-analyses confirmed the increased prevalence of HCC in overweight/obese individuals, ranging from 17% to 89%,[12] with an average 24% increase in risk of liver cancer for each 5 kg/m² increase in BMI.[13] A recent systematic review of 10 cohort studies including more than 7 million participants found a positive association between obesity and risk of HCC in the majority (relative risks ranging from 1.4 to 4.1), no association in 2, and an inverse association only in 1.[14]

Overwhelming evidence supports a link between obesity and HCC, even though these studies are burdened with several limitations, such as the lack of adjustment for potential confounders (viral hepatitis and/or alcohol intake) or of categorization according to age, gender, ethnic background, and other risk factors, which often precludes the comparison between diverse populations.

Unfortunately, only a few studies have investigated the role of visceral adiposity in HCC development. In the EPIC study the waist-to-hip ratio (WHR), a rough estimate of abdominal fat, was the anthropometric measure of adiposity that better predicted the incidence of HCC over a follow-up of 8.6 years and conferred a 3-fold HCC risk to subjects in the upper tertile of WHR.[15] In another study, the recurrence of HCC after radiofrequency ablation was almost 2-fold higher in patients with increased VF assessed by CT after adjustment for other confounders.[16] Despite this intriguing preliminary evidence, the role of visceral rather than generalized adiposity in HCC risk remains an open question, and is certainly deserving of ad hoc studies.

	Measure (95% CI): Men	Measure (95% CI): Women	Measure (95% CI): All
Table 1			
HCC risks for overweight and obesity			
Authors,[Ref.] Year	Measure (95% CI): Men	Measure (95% CI): Women	Measure (95% CI): All
Wolk et al,[56] 2001	SIR	SIR	SIR
Overweight	—	—	—
Obesity	3.60 (2.00–6.00)	1.70 (1.10–2.50)	2.4 (1.6–3.4)
Nair et al,[57] 2002	—	—	RR
Overweight	—	—	—
Obesity	—	—	1.65 (1.22–2.22)
Calle et al,[5] 2003	RR	RR	—
Overweight	1.13 (0.94–1.34)	1.02 (0.80–1.31)	—
Obesity	2.41 (1.92–3.01)	1.47 (1.08–2.00)	—
Pan et al,[58] 2004	OR	OR	OR
Overweight	0.99 (0.72–1.38)	0.61 (0.35–1.07)	0.89 (0.68–1.17)
Obesity	1.30 (0.85–1.97)	0.94 (0.48–1.84)	1.17 (0.83–1.66)
Kuriyama et al,[59] 2005	RR	RR	—
Overweight	0.91 (0.52–1.59)	1.13 (0.57–2.27)	—
Obesity	—	—	—
Batty et al,[60] 2005	RR	—	—
Overweight	0.99 (0.53–1.88)	—	—
Obesity	3.76 (1.36–10.4)	—	—
Oh et al,[61] 2005	RR	—	—
Overweight	1.05 (0.97–1.14)	—	—
Obesity	1.56 (1.15–2.12)	—	—
Rapp et al,[62] 2005	HR	—	—
Overweight	1.32 (0.73–2.37)	—	—
Obesity	1.67 (0.75–3.72)	—	—
Samanic et al,[63] 2006	RR	—	—
Overweight	1.29 (1.00–1.68)	—	—
Obesity	3.62 (2.62–5.00)	—	—
Chen et al,[33] 2008	—	—	RR
Overweight	—	—	0.86 (0.42–1.74)
Obesity	—	—	2.36 (0.91–6.17)
Polesel et al,[64] 2009	—	—	OR
Overweight	—	—	1.0 (0.5–1.9)
Obesity	—	—	1.9 (0.9–3.9)
Renehan et al,[13] 2008	RR	RR	—
For 5 kg/m² increase	1.24 (0.95–1.62)	1.07 (0.55–2.08)	—

Abbreviations: HR, hazard ratio; OR, odds ratio; RR, relative risk; SIR, standardized incidence ratio.
  Data from Refs.[5,13,33,56–64]

HEPATOCELLULAR CARCINOMA AND OBESITY IN THE SETTING OF NONALCOHOLIC FATTY LIVER DISEASE

Although obesity per se exerts a carcinogenic potential, the risk of HCC development can be mainly attributed to the simultaneous presence of nonalcoholic fatty liver disease (NAFLD). In fact, NAFLD affects up to 90% of obese individuals, including 25% with nonalcoholic steatohepatitis (NASH), the most aggressive and potentially progressive form of the wide histologic spectrum of NAFLD.

The evidence that HCC is a possible complication of NAFLD derives from heterogeneous studies performed in subjects with a clinical diagnosis of NAFLD (by unexplained elevated serum transaminases or by ultrasonography), with biopsy-proven evidence of NAFLD/NASH, or with NASH-related or cryptogenic cirrhosis (**Table 2**).

NAFLD was the most common underlying etiologic risk factor for HCC (59%) in a United States population–based study, with a cumulative incidence of 0.3% over a 6-year follow-up compared with 0.6% in HCV-related liver disease.[17] The cumulative HCC mortality rates in NAFLD ranged from 0.25% to 2.3% over a time frame of 8.3 to 13.7 years in 2 further studies.[18,19] An elevated absolute risk of HCC (3%–6% over 8.2–21 years of follow-up) in these patients has been further described by other studies,[20,21] but not universally confirmed.[22,23]

As expected, the risk of HCC is more elevated when examining NAFLD patients with advanced liver disease. In the largest prospective community-based study performed thus far,[24] after a mean follow-up of 7.6 years only 0.5% patients developed HCC, but the rate among cirrhotic patients was 2 of 21 (10%). In a retrospective case-control study,[25] cryptogenic cirrhosis represented the fourth-ranked cause of HCC.

In general, the relative HCC risk and the HCC mortality rate in NASH-related and cryptogenic cirrhosis cohorts are lower in comparison with patients with viral or alcohol-related cirrhosis. These findings reflect the slower progression of NASH in comparison with other liver diseases, although observation periods of limited length can underestimate the incidence of HCC. Two longitudinal studies on the natural history of NASH-related cirrhosis in United States[26] and Japanese[24] populations found a lower mortality rate for liver-related causes, but an increased cardiovascular mortality compared with HCV cirrhotics. Nevertheless, HCC was the cause of 47% of deaths in NASH patients, representing an independent risk factor for mortality (hazard ratio [HR] 7.96). In another cohort study, the standardized incidence rate for HCC in NASH-related or cryptogenic cirrhosis was lower than for alcohol-related cirrhosis, but similar to that observed for HCV-related HCC (43 in 100,000 person-years for cryptogenic and HCV cirrhosis–related HCC vs 71 in 100,000 person-years for alcoholic cirrhosis–related HCC).[27] In patients referred for liver transplant evaluation, the annual cumulative risk of HCC can be as high as 2.6% per year in NASH cirrhosis, compared with 4.0% in HCV cirrhosis.[28]

Of importance, the lower rates of HCC incidence are outweighed by the much larger spread of NAFLD compared with other causes of chronic liver disease, thus foreseeing the future trends of HCC in the general population along with its important implications. Moreover, the insidious and indolent course of NAFLD may delay the diagnosis of HCC, limiting the possibility of therapeutic interventions.[29] A synchronous or metachronous development of multicentric HCCs has been described in the NASH setting, especially in older patients with type 2 diabetes and cirrhosis.[30] Older age and concurrent metabolic or vascular disease frequently occurring in NAFLD can further limit the possibility of potentially curative treatments, such as orthotopic liver transplantation (OLT).

HEPATOCELLULAR CARCINOMA IN NONCIRRHOTIC LIVER WITH NONALCOHOLIC FATTY LIVER DISEASE

In general, most cases of HCC are diagnosed in patients affected by long-standing cirrhosis, but HCCs arising in noncirrhotic livers having MS as the only risk have been consistently described in recent years. In a cohort of HCC patients with MS, the tumor

Table 2
Principal case reports and case series of NAFLD/NASH/MS-related HCC

Authors,[Ref.] Year	No. of NAFLD/MS-related HCC	Mean Age at Diagnosis of HCC	Gender	Overweight/Obesity (Yes/No; %)	Tumor	Liver Histology (METAVIR Score)
Regimbeau et al,[65] 2004	18	66	18 M	Yes (50%)	14 single/4 multifocal	4 cirrhotic/14 noncirrhotic (F2–F3)
Iannaccone et al,[66] 2007	22	64.5	22 M	Yes (55%)	21 single/1 multifocal	6 cirrhotic/16 noncirrhotic (F0–F3)
Ohki et al,[16] 2009	62	68.5	40 M/22 F	Yes (44%)	40 single/22 multifocal	38 cirrhotic/24 noncirrhotic (NA)
Paradis et al,[31] 2009	31	67.4	30 M/1 F	Yes (80%)	24 single/7 multifocal	20 F0–F2/11 F3–F4
Hashimoto et al,[67] 2009	34	70 (median)	21 M/13 F	Yes (62%)	Among noncirrhotics, 3 single/1 multifocal	30 cirrhotic/4 noncirrhotic (F1–F2)
Yasui et al,[32] 2011	87	72	54 M/33 F	Yes (61.5%)	65 single/22 multifocal	44 cirrhotic/43 noncirrhotic (F1–F3)
Ertle et al,[68] 2011	36	68.6	32 M/4 F	Yes (95%)	NR	19 cirrhotic/17 noncirrhotic (F0–F3)
Tokushige et al,[69] 2011	292	72 (median)	181 M/111 F	Yes (66%)	NR	181 cirrhotic/111 noncirrhotic (NR)

Abbreviations: F, female; M, male; NR/NA, not reported/not available.
Data from Refs.[16,32,65–69]

developed in a background liver without significant fibrosis in two-thirds of cases, compared with less than one-third in those with an overt cause of liver disease.[31] Other reports confirmed this first observation. To date, the largest group of noncirrhotic NAFLD with HCC has been described in a Japanese study, where half of the 87 cases of HCC occurring in patients with histologically confirmed NASH had no established cirrhosis.[32]

The development of HCC in the setting of NAFLD/NASH without advanced fibrosis is a worrisome issue of increasing importance, because of the rising incidence of MS and its components. This trend has important implications in terms of planning screening programs to prevent the occurrence of HCC, particularly in the obese and diabetic populations, because of the synergistic carcinogenic effect. Better understanding of the risk factors linked to the development of HCC in noncirrhotic livers may help to identify patients at high risk and to set up strategies for screening and surveillance.

OBESITY AS A RISK FACTOR FOR HEPATOCELLULAR CARCINOMA ARISING IN CHRONIC LIVER DISEASE OF DIFFERENT ETIOLOGY

Overweight and obesity are also risk factors for HCC in patients with viral or alcohol-related chronic liver disease, but the extent to which this is caused by the concurrent presence of NAFLD has not been clearly defined. In a Taiwanese population study, obesity was associated with a 4-fold risk of HCC in anti-HCV seropositive subjects and with a 2-fold risk in patients without viral infections, after controlling for other risk factors. Of note, the presence of both obesity and diabetes increased more than 100-fold the risk of HCC in HBV or HCV carriers, indicating a possible synergistic effect of metabolic factors and viral hepatitis.[33] Similar conclusions were drawn in a cohort study of patients with chronic hepatitis C, where obesity was identified as an independent risk factor for HCC (HR 3.10; 95% confidence interval [CI] 1.41–6.81).[34] Alcohol intake and obesity can have a multiplicative effect on the risk of incident HCC, as observed in male patients with hepatitis B infection (HR 3.41; 95% CI 1.25–9.27).[35] By contrast, obesity does not increase the risk for surgery-related adverse events after hepatic resection,[36] but the long-term prognosis of these patients may be burdened with a poorer oncologic outcome, a lower survival rate, and a shorter time to recurrence. Among HCV patients who underwent OLT because of HCC, the cancer recurrence was doubled in the presence of obesity.[37] Recently, a histologic subtype of HCC, termed steatohepatitic hepatocellular carcinoma, has been described in approximately 13% of explant livers with chronic hepatitis C and in the nonneoplastic liver features resembling steatohepatitis, including steatosis, ballooning of malignant hepatocytes, Mallory-Denk bodies, and pericellular fibrosis.[38] Certainly the prevalence of NAFLD in HBV/HCV-related chronic liver disease can be as high as in the general population, and the synergistic effect with alcohol can be explained by common pathways of liver damage. Thus, the main effort should be directed toward prevention and treatment of metabolic derangements also in patients with viral chronic hepatitis, firstly by promoting healthful dietary practices and physical activity.

MECHANISMS OF HEPATOCELLULAR CARCINOMA CARCINOGENESIS IN OBESITY

In the cirrhotic liver, chromosomal instability and selection of premalignant clones are favored by expansion of liver progenitor cells. In the setting of obesity, both a dysfunctional adipose tissue (which leads to lipid accumulation in multiple ectopic sites, including the liver) and the pathophysiologic mechanisms leading to NASH might have a superimposed carcinogenic potential, even in precirrhotic stages.[29]

Among potential mediators, lipotoxicity and oxidative stress, an imbalance in the relative proportion of proinflammatory/anti-inflammatory cytokines, stimulation of the insulin-like growth factor 1 (IGF-1) axis by hyperinsulinemia, and gut microbiota are being actively investigated because they may stimulate cellular proliferation or favor epigenetic aberrations (**Fig. 3**).

Lipotoxicity is generally attributed to products of free fatty acid metabolism, consisting of high levels of reactive oxygen species and other toxic intermediates caused by increased fatty acid oxidation in the mitochondria, endoplasmic reticulum, and peroxisomes in the ectopic sites of fat accumulation, including the liver.[39] The chronic deregulation of redox homeostasis may favor tumorigenesis indirectly, through

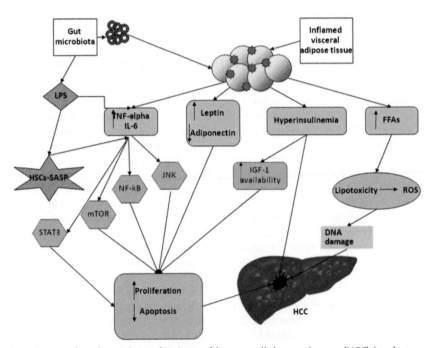

Fig. 3. Proposed pathogenic mechanisms of hepatocellular carcinoma (HCC) in obese persons. Hypertrophic and inflamed visceral adipose tissue increases the secretion of proinflammatory adipokines (tumor necrosis factor [TNF]-α, interleukin [IL]-6, leptin), and reduces the release of adiponectin; this accelerates the cell-cycle progression and downregulates proapoptotic pathways, inducing proliferation, invasion, migration, and angiogenesis. Insulin resistance leads to hyperinsulinemia and increased release from adipose tissue of free fatty acids (FFAs). These mechanisms favor the development of hepatic steatosis and promote an inflammatory response within the liver. Hyperinsulinemia, in turn, increases the levels of bioavailable insulin-like growth factor 1 (IGF-1). Insulin and IGF-1 signals promote cellular proliferation and inhibit apoptosis in many tissue types, including the liver. Increased hepatic mitochondrial production of reactive oxygen species (ROS) modulates the expression of genes involved in hepatocarcinogenesis. Finally, alterations of intestinal microbiota, associated with obesity, lead to an increased translocation of lipopolysaccharide (LPS), triggering inflammatory response through toll-like receptors (TLRs), contributing to hepatic inflammation and fibrosis. LPS-dependent TLR4 activation may contribute to HCC promotion by increasing proliferative and antiapoptotic signals. HSCs, hepatic stellate cells; mTOR, mammalian target of rapamycin; NF-kB, nuclear factor κB; SASP, senescence-associated secretory phenotype; STAT3, signal transducer and activator of transcription 3.

inflammatory response and proliferation, or directly, by inducing cancer-promoting mutations.[29] Of interest, a single gene linking oxidative stress to NASH and hepatic tumors has been identified. Liver-specific inactivation of *Nrf1*, a transcription factor essential for embryonic development involved in antioxidant response, sensitizes hepatocytes to oxidative stress and leads to unequivocal features of progressing NAFLD, starting from histologic evidence of apoptotic cells and progressing to steatosis, fibrosis, and finally to the appearance of hepatic tumors.[40] During the neoplastic process, epithelial hyperplasia and dysplasia generally precede cancer, and the development of liver tumors is linked to the activation and proliferation of adult liver progenitor (oval) cells.[41] Cell hyperplasia is present in the earliest stages of NAFLD in *ob/ob* mice, suggesting that metabolic abnormalities, rather than cirrhosis, may initiate the hepatic hyperplastic/neoplastic changes.[41]

Adipokines may contribute to the regulation of immune response (leptin, adiponectin), inflammatory response (tumor necrosis factor [TNF]-α, interleukin [IL]-6, serum amyloid A, adiponectin), and angiogenesis (vascular endothelial growth factor 1).[42] Adiponectin, whose secretion is reduced in obesity and insulin-resistant states, exhibits several antitumor properties through an antiproliferative, antiangiogenic, and proapoptotic action.[43] Adiponectin can also inhibit the phosphorylation of the mammalian target of rapamycin (mTOR), an important regulator of cell and tumor growth.[44] Leptin promotes hepatic neovascularization in the presence of vascular endothelial growth factor,[45] and seems to have both proliferative and antiapoptotic effects on HCC cells, by accelerating the cell-cycle progression and downregulating proapoptotic pathways.[46] However, several studies have reported opposite effects of leptin in HCC growth, and its role in tumorigenesis is still uncertain. TNF-α, another proinflammatory cytokine increased in obesity, is a potent activator of pro-oncogenic pathways.[47]

Cellular pathways transducing the signal of insulin, including the IRS/PI3K/Akt and RAS/MAPK axis, are intimately linked to proliferative pathways that are not blunted in obesity, and can be stimulated by the compensatory hyperinsulinemia. Insulin per se seems to have tumorigenic properties, through its receptors expressed in human neoplasms.[48] Insulin also promotes the synthesis and biological activity of IGF-1, a peptide hormone that regulates energy-dependent growth processes, through stimulation of cell proliferation and inhibition of apoptosis.[49] Changes in the expression pattern of components of the IGF system were observed in patients with HCC, in human hepatoma cell lines as well as in rodent models of hepatocarcinogenesis. The antisense oligonucleotides anti–IGF-1 and anti–IGF-2 selectively inhibited the growth of human hepatoma cell lines and decreased the growth rate of rat HCC in vivo and in vitro.[50]

Both dietary and genetic obesity may favor HCC by altering signal transduction pathways that modulate cell proliferation independent of liver damage, in particular through downregulation of autophagy by IL-6–mediated inhibition of AMPK and activation of TORC1.[51] Conversely, treatment with the antidiabetic drug metformin, which stimulates autophagy through activation of AMPK, is associated with a reduced risk of HCC among diabetics.[52]

Alterations of the intestinal microbiota are associated with obesity, and contribute to both systemic and hepatic inflammation through increased translocation of bacterial components (lipopolysaccharides [LPS]) and activation of the toll-like receptors (TLRs). LPS-dependent TLR4 activation is also able to promote the development of HCC in animal models by inducing compensatory proliferation in hepatocytes and preventing apoptosis of tumor cells.[53] Conversely, treatment with antibiotics or gut sterilization can decrease plasma levels of LPS, hepatic levels of TNF-α, and IL-6 mRNAs, along with a decrease in the number and size of tumors.[54] Gut bacteria are also able to promote obesity-associated HCC development by modulating cellular senescence and inducing a senescence-associated secretory phenotype (SASP) in hepatic stellate cells.[55] This process may be important in HCC arising from noncirrhotic livers, and signs of cellular senescence and SASP were observed in HCC arising in NASH.[55]

SUMMARY

Obesity is becoming a serious public health problem in the Western world, eliciting metabolic and cardiovascular disorders and increasing the risk of cancer. Among all cancers HCC is strongly enhanced by obesity, mainly through its close association with NAFLD/NASH. Even though NAFLD has a more indolent course than virus-related or alcohol-related chronic liver disease, HCC represents a frequent complication of NASH-related cirrhosis. The delay in diagnosis, older age, and the presence of relevant comorbidities limit the possibility of therapeutic intervention. A considerable number of NAFLD-associated HCC cases develop in noncirrhotic livers in patients with multiple metabolic risk factors, mainly obesity and type 2 diabetes. In consideration of the large spread of obesity and its complications in the general population, this issue will become a future challenge for public health, in terms of planning screening and surveillance programs to prevent the occurrence of HCC.

Better understanding of the genetic and biological determinants of hepatocyte growth and differentiation in the setting of obesity will help to identify new targets for therapeutic interventions. Until then, greater efforts should be directed toward the promotion of community awareness and a healthful life, starting from childhood.

REFERENCES

1. World Health Organization. Obesity 2008. Available at: http://www.who.int/topics/ obesity/en/. Accessed October 22, 2009.
2. Ogden CL, Carroll MD, Flegal KM. High body mass index for age among US children and adolescents, 2003-2006. JAMA 2008;299:2401–5.
3. Nader PR, O'Brien M, Houts R, et al. Identifying risk for obesity in early childhood. Pediatrics 2006;118:e594–601.
4. Singh AS, Mulder C, Twisk JW, et al. Tracking of childhood overweight into adulthood: a systematic review of the literature. Obes Rev 2008;9:474–88.
5. Calle EE, Rodriguez C, Walker-Thurmond K, et al. Overweight, obesity, and mortality from cancer in a prospectively studied cohort of U.S adults. N Engl J Med 2003;348:1625–38.
6. Vongsuvanh R, George J, Qiao L, et al. Visceral adiposity in gastrointestinal and hepatic carcinogenesis. Cancer Lett 2013;330:1–10.
7. Boeing H. Obesity and cancer—the update 2013. Best Pract Res Clin Endocrinol Metab 2013;27:219–27.
8. El-Serag HB. Hepatocellular carcinoma. N Engl J Med 2011;365:1118–22.
9. Welzel TM, Graubard BI, Zeuzem S, et al. Metabolic syndrome increases the risk of primary liver cancer in the United States: a study in the SEER-Medicare database. Hepatology 2011;54:463–71.
10. Alberti KG, Zimmet P, Shaw J. Metabolic syndrome—a new world-wide definition. A consensus statement from the International Diabetes Federation. Diabet Med 2006;23:469–80.
11. Bugianesi E, Vanni E, Marchesini G. NASH and the risk of cirrhosis and hepatocellular carcinoma in type 2 diabetes. Curr Diab Rep 2007;7:175–80.
12. Larsson SC, Wolk A. Overweight, obesity and risk of liver cancer: a meta-analysis of cohort studies. Br J Cancer 2007;97:1005–8.

13. Renehan AG, Tyson M, Egger M, et al. Body-mass index and incidence of cancer: a systematic review and meta-analysis of prospective observational studies. Lancet 2008;371:569–78.

14. Saunders D, Seidel D, Allison M, et al. Systematic review: the association between obesity and hepatocellular carcinoma—epidemiological evidence. Aliment Pharmacol Ther 2010;31:1051–63.

15. Schlesinger S, Aleksandrova K, Pischon T, et al. Abdominal obesity, weight gain during adulthood and risk of liver and biliary tract cancer in a European cohort. Int J Cancer 2013;132:645–57.

16. Ohki T, Tateishi R, Shiina S, et al. Visceral fat accumulation is an independent risk factor for hepatocellular carcinoma recurrence after curative treatment in patients with suspected NASH. Gut 2009;58:839–44.

17. Sanyal A, Poklepovic A, Moyneur E, et al. Population-based risk factors and resource utilization for HCC: US perspective. Curr Med Res Opin 2010;26: 2183–91.

18. Matteoni CA, Younossi ZM, Gramlich T, et al. Nonalcoholic fatty liver disease: a spectrum of clinical and pathological severity. Gastroenterology 1999;116:1413–9.

19. Ekstedt M, Franzén LE, Mathiesen UL, et al. Long-term follow-up of patients with NAFLD and elevated liver enzymes. Hepatology 2006;44:865–73.

20. Söderberg C, Stål P, Askling J, et al. Decreased survival of subjects with elevated liver function tests during a 28-year follow-up. Hepatology 2010;51: 595–602.

21. Arase Y, Kobayashi M, Suzuki F, et al. Difference in malignancies of chronic liver disease due to non-alcoholic fatty liver disease or hepatitis C in Japanese elderly patients. Hepatol Res 2012;42:264–72.

22. Dam-Larsen S, Becker U, Franzmann MB, et al. Final results of a long-term, clinical follow-up in fatty liver patients. Scand J Gastroenterol 2009;44:1236–43.

23. Ong JP, Pitts A, Younossi ZM. Increased overall mortality and liver-related mortality in non-alcoholic fatty liver disease. J Hepatol 2008;49:608–12.

24. Yatsuji S, Hashimoto E, Tobari M, et al. Clinical features and outcomes of cirrhosis due to non-alcoholic steatohepatitis compared with cirrhosis caused by chronic hepatitis C. J Gastroenterol Hepatol 2009;24:248–54.

25. Bugianesi E, Leone N, Vanni E, et al. Expanding the natural history of nonalcoholic steatohepatitis: from cryptogenic cirrhosis to hepatocellular carcinoma. Gastroenterology 2002;123:134–40.

26. Sanyal AJ, Banas C, Sargeant C, et al. Similarities and differences in outcomes of cirrhosis due to nonalcoholic steatohepatitis and hepatitis C. Hepatology 2006;43:682–9.

27. Sorensen HT, Friis S, Olsen JH, et al. Risk of liver and other types of cancer in patients with cirrhosis: a nationwide cohort study in Denmark. Hepatology 1998; 28:921–5.

28. Ascha MS, Hanouneh IA, Lopez R, et al. The incidence and risk factors of hepatocellular carcinoma in patients with nonalcoholic steatohepatitis. Hepatology 2010;51:1972–8.

29. Bugianesi E. Non-alcoholic steatohepatitis and cancer. Clin Liver Dis 2007;11: 191–207.

30. Kawai H, Nomoto M, Suda T, et al. Multicentric occurrence of hepatocellular carcinoma with nonalcoholic steatohepatitis. World J Hepatol 2011;3:15–23.

31. Paradis V, Zalinski S, Chelbi E, et al. Hepatocellular carcinomas in patients with metabolic syndrome often develop without significant liver fibrosis: a pathological analysis. Hepatology 2009;49:851–9.

32. Yasui K, Hashimoto E, Komorizono Y, et al. Characteristics of patients with nonalcoholic steatohepatitis who develop hepatocellular carcinoma. Clin Gastroenterol Hepatol 2011;9:428–33.
33. Chen CL, Yang HI, Yang WS, et al. Metabolic factors and risk of hepatocellular carcinoma by chronic hepatitis B/C infection: a follow-up study in Taiwan. Gastroenterology 2008;135:111–21.
34. Ohki T, Tateishi R, Sato T, et al. Obesity is an independent risk factor for hepatocellular carcinoma development in chronic hepatitis C patients. Clin Gastroenterol Hepatol 2008;6:459–64.
35. Loomba R, Yang H, Su J, et al. Obesity and alcohol synergize to increase the risk of incident hepatocellular carcinoma in men. Clin Gastroenterol Hepatol 2010;8:891–8.
36. Nishikawa H, Arimoto A, Wakasa T, et al. The relation between obesity and survival after surgical resection of hepatitis C virus-related hepatocellular carcinoma. Gastroenterol Res Pract 2013;2013:430438.
37. Mathur A, Franco ES, Leone JP, et al. Obesity portends increased morbidity and earlier recurrence following liver transplantation for hepatocellular carcinoma. HPB (Oxford) 2013;15:504–10.
38. Salomao M, Remotti H, Vaughan R, et al. The steatohepatitic variant of hepatocellular carcinoma and its association with underlying steatohepatitis. Hum Pathol 2012;43:737–46.
39. Unger RH, Clark GO, Scherer PE, et al. Lipid homeostasis, lipotoxicity and the metabolic syndrome. Biochim Biophys Acta 2010;1801:209–14.
40. Xu Z, Chen L, Leung L, et al. Liver-specific inactivation of the Nrf1 gene in adult mouse leads to nonalcoholic steatohepatitis and hepatic neoplasia. Proc Natl Acad Sci U S A 2005;102:4120–5.
41. Yang SQ, Lin HZ, Hwang J, et al. Hepatic hyperplasia in noncirrhotic fatty livers is obesity-related hepatic steatosis a premalignant condition? Cancer Res 2001; 61:5016–23.
42. Rajala MW, Scherer PE. Minireview: the adipocyte—at the crossroads of energy homeostasis, inflammation, and atherosclerosis. Endocrinology 2003;144: 3765–73.
43. Roberts DL, Dive C, Renehan AG. Biological mechanisms linking obesity and cancer risk: new perspectives. Annu Rev Med 2010;61:301–16.
44. Saxena NK, Fu PP, Nagalingam A, et al. Adiponectin modulates C-jun N-terminal kinase and mammalian target of rapamycin and inhibits hepatocellular carcinoma. Gastroenterology 2010;139:1762–73.
45. Kitade M, Yoshiji H, Kojima H, et al. Leptin mediated neovascularization is a prerequisite for progression of nonalcoholic steatohepatitis in rats. Hepatology 2006;44:983–91.
46. Chen C, Chang YC, Liu CL, et al. Leptin induces proliferation and anti-apoptosis in human hepatocarcinoma cells by up-regulating cyclin D1 and down-regulating Bax via a Janus kinase 2-linked pathway. Endocr Relat Cancer 2007;14:513–29.
47. Marra F, Bertolani C. Adipokines in liver diseases. Hepatology 2009;50:957–69.
48. Pollak M. Insulin and insulin-like growth factor signaling in neoplasia. Nat Rev Cancer 2008;8:915–28.
49. Ish-Shalom D, Christoffersen CT, Vorwerk P, et al. Mitogenic properties of insulin and insulin analogues mediated by the insulin receptor. Diabetologia 1997; 40(Suppl 2):S25–31.
50. Alexia C, Fallot G, Lasfer M, et al. An evaluation of the role of insulin-like growth factors (IGF) and of type-I IGF receptor signalling in hepatocarcinogenesis and

in the resistance of hepatocarcinoma cells against drug-induced apoptosis. Biochem Pharmacol 2004;68:1003–15.

51. Park EJ, Lee JH, Yu G, et al. Dietary and genetic obesity promote liver inflammation and tumorigenesis by enhancing IL-6 and TNF expression. Cell 2010; 140:197–208.

52. Donadon V, Balbi M, Mas MD, et al. Metformin and reduced risk of hepatocellular carcinoma in diabetic patients with chronic liver disease. Liver Int 2010;30: 750–8.

53. Yu XL, Yan HX, Liu Q, et al. Endotoxin accumulation prevents carcinogen-induced apoptosis and promotes liver tumorigenesis in rodents. Hepatology 2010;52:1322–33.

54. Dapito DH, Mencin A, Gwak GY, et al. Promotion of hepatocellular carcinoma by the intestinal microbiota and TLR4. Cancer Cell 2012;21:504–16.

55. Yoshimoto S, Loo TM, Atarashi K, et al. Obesity-induced gut microbial metabolite promotes liver cancer through senescence secretome. Nature 2013;499: 97–101.

56. Wolk A, Gridley G, Svensson M, et al. A prospective study of obesity and cancer risk (Sweden). Cancer Causes Control 2001;12:13–21.

57. Nair S, Mason A, Eason J, et al. Is obesity an independent risk factor for hepatocellular carcinoma in cirrhosis? Hepatology 2002;36:150–5.

58. Pan SY, Johnson KC, Ugnat AM, et al. Association of obesity and cancer risk in Canada. Am J Epidemiol 2004;159:259–68.

59. Kuriyama S, Tsubono Y, Hozawa A, et al. Obesity and risk of cancer in Japan. Int J Cancer 2005;113:148–57.

60. Batty GD, Shipley MJ, Jarrett RJ, et al. Obesity and overweight in relation to organ-specific cancer mortality in London (UK): findings from the original Whitehall study. Int J Obes 2005;29:1267–74.

61. Oh SW, Yoon YS, Shin SA. Effects of excess weight on cancer incidences depending on cancer sites and histologic findings among men: Korea National Health Insurance Corporation Study. J Clin Oncol 2005;23:4742–54.

62. Rapp K, Schroeder J, Klenk J, et al. Obesity and incidence of cancer: a large cohort study of over 145,000 adults in Austria. Br J Cancer 2005;93:1062–7.

63. Samanic C, Chow WH, Gridley G, et al. Relation of body mass index to cancer risk in 362,552 Swedish men. Cancer Causes Control 2006;17:901–9.

64. Polesel J, Zucchetto A, Montella M, et al. The impact of obesity and diabetes mellitus on the risk of hepatocellular carcinoma. Ann Oncol 2009;20:353–7.

65. Regimbeau JM, Colombat M, Mognol P, et al. Obesity and diabetes as a risk factor for hepatocellular carcinoma. Liver Transpl 2004;10(2 Suppl 1):S69–73.

66. Iannaccone R, Piacentini F, Murakami T, et al. Hepatocellular carcinoma in patients with nonalcoholic fatty liver disease: helical CT and MR imaging findings with clinical-pathologic comparison. Radiology 2007;243:422–30.

67. Hashimoto E, Yatsuji S, Tobari M, et al. Hepatocellular carcinoma in patients with nonalcoholic steatohepatitis. J Gastroenterol 2009;44(Suppl 19):89–95.

68. Ertle J, Dechene A, Sowa JP, et al. Nonalcoholic fatty liver disease progresses to hepatocellular carcinoma in the absence of apparent cirrhosis. Int J Cancer 2011;128:2436–43.

69. Tokushige K, Hashimoto E, Horie Y, et al. Hepatocellular carcinoma in Japanese patients with nonalcoholic fatty liver disease, alcoholic liver disease, and chronic liver disease of unknown etiology: report of the nationwide survey. J Gastroenterol 2011;46:1230–7.

Impact of Nutrition and Obesity on Chronic Liver Disease

Vignan Manne, MD[a], Sammy Saab, MD, MPH, AGAF[a,b],*

KEYWORDS

- Malnutrition • Obesity • Chronic liver disease • Protein-calorie malnutrition
- Nonalcoholic fatty liver disease

KEY POINTS

- The liver is a central organ in total body nutrition, playing a role in the metabolism of all major macronutrient groups as well as multiple micronutrients
- Malnutrition has been implicated in causing liver disease and is a common complication, seen in up to 90% of patients with liver disease.
- Obesity is associated with the formation of nonalcoholic fatty liver disease (NAFLD), considered to be the hepatic manifestation of metabolic syndrome, and has been shown to be a risk factor for progression of chronic liver disease.
- Assessment of nutritional status is still a topic of debate, but measures commonly used include clinical signs, blood tests, and anthropometric assessments such as hand-grip strength.
- The management of obesity and malnutrition is important, as it has been shown to increase insulin sensitivity, decrease hepatic steatosis, and have a positive impact on the management of other liver diseases.

INTRODUCTION

Malnutrition, or undernutrition, and obesity are at opposite ends of a spectrum that has an enormous impact on all aspects of liver diseases. Patients with chronic liver disease develop some form of malnutrition that becomes more recognizable as the liver disease progresses.[1–3] Cases of malnutrition can be found in 65% to 90% of all patients with advanced liver disease and in almost 100% of liver transplantation candidates.[4,5] Specific micronutrient deficiencies are common in patients with liver disease, albeit less obvious than signs seen in protein deficiencies such as muscle wasting.[6]

[a] Department of Surgery, University of California, Los Angeles, 200 Medical Plaza, Suite 214, Los Angeles, CA 90095, USA; [b] Department of Medicine, University of California, Los Angeles, 200 Medical Plaza, Suite 214, Los Angeles, CA 90095, USA
* Corresponding author. Pfleger Liver Institute, UCLA Medical Center, 200 Medical Plaza, Suite 214, Los Angeles, CA 90095.
E-mail address: SSaab@mednet.ucla.edu

Clin Liver Dis 18 (2014) 205–218
http://dx.doi.org/10.1016/j.cld.2013.09.008
1089-3261/14/$ – see front matter © 2014 Elsevier Inc. All rights reserved.

Micronutrients, such as fat-soluble and water-soluble vitamins or various minerals, which are seen to be deficient in liver disease, lead to unique complications based on specific deficiencies.[7–13] These micronutrients and other nutrient deficiencies are being increasingly recognized as sequelae of liver disease.[14,15]

At the opposite end of the spectrum, obesity has also been shown to have significant effects on different stages of liver disease. The rate of obesity in the United States has been increasing over the past 3 decades. Obesity in adults has more than doubled in the period between 1970 and 2008, from 15% in the 1970s to 35% in 2008.[16] Equally important, obesity has almost tripled in the pediatric population from 15% in the 1970s to 48% in 2008.[16] These trends have been used to explain the exponential increase in nonalcoholic fatty liver disease (NAFLD) as a common cause of liver disease worldwide in both adult and pediatric populations.[12,17] Not only does obesity cause fatty liver, it also has been shown to increase morbidity and mortality in other existing liver conditions such as viral hepatitis or liver transplantation, and weight loss by itself has been shown to improve treatment outcomes in various hepatic conditions.[18] Indeed, morbid obesity is seen as such a poor prognostic factor for liver transplantation that many transplantation centers use a cutoff value above which they will not consider such candidates.

The myriad effects of the opposing ends of the nutrition spectrum have led to a wealth of research aimed at elucidating the exact mechanisms of how they cause liver damage. In this article, the role of the liver in nutrient and energy metabolism is discussed, as well as the known and possible effects of specific nutrient deficiencies and obesity.

ROLE OF THE LIVER IN NUTRIENT METABOLISM

In metabolism, the liver serves as an intermediary between dietary and endogenous sources of energy and the extrahepatic organs that use such energy.[19] The liver accomplishes this role by contributing to the synthesis, storage, or breakdown of most of the major macronutrients used by the body. In Western society these major macronutrient groups include carbohydrates, fats, and protein, and the major micronutrient groups include electrolytes, trace elements, and vitamins.[20] The liver also plays a role in the transport and storage of multiple micronutrients, and has various other functions (**Table 1**).

Gluconeogenesis, cholesterol synthesis, fatty acid oxidation, amino acid oxidation, ureagenesis, and bile acid production comprise just a fraction of the many functions performed by the liver.[19,21–23] The heterogeneity of these functions requires the liver to be organized in a heterogeneous pattern, allowing for different areas of the liver to specialize in a few of these functions so that other sites can specialize in various other functions.[24]

MALNUTRITION AND CHRONIC LIVER DISEASE

The fundamentals of how malnutrition occurs in and causes liver disease are 3-fold in nature. Chronic liver disease increases the energy and nutritional requirements of the body because liver disease can induce a hypermetabolic state that increases the resting expenditures of the body.[25–31] Patients with liver disease also have issues with increased nutrient losses from the body because of malabsorption resulting from decreased bile production, diarrhea, or other causes (**Table 2**). The third fundamental cause of malnutrition in patients with liver disease arises from patients having either a decreased intake of nutritional substances or an absolute decrease in food intake.[32,33] Mechanisms through which patients have decreased dietary intake are

Table 1
Role of liver in metabolism

Nutrient Group	Select Liver Functions
Protein	Synthesis of plasma proteins (transferrin, albumin, ceruloplasmin, etc) Deamination of amino acids to make urea Transamination and synthesis of amino acids Oxidation of amino acids
Carbohydrates	Gluconeogenesis Glycogenesis Glycogenolysis
Fat	Production of bile for solubilization and fat storage Synthesis of cholesterol and triglycerides Uptake and oxidation of fatty acids Synthesis of lipoproteins
Vitamins	Uptake and storage of multiple vitamins (A, D, E, B_{12}, K) Enzymatic activation of vitamins (B_6, B_1, D, folic acid) Vitamin transport (A, B_{12}, etc) through carrier proteins synthesized by liver
Minerals	Storage site for multiple minerals (zinc, iron, copper, etc)

Table 2
Select nutrient deficiencies and their relation to liver disease

Nutrient Group	Relation to Liver	Some Associated Signs/Symptoms
Protein	Decreased synthesis and transportation in liver disease	Muscle wasting Edema/ascites
Fat	Decreased absorption in liver disease	Scaly skin Soft/brittle nails
Vitamins		
Vitamin B_1 (thiamine)	Increased requirement in liver disease, especially alcoholic liver disease	Cheilosis
Vitamin B_6 (pyridoxine)	Increased degradation in liver disease	Weakness
Vitamin B_{12} (cyanocobalamin)	Malabsorption seen in liver disease	Neuropathy
Folate	Deficiency seen in liver disease	Anemia
Fat-soluble vitamins (A, D, E, K)	Malabsorption in liver disease	Night blindness Keratosis Osteoporosis Neuropathy Increased risk of bleeding
Minerals		
Zinc	Malabsorption and increased requirement in liver disease, thought to be a risk factor for encephalopathy[52,53]	Risk of infections Taste and smell changes Slow wound healing
Magnesium	Deficiency seen in liver disease	Taste changes

Data from Morrison S. Clinical nutrition physical examination. Support Line 1997;19(2):16–8; and Jeejeebhoy KN. Nutritional assessment. Gastroenterol Clin North Am 1998;27(2):347–69.

attributed to a multitude of factors, ranging from simple nausea and loss of taste to early satiety secondary to gastroparesis, ascites, bacterial overgrowth, or abnormal small-bowel motility.[34–36] Another major reason for decreased intake is the diet restrictions that must be followed by a person with chronic liver disease.

A common form of malnutrition seen in patients is referred to as protein-calorie malnutrition (PCM), the deficiency of protein and/or calories relative to a person's needs. PCM includes clinical syndromes such as Kwashiorkor, a deficiency of protein intake that is not commonly seen in the developed world but can lead to ascites, hepatomegaly, and NAFLD.[32] There is an abundance of evidence detailing the development of fatty liver possibly arising from derangements in lipoprotein synthesis, such as in patients with Kwashiorkor.[37,38] The proposed aberration in hepatic synthesis of lipoproteins is directly related to the fundamental principle regarding the decreased proportion of protein in one's diet leading to the development of liver disease, as amino acids are a major energy source for the liver.[19]

PCM can occur at any stage of liver disease. The clinical presentation is heterogeneous, and does not have specific histologic or biochemical parameters.[4] PCM is caused by a combination of all 3 principles: increased protein loss due to malabsorption, hypermetabolism of the liver, and decreased dietary intake.[26,30,39,40] Some of the most significant findings seen in patients with PCM are cachexia and muscle wasting that can sometimes be masked by the edema normally seen in liver disease.[6,40]

The importance of the liver in fatty acid metabolism, from the production of bile to the synthesis of cholesterol, makes it such that hepatic dysfunction can be assumed to also lead to disorders in fatty acid metabolism. Polyunsaturated fatty acid (PUFA) deficiency is one such characteristic that is commonly seen in cirrhotic patients.[14,33,41] The reason for PUFA deficiency in patients with liver disease is related to the synthesis of PUFAs from fatty acid precursors in the liver.[42] PUFAs are important constituents of plasma membranes that increase the fluidity of these membranes, and can also be used as a component of secondary messaging systems within the body.[42] Although the deficiency of PUFAs is worth noting, the consequences of this deficiency are still unknown.[43]

Micronutrient deficiencies are also commonly seen in liver disease, and are also associated with many complications. Fat-soluble vitamins can become deficient in patients with liver disease, especially cholestatic liver disease, because of decreased bile production, decreased oral intake, derangement in hepatic synthesis of carrier proteins for transport, and other causes.[44] Vitamin D is another fat-soluble vitamin affected by liver disease. Recent studies have shown that vitamin D is used in the body for roles outside of simple calcium regulation, including anti-inflammatory, anti-fibrotic, and immunomodulatory roles.[13] In one study, more than 90% of patients with advanced liver disease were recorded to be deficient in vitamin D.[45] Vitamin D deficiency is a common complication of liver disease that has been associated with osteoporosis in cirrhosis for some time.[9] The proposed mechanism of vitamin D deficiency involves a defect in hepatic synthesis.[8] Vitamin E is a fat-soluble vitamin well known for its antioxidant properties. In one study this vitamin was deficient in nearly half of all the cirrhotic patients in the cohort.[46] Studies have suggested a link between vitamin E deficiency and the progression of NAFLD to nonalcoholic steatohepatitis (NASH).[47] The final fat-soluble vitamin is vitamin K, which is used in the synthesis of clotting factors. Vitamin K deficiency usually manifests as bleeding. The effects of liver disease on vitamin K are less well studied, but it has been recommended that for patients with impaired prothrombin time and/or International Normalized Ratio, vitamin K supplementation can be considered.[48]

Water-soluble vitamin deficiencies also commonly occur in liver disease. The liver is required for the activation and transport of vitamin B_1 and B_6, and other vitamins.[7] Thiamine (vitamin B_1) deficiency is a well-recognized complication of alcoholic liver disease (ALD) leading to the Wernicke encephalopathy and Korsakoff syndrome. Thiamine deficiency can also be seen in other chronic liver diseases along with other water-soluble vitamin deficiencies such as niacin (B_3), ascorbic acid (C), and pyridoxine (B_6) deficiency.[7] Rossouw and colleagues[7] showed that 88% of patients with decompensated chronic liver disease had deficiencies of all the aforementioned, and a variable number of patients with alcoholic and nonalcoholic liver disease had variable rates of deficiencies in these vitamins. Cyanocobalamin (B_{12}) and folate (B_2) have also been found to be deficient in patients with liver disease. The blood test for B_{12} is usually falsely elevated because of the inclusion of endogenous metabolically inactive forms of cobalamin, even though tissue stores usually are depleted.[49]

Many minerals are also affected in patients with liver disease. Indeed one of the possible explanations as to why patients have decreased dietary intake in liver disease has been linked to zinc or magnesium deficiencies, which cause dysgeusia or altered taste sensation.[35] Zinc deficiency generally has been associated with ALD for some time. Zinc deficiency is thought to be partially due to the same principles stated earlier of decreased intake, increased losses due to malabsorption, an increased dietary requirement and, possibly, diuretic induced.[33,44,50] Zinc deficiency leads to many complications including altered taste and smell, immune dysfunction, and altered protein metabolism,[44,51] and has also been thought to precipitate hepatic encephalopathy.[52,53] Magnesium deficiency affects a person's appetite, and magnesium levels have been shown to be an independent predictor of muscle strength.[54] Whether this is due to cirrhosis or heavy alcohol use is still debated, and whether magnesium supplementation is truly useful is also under debate.[55,56] Other minerals, such as selenium, are affected by liver disease but with less obvious effects.[51]

The complications and deficiencies of nutrients seen in liver disease and the severity of malnutrition do not seem to be directly related to the etiology of liver disease.[57] That being said, there is some controversy as to whether ALD leads to poorer nutritional status in comparison with other causes of liver disease.[57] Thuluvath and Triger[58] and Caregaro and colleagues[59] have reported that there is no difference in the prevalence and severity of malnutrition seen in patients with ALD in comparison with viral liver disease, but Caly and colleagues[60] found that patients with ALD cirrhosis seemed to have poorer nutritional status when compared with hepatitis C virus cirrhosis. These conflicting data indicate that the effects, prevalence, and severity of malnutrition in chronic liver disease require further study and assessment.

OBESITY AND CHRONIC LIVER DISEASE

If malnutrition is one extreme of the nutrition spectrum, it follows that obesity would be on the opposite extreme. Obesity can lead to a variety of health complications such as hypertension, diabetes, increased cardiovascular risk, and metabolic syndrome, and has even been linked to higher rates of multiple cancers including liver cancer.[61] To address this problem the American Medical Association has recently classified obesity as a disease, perhaps to give physicians an incentive to discuss the complicated and sensitive subject of weight-related health issues with their patients.[62] Obesity has many different causes, from genetics to environmental and psychosocial factors.

The current increased incidence of obesity is most likely related to the trend of decreased physical activity and increased caloric intake seen in the United States, although genetics also play a role in its development, given the increased rates of obesity seen among family members.[63,64]

Obesity has been implicated as a risk factor for the development of liver disease. Some population-based studies have shown that almost one-third of the adult population of the United States has hepatic steatosis to some extent.[65]

The mechanism of how obesity leads to NAFLD is not yet clear, but important issues to note are that the accumulation of triglycerides in the liver occurs through several pathways.[66,67] Another important factor believed to play a major role in the development of fatty liver is the development of insulin resistance.[63,68–75] In fact, NAFLD is considered to be the hepatic component of the metabolic syndrome.[76] The increased uptake and synthesis of free fatty acids (FFAs) in the liver, through the mechanism of inducing free oxygen radicals, can have a direct toxic effect on the liver besides causing hepatic steatosis. Other major targets of research in the development of NAFLD include the study of hormones called adipokines. One such hormone, adiponectin, is secreted by adipose tissue that, along with other functions, enhances lipid clearance from the plasma and increases β-oxidation of fatty acids in muscle.[77] Low adiponectin levels have been associated with the presence of NAFLD, hepatic fibrosis, and metabolic syndrome.[78] Even though obese patients have increased amounts of adipose tissue, there appear to be decreased levels of adiponectin.[79] Another interesting piece of evidence of obesity's effect comes from Viljanen and colleagues,[80] who were able to demonstrate that rapid weight loss directly affected the liver in that it decreased FFA uptake, increased insulin sensitivity, and decreased liver triglyceride content by almost 60%.

As well as being a risk factor for the development of NAFLD, obesity has also been shown to be a risk factor for the progression of NAFLD to NASH, and finally to cirrhosis.[81] In a study conducted on overweight individuals by Ratziu and colleagues,[81] 30% of patients with abnormal liver function tests in which liver biopsies were collected had septal fibrosis, and 11% of those patients had silent cirrhosis, proving that simply being overweight can cause liver damage.

Obesity is not only associated with the development of liver disease in NAFLD, but also adversely affects the progression, treatment, and complication rates of other liver diseases. Everhart and colleagues[82] demonstrated that there was an association between several weight-related measures, such as insulin resistance, and progression of liver disease in patients with hepatitis C. Other liver diseases can also be affected by steatosis, such as ALD, hemochromatosis, or other forms of viral hepatitis.[83,84] As obesity is a risk factor for the progression of liver disease to cirrhosis, it can also be extrapolated as a risk factor for liver cancers. It has been shown that in the United States, obesity can almost double the risk of contracting hepatocellular carcinoma.[85]

Liver transplant recipients are also affected by the presence of obesity. Multiple epidemiologic studies have shown that liver transplantation increases the risk of the metabolic syndrome, with reported rates ranging from 48% to 53%.[86–89] Although the risk of metabolic syndrome and related comorbidities that occur in liver transplantation is multifactorial, the role of obesity cannot be understated, and counseling regarding the management of obesity should be initiated in patients undergoing, or who are planning to undergo, liver transplantation.[18] The multiple detrimental roles that obesity plays in chronic liver disease makes it an imminent health issue that should be aggressively addressed to both decrease rates of liver disease and increase treatment successes.

ASSESSMENT OF NUTRITIONAL STATUS

The undeniable importance of a patient's nutritional status makes the accurate assessment of such status equally important. However, many factors complicate the assessment of nutritional status among patients with chronic liver disease, especially cirrhosis.[6] Many common parameters for nutritional assessment may not be as useful. Weight, for example, is usually decreased among malnourished patients with healthy livers, but may be increased in patients with chronic liver disease because of edema and ascites, even though lean body mass is decreased. Methods such as food-frequency questionnaires, food diaries, or calorie counting are effective first tools for the assessment of a patient's dietary history.[90–93]

Many of the anthropomorphic measures are not performed in clinical practice (**Table 3**).[94,95] Potential limitations can include problems such as poor interobserver reproducibility or possible overestimation owing to third-spacing of fluid.[2] One commonly used measure is the hand-grip strength, which is used to detect for the presence of malnutrition.[6,96] Another important tool used to estimate a patient's nutritional status is the Subjective Global Assessment (SGA).[97] This method is a subjective assessment based on a clinician's knowledge and experience in the context of specific variables. Laboratory testing is also useful in assessing nutritional status. Tests such as serum albumin, retinol-binding protein, transferrin, and others can be useful for detecting deficiencies seen in liver disease.[94] Alterations can occur on conventional laboratory testing of patients with chronic liver disease, because the underlying disease makes difficult the distinction between whether the abnormal test was due to the liver disease or the nutritional status.[6,98] The combination of laboratory values and physical measurements has been led to the creation of the Prognostic Nutritional Index (PNI). This index is obtained by plugging into a formula the laboratory values of albumin, transferrin, and lymphocyte score with the anthropomorphic measure of triceps skin-fold thickness; the higher the PNI, the higher the risk of malnutrition. The use of this index is controversial because studies have shown that objective measurements such as this underestimate the true prevalence of malnutrition in patients.[96,99]

GENERAL MANAGEMENT STRATEGIES FOR POOR NUTRITIONAL STATUS IN CHRONIC LIVER DISEASE

The management of obesity and malnutrition in chronic liver disease sounds simple in theory. Modifying dietary and lifestyle habits of patients should correct the issue, but the full effects of this therapy have not been fully elucidated.

With obesity implicated as a risk factor for developing NAFLD, it follows that treating this condition by losing weight should help reduce the risk of NAFLD. Indeed, many studies have shown that weight loss and increased physical activity can lead to

Table 3
Common anthropometric measurements in liver disease

Tool	Measured
Mid-arm muscle circumference (MAMC)	Assesses muscle mass
Skin-fold thickness (triceps, biceps, etc)	Assesses body fat
Hand-grip strength (HGS)	Assesses strength as a measure of malnutrition
Body cell mass (BCM)	Assesses body composition
Body mass index (BMI)	Measures the weight
Waist circumference	Measures abdominal adiposity

improvement in liver enzymes and liver histology in patients with NAFLD.[76,100–105] Other clinically beneficial effects on the liver of weight loss have included decreased fatty acid uptake and storage, and increased insulin sensitivity.[80] One study showed that weight loss in excess of 0.28 kg/d can lead to portal fibrosis, whereas patients with weight loss of 0.15 kg/d did not have the same histologic issues, suggesting that rapid weight loss can in fact be detrimental to the liver as opposed to more gradual weight loss.[104] Another issue is that other studies have not shown the same improvement in liver histology after weight loss, and have reported even worsening inflammation in NAFLD with a low-fat and low-calorie diet, indicating that further research to evaluate the best method of treatment needs to be conducted.[106,107]

Another avenue for weight loss in patients, and a common practice today in obese individuals, is bariatric surgery. Multiple studies have been done to evaluate whether bariatric surgery aids in the healing process of NAFLD. Just as for the effect of diet change, the evidence here is also conflicting. One review noted that most studies showed an improvement in liver inflammation and fibrosis, but several studies showed a worsening in fibrosis.[108,109] Further data are needed to fully understand whether bariatric surgery will be useful for patients with liver disease.

The case for treating malnutrition in chronic liver disease is more complicated than with obesity, in that questions arise as to whether any deficiency seen should be corrected or if specific deficiencies are more important than others. A Cochrane review meta-analysis of available data has found that there is no clear morbidity or mortality benefit in nutrition supplementation, meaning other than the food a patient eats, of any kind, orally, enteral, or parenteral, even when specific nutrient deficiencies have been identified and can be corrected.[110] This finding throws into question whether nutrient supplementation should even be attempted. Although there is a good case for the supplementation of certain nutrients, such as vitamins D or E, further study is required to demonstrate such a benefit.[13,111–113]

SUMMARY

As both malnutrition and obesity have a significant impact on the development and exacerbation of liver disease, it is important to further the understanding of the exact impact of the different nutrients on the liver and the role played by the liver in metabolism. Much of what is known about the impact of these 2 conditions has not kept up with the times, with most of the information still shrouded in mystery. The pathogenesis of how the liver is affected by these 2 conditions is well accepted throughout the medical community, but without specific assessment and treatment guidelines there is still much variation in how these conditions are tackled by different physicians and institutions. Further research into discovering the potential value of treating these 2 conditions in liver disease will pave the way for developing the necessary guidelines. Standardizing treatment to follow specific guidelines should be useful in furthering the approach to treating chronic liver disease.

REFERENCES

1. Merli M, Riggio O, Dally L. PINC. Does malnutrition affect survival in cirrhosis? Hepatology 1996;23(5):1041–6.
2. Prijatmoko D, Strauss BJ, Lambert JR, et al. Early detection of protein depletion in alcoholic cirrhosis: role of body composition analysis. Gastroenterology 1993; 105(6):1839–45.
3. McCullough AJ, Bugianesi E. Protein calorie malnutrition and the etiology of cirrhosis. Am J Gastroenterol 1997;92(5):734–8.

4. Lautz HU, Selberg O, Korber J, et al. Protein calorie malnutrition in liver cirrhosis. Clin Investig 1992;70(6):478–86.
5. DiCecco SR, Wieners EJ, Wiesner RH, et al. Assessment of nutritional status of patients with end stage liver disease undergoing liver transplantation. Mayo Clin Proc 1989;64(1):95–102.
6. Henkel AS, Buchman AL. Nutritional support in patients with chronic liver disease. Nat Clin Pract Gastroenterol Hepatol 2006;3(4):202–9.
7. Rossouw JE, Labadarios D, Davis M, et al. Water-soluble vitamins in severe liver disease. S Afr Med J 1978;54(5):183–6.
8. Mawer EB, Klass HJ, Warnes TW, et al. Metabolism of vitamin D in patients with primary biliary cirrhosis and alcoholic liver disease. Clin Sci (Lond) 1985;69(5): 561–70.
9. Mobarhan SA, Russell RM, Recker RR, et al. Metabolic bone disease in alcoholic cirrhosis: a comparison of the effect of vitamin D2, 25-hydroxyvitamin D, or supportive treatment. Hepatology 1984;4(2):266–73.
10. Gruengreiff K, Gruengreiff S, Reinhold D. Zinc deficiency and hepatic encephalopathy: results of a long term follow-up on zinc supplementation. J Trace Elem Exp Med 2000;13(1):21–31.
11. Collier JD, Ninkovic M, Compston JE. Guidelines on the management of osteoporosis associated with chronic liver disease. Gut 2002;50(Suppl 1):i1–9.
12. Tsouka A, Mclin VA. Complications of chronic liver disease. Clin Res Hepatol Gastroenterol 2012;36(3):262–7.
13. Kitson MT, Roberts SK. D-livering the message: the importance of vitamin D status in chronic liver disease. J Hepatol 2012;57(4):897–909.
14. Duerksen DR, Nehra V, Palombo JD, et al. Essential fatty acid deficiencies in patients with chronic liver disease are not reversed by short-term intravenous lipid supplementation. Dig Dis Sci 1999;44(7):1342–8.
15. Vos MB, Ryan C, Patricia B, et al, the NASH CRN Research Group. Correlation of vitamin E, uric acid and diet composition with histologic features of pediatric nonalcoholic fatty liver disease. J Pediatr Gastroenterol Nutr 2012;54(1):90–6.
16. Dietary guidelines for Americans. 2010. Available at: www.dietaryguidelines. gov. Accessed July 7, 2013.
17. Diehl AM. Hepatic complications of obesity. Gastroenterol Clin North Am 2010; 39(1):57–68.
18. Nobili V, Carter-Kent C, Feldstein AE. The role of lifestyle changes in the management of chronic liver disease. BMC Med 2011;9:70.
19. Muller MJ. Hepatic energy and substrate metabolism: a possible metabolic basis for early nutritional support in cirrhotic patients. Nutrition 1998;14(1):30–8.
20. Jungermann K, Kietzmann T. Zonation of parenchymal and nonparenchymal metabolism in the liver. Annu Rev Nutr 1996;16:179–203.
21. Sherlock S. Carbohydrates changes in liver disease. Am J Clin Nutr 1970;22(4): 462–6.
22. Tavill AS. The synthesis and degradation of liver-produced proteins. Gut 1972; 13(3):225–41.
23. Hasse J. Nutrition and liver disease: complex connections. Nutr Clin Pract 2013; 28(1):12–4.
24. Racine-Samson L, Scoazec JY, D'Errico A, et al. The metabolic organization of the adult human liver: a comparative study of normal, fibrotic, and cirrhotic liver tissue. Hepatology 1996;24(1):104–13.
25. Merli M, Riggio O, Romiti A, et al. Basal energy production rate and substrate use in stable cirrhotic patients. Hepatology 1990;12(1):106–12.

26. Green JH, Bramley PN, Losowsky MS. Are patients with primary biliary cirrhosis hypermetabolic? A comparison between patients before and after liver transplantation and controls. Hepatology 1991;14(3):464–72.
27. Shanbhogue RL, Bistrian BR, Jenkins RL, et al. Resting energy expenditure in patients with end-stage liver disease and in normal population. JPEN J Parenter Enteral Nutr 1987;11(3):305–8.
28. Schneeweiss B, Graninger W, Ferenci P, et al. Energy metabolism in patients with acute and chronic liver disease. Hepatology 1990;11(3):387–93.
29. Muller MJ, Boker KH, Selberg O. Are patients with liver cirrhosis hypermetabolic? Clin Nutr 1994;13(3):131–44.
30. Muller MJ, Bottcher J, Selberg O, et al. Hypermetabolism in clinically stable patients with liver cirrhosis. Am J Clin Nutr 1999;69(6):1194–201.
31. Delissio M, Goodyear LJ, Fuller S, et al. Effects of treadmill exercise on fuel metabolism in hepatic cirrhosis. J Appl Physiol 1991;70(1):210–5.
32. Grover Z, Ee LC. Protein energy malnutrition. Pediatr Clin North Am 2009;56(5): 1055–68.
33. O'Brien A, Williams R. Nutrition in end-stage liver disease: principles and practice. Gastroenterology 2008;134:1729–40.
34. Thuluvath PJ, Triger DR. Autonomic neuropathy in chronic liver disease. Q J Med 1989;72(268):737–47.
35. Madden AM, Bradbury W, Morgan MY. Taste perception in cirrhosis: its relationship to circulating micronutrients and food preferences. Hepatology 1997;26(1):40–8.
36. Quigley EM. Gastrointestinal dysfunction in liver disease and portal hypertension. Gut-liver interaction revisited. Dig Dis Sci 1996;41(3):557–61.
37. Truswell AS, Hansen JD, Watson CE, et al. Relation of serum lipids and lipoproteins to fatty liver in Kwashiorkor. Am J Clin Nutr 1969;22(5):568–76.
38. Flores H, Pak N, Maccioni A, et al. Lipid transport in Kwashiorkor. Br J Nutr 1970; 24(4):1005–11.
39. Dolz C, Raurich JM, Ibanez J, et al. Ascites increases the resting energy expenditure in liver cirrhosis. Gastroenterology 1991;100(3):738–44.
40. Peng S, Plank LD, McCall JL, et al. Body composition, muscle function, and energy expenditure in patients with liver cirrhosis: a comprehensive study. Am J Clin Nutr 2007;85(5):1257–66.
41. Cabre E, Periago JL, Abad-Lacruz A, et al. Plasma fatty acid profile in advanced cirrhosis: unsaturation deficit of lipid fractions. Am J Gastroenterol 1990;85(12): 1597–604.
42. Cabre E, Gassull MA. Polyunsaturated fatty acid deficiencies in liver diseases: pathophysiological and clinical significance. Nutrition 1996;12:542–8.
43. Cabre E, Gassull MA. Feeding long-chain PUFA to advanced cirrhotics: is it worthwhile? Nutrition 1999;15:322–4.
44. Johnson TM, Overgard EB, Cohen AE, et al. Nutrition assessment and management in advanced liver disease. Nutr Clin Pract 2013;28(1):15–29.
45. Arteh J, Narra S, Nair S. Prevalence of vitamin D deficiency in chronic liver disease. Dig Dis Sci 2010;55(9):2624–8.
46. Look MP, Reichel C, Von Falkenhausen M, et al. Vitamin E status in patients with liver cirrhosis: normal or deficient? Metabolism 1999;48(1):86–91.
47. Cankutaran M, Kav T, Yavuz B, et al. Serum vitamin E levels and its relation to clinical features in nonalcoholic fatty liver disease with elevated ALT levels. Acta Gastroenterol Belg 2006;69(1):5–11.
48. Kowdley KV, Emond MJ, Sadowsky JA, et al. Plasma vitamin K1 level is decreased in primary biliary cirrhosis. Am J Gastroenterol 1997;92(11):2059–61.

49. Baker H, Leevy CB, DeAngelis B, et al. Cobalamin (Vitamin B_{12}) and holotran-scobalamin changes in plasma and liver tissues in alcoholics with liver disease. J Am Coll Nutr 1998;17(3):235–8.
50. Cheung K, Lee SS, Raman M. Prevalence and mechanisms of malnutrition in patients with advanced liver disease, and nutrition management strategies. Clin Gastroenterol Hepatol 2012;10(2):117–25.
51. Lin CC. Selenium, iron, copper, zinc levels and copper-to-zinc ratios in serum of patients at different stages of viral hepatic diseases. Biol Trace Elem Res 2006; 109(1):15–24.
52. van der Rijt CC, Schalm SW, Schat H, et al. Overt hepatic encephalopathy precipitated by zinc deficiency. Gastroenterology 1991;100(4):1114–8.
53. Rahelic D, Kujundzic M, Romic Z, et al. Serum concentrations of zinc, copper, manganese, and magnesium in patients with liver cirrhosis. Coll Antropol 2006;30(3):523–8.
54. Aargaard NK, Andersen H, Vilstrup H, et al. Muscle strength, Na,K-pumps, magnesium and potassium in patients with alcoholic liver cirrhosis—relation to spironolactone. J Intern Med 2002;252(1):56–63.
55. Aargaard NK, Andersen H, Vilstrup H, et al. Decreased muscle strength and contents of Mg and Na,K-pumps in chronic alcoholics occur independently of cirrhosis. J Intern Med 2003;253(3):359–66.
56. Aargaard NK, Andersen H, Vilstrup H, et al. Magnesium supplementation and muscle function in patients with alcoholic liver disease: a randomized-placebo-controlled trial. Scand J Gastroenterol 2005;40(8):972–9.
57. Cabre E, Gassull MA. Nutrition in liver disease. Curr Opin Clin Nutr Metab Care 2005;8(5):545–51.
58. Thuluvath PJ, Triger DR. Evaluation of nutritional status by using anthropometry in adults with alcoholic and non-alcoholic liver disease. Am J Clin Nutr 1994;60: 269–73.
59. Caregaro L, Alberino F, Amodio P, et al. Malnutrition in alcoholic and virus-related cirrhosis. Am J Clin Nutr 1996;63(4):602–9.
60. Caly WR, Strauss E, Carrilho FJ, et al. Different degrees of malnutrition and immunological alterations according to aetiology of cirrhosis: a prospective and sequential study. Nutr J 2003;2:10.
61. Calle EE, Rodriguez C, Walker-Thurmond K, et al. Overweight, obesity, and mortality from cancer in a prospectively studied cohort of US adults. N Engl J Med 2003;348(17):1625–38.
62. Frellick M. AMA declares obesity a disease. Medscape Medical News 2013. Available at: http://www.medscape.com/viewarticle/806566. Accessed July 17, 2013.
63. Willner IR, Waters B, Patil SR, et al. Ninety patients with nonalcoholic steatohepatitis: insulin resistance, familial tendency, and severity of disease. Am J Gastroenterol 2001;96(10):2957–61.
64. Lyon HN, Hirschorn JN. Genetics of common forms of obesity: a brief review. Am J Clin Nutr 2005;82(1):2155–75.
65. Browning JD, Szczepaniak LS, Dobbins R, et al. Prevalence of hepatic steatosis in an urban population in the United States: impact of ethnicity. Hepatology 2004;40(6):1387–95.
66. Donnelly KL, Smith CI, Schwarzenberg SJ, et al. Sources of fatty acids stored in liver and secreted via lipoproteins in patients with nonalcoholic fatty liver disease. J Clin Invest 2005;115(5):1343–51.
67. Bjorntorp P. Abdominal obesity and the metabolic syndrome. Ann Med 1992; 24(6):465–8.

68. Sheth SG, Gordon FD, Chopra S. Nonalcoholic steatohepatitis. Ann Intern Med 1997;126(2):137–45.
69. Sanyal AJ, Campbell-Sargent C, Mirshahi F, et al. Nonalcoholic steatohepatitis: association of insulin resistance and mitochondrial abnormalities. Gastroenterology 2001;120(5):1183–92.
70. Chitturi S, Abeygunasekara S, Farrell GC, et al. NASH and insulin resistance: insulin hypersecretion and specific association with the insulin resistance syndrome. Hepatology 2002;35(2):373–9.
71. Pagano G, Pacini G, Musso G, et al. Nonalcoholic steatohepatitis, insulin resistance, and metabolic syndrome: further evidence for an etiologic association. Hepatology 2002;35(2):367–72.
72. Marchesini G, Brizi M, Morselli-Labate AM, et al. Association of nonalcoholic fatty liver disease with insulin resistance. Am J Med 1999;107(5):450–5.
73. Hamaguchi M, Kojima T, Takeda N, et al. The metabolic syndrome as a predictor of nonalcoholic fatty liver disease. Ann Intern Med 2005;143(10):722–8.
74. Marchesini G, Brizi M, Bianchi G, et al. Nonalcoholic fatty liver disease: a feature of the metabolic syndrome. Diabetes 2001;50(8):1844–50.
75. Gholam PM, Flancbaum L, Machan JT, et al. Nonalcoholic fatty liver disease in severely obese subjects. Am J Gastroenterol 2007;102(2):399–408.
76. Oza N, Eguchi Y, Mizuta T, et al. A pilot trial of body weight reduction for nonalcoholic fatty liver disease with a home-based lifestyle modification intervention delivered in collaboration with interdisciplinary medical staff. J Gastroenterol 2009;44(12):1203–8.
77. Xu A, Wang Y, Keshaw H, et al. The fat-derived hormone adiponectin alleviates alcoholic and nonalcoholic fatty liver disease in mice. J Clin Invest 2003;112(1):91–100.
78. Savvidou S, Hytiroglou P, Orfanau-Koumerkeridou H, et al. Low serum adiponectin levels are predictive of advanced hepatic fibrosis in patients with NAFLD. J Clin Gastroenterol 2009;43(8):765–72.
79. Arita Y, Kihara S, Ouchi N, et al. Paradoxical decrease of an adipose-specific protein, adiponectin, in obesity. Biochem Biophys Res Commun 1999;257(1):79–83.
80. Viljanen AP, Iozzo P, Borra R, et al. Effect of weight loss on liver free fatty acid uptake and hepatic insulin resistance. J Clin Endocrinol Metab 2009;94(1):50–5.
81. Ratziu V, Giral P, Charlotte F, et al. Liver fibrosis in overweight patients. Gastroenterology 2000;118:1117–23.
82. Everhart JE, Lok AS, Kim HY, et al, HALT-C trial group. Weight-related effects on disease progression in the hepatitis C antiviral long-term treatment against cirrhosis trial. Gastroenterology 2009;137(2):549–57.
83. Powell EE, Jonsson JR, Clouston AD. Steatosis: co-factor in other liver diseases. Hepatology 2005;42(1):5–13.
84. Persico M, Iolascon A. Steatosis as a co-factor in chronic liver diseases. World J Gastroenterol 2010;16(10):1171–6.
85. Welzel TM, Graubard BI, Zeuzem S, et al. Metabolic syndrome increases the risk of primary liver cancer in the United States: a study in the SEER-Medicare database. Hepatology 2011;54(2):463–71.
86. Laish I, Braun M, Mor E, et al. Metabolic syndrome in liver transplant recipients: prevalence, risk factors, and association with cardiovascular events. Liver Transpl 2011;17(1):15–22.
87. Laryea M, Watt KD, Molinari M, et al. Metabolic syndrome in liver transplant recipients: prevalence and association with major vascular events. Liver Transpl 2007;13(8):1109–14.

88. Francioso S, Angelico F, Baiocchi L, et al. High prevalence of metabolic syndrome and long-term survival after liver transplantation. J Hepatol 2008;14:S82.
89. Bianchi G, Marchesini G, Marzocchi R, et al. Metabolic syndrome in liver transplantation: relation to etiology and immunosuppression. Liver Transpl 2008;14: 1648–54.
90. Mueller CM. The American Society for Parenteral and Enteral Nutrition (A.S.P.E.N) adult nutrition support core curriculum. 2nd edition. Silver Spring (MD): American Society for Parenteral and Enteral Nutrition; 2012.
91. Schatzkin A, Kipnis V, Carroll RJ, et al. Comparison of a food frequency questionnaire with a 24-hour recall for use in an epidemiological cohort study: results from the biomarker-based Observing Protein and Energy Nutrition (OPEN) study. Int J Epidemiol 2003;32(6):1054–62.
92. Brunner E, Stallone D, Juneja M, et al. Dietary Assessment in Whitehall II: comparison of 7 d diet diary and food-frequency questionnaire and validity against biomarkers. Br J Nutr 2001;86(3):405–14.
93. Krall EA, Dwyer JT. Validity of a food frequency questionnaire and a food diary in a short-term recall situation. J Am Diet Assoc 1987;87(10):1374–7.
94. McCullough AJ, Mullen KD, Smanik EJ, et al. Nutrition therapy and liver disease. Gastroenterol Clin North Am 1989;18:619–41.
95. Carvalha L, Parise ER. Evaluation of nutritional status of non hospitalized patients with liver cirrhosis. Arq Gastroenterol 2006;43:269–74.
96. Alvares-Da-Silva MR, Reverbel da Silveira T. Comparison between handgrip strength, subjective global assessment, and prognostic nutritional index in assessing malnutrition and predicting clinical outcome in cirrhotic outpatients. Nutrition 2005;21(2):113–7.
97. Detsky AS, McLaughlin JR, Baker JP, et al. What is subjective global assessment of nutritional status? JPEN J Parenter Enteral Nutr 1987;11(1):8–13.
98. Chadalavada R, Sappati Biyyani RS, Maxwell J, et al. Nutrition in hepatic encephalopathy. Nutr Clin Pract 2010;25(3):257–64.
99. Baker JP, Detsky AS, Wesson DE, et al. Nutritional assessment: a comparison of clinical judgment and objective measurements. N Engl J Med 1982;306(16): 969–72.
100. Hickman IJ, Jonsson JR, Prins JB, et al. Modest weight loss and physical activity in overweight patients with chronic liver disease results in sustained improvements in alanine aminotransferase, fasting insulin, and quality of life. Gut 2004;53(3):413–9.
101. Dixon JB, Bathal PS, Hughes NR, et al. Nonalcoholic fatty liver disease: improvement in liver histological analysis with weight loss. Hepatology 2004; 39(6):1647–54.
102. Peterson KF, Dufour S, Befroy D, et al. Reversal of nonalcoholic hepatic steatosis, hepatic insulin resistance, and hyperglycemia by moderate weight reduction in patients with type 2 diabetes. Diabetes 2005;54(3):603–8.
103. Promrat K, Kleiner DE, Niemeier HM, et al. Randomized controlled trial testing the effects of weight loss on nonalcoholic steatohepatitis. Hepatology 2010; 51(1):121–9.
104. Keating SE, Hackett DA, George J, et al. Exercise and nonalcoholic fatty liver disease: a systematic review and meta-analysis. J Hepatol 2012;57(1): 157–66.
105. Larson-Meyer DE, Heilbronn LK, Redman LM, et al. Effect of calorie restriction with or without exercise on insulin sensitivity, beta-cell function, fat-cell size, and ectopic lipid in overweight subjects. Diabetes Care 2006;29:1337–44.

106. Solga S, Alkhuraishe AR, Clark JM, et al. Dietary composition and nonalcoholic fatty liver disease. Dig Dis Sci 2004;49(10):1578–83.
107. Ueno T, Sugawara H, Sujaku K, et al. Therapeutic effects of restricted diet and exercise in obese patients with fatty liver. J Hepatol 1997;27(1):103–7.
108. Chavez-Tapia NC, Tellez-Avila FI, Barrientos-Gutierrez T, et al. Bariatric surgery for nonalcoholic steatohepatitis in obese patients. Cochrane Database Syst Rev 2010;(1):CD007340.
109. Stephen S, Baranova A, Younossi ZM. Nonalcoholic fatty liver disease and bariatric surgery. Expert Rev Gastroenterol Hepatol 2012;6(2):163–71.
110. Koretz RL, Avenell A, Lipman TO. Nutritional support for liver disease. Cochrane Database Syst Rev 2012;(5):CD008344.
111. Sanyal AJ, Mofrad PS, Contos MJ, et al. A pilot study of vitamin E versus vitamin E and pioglitazone for the treatment of nonalcoholic steatohepatitis. Clin Gastroenterol Hepatol 2004;2(12):1107–15.
112. Harrison SA, Torgerson S, Hayashi P, et al. Vitamin E and vitamin C treatment improves fibrosis in patients with nonalcoholic steatohepatitis. Clin Gastroenterol Hepatol 2004;2(12):1107–15.
113. Lavine JE. Vitamin E treatment of nonalcoholic steatohepatitis in children: a pilot study. J Pediatr 2000;136(6):734–8.

Obesity, Nutrition, and Liver Disease in Children

Ariel E. Feldstein, MD[a,b,*], Dana Patton-Ku, MD[a,b],
Kerri N. Boutelle, PhD[a,c,d]

KEYWORDS

- Obesity • Nutrition • Liver disease • Children

KEY POINTS

- One-third of children in the United States are overweight or obese.
- Overweight children can suffer from a host of comorbid conditions and should be screened appropriately.
- Making the diagnosis of nonalcoholic or metabolic fatty liver disease in children remains difficult, given the impracticality of liver biopsy and the lack of reliable biomarkers.
- The gold standard for childhood weight loss is family-based behavioral therapy, with 30% of children no longer overweight at 10-year follow-up.
- Pharmacologic intervention for weight loss is limited in children and for liver disease is limited to those children with nonalcoholic steatohepatitis.

SCOPE OF THE PROBLEM
Epidemiology of Obesity

Children have natural weight fluctuations as they grow, therefore defining overweight in youth requires standardized growth charts that account for sex and age. Currently, for children aged 2 to 18 years, overweight is defined as a body mass index (BMI, calculated as weight in kilograms divided by the square of height in meters) in the

Funding: the work was funded by NIH (DK076852 and DK082451 to AEF), T32 DK007202-37 (DPK) and (DK075861, HL112042 DK094475 to KNB).
Disclosure of Financial and Competing Interests: Dr Feldstein reports that he is named as coinventor on pending and issued patents filed by the Cleveland Clinic and University of California San Diego that refer to the use of biomarkers in fatty liver disorders. Dr Patton-Ku and Dr Boutelle have no financial disclosures.
[a] Division of Pediatric Gastroenterology, Hepatology, and Nutrition, Rady Children's Hospital, 3020 Children's Way, San Diego, CA 92123, USA; [b] Division of Pediatric Gastroenterology, Hepatology, and Nutrition, University of California, San Diego, 9500 Gilman Drive, MC 0984, La Jolla, CA 92093, USA; [c] Department of Pediatrics, University of California, San Diego, 9500 Gilman Drive, 0874 La Jolla, CA 92093-0874, USA; [d] Department of Psychiatry, University of California, San Diego, 9500 Gilman Drive, 0874 La Jolla, CA 92093-0874, USA
* Corresponding author. Division of Pediatric Gastroenterology, Hepatology, and Nutrition, University of California, San Diego.
E-mail address: afeldstein@ucsd.edu

85th percentile or greater and obesity is BMI in the 95th percentile or greater, adjusted for sex and age.[1] In children younger than 2 years, a weight-for-length value greater than 95th percentile for age and sex is categorized as overweight. There are no normative data for BMI in this age group. Recent data from the 2009 to 2010 National Health and Nutrition Examination Survey showed that 31.8% of children aged 2 to 19 years were overweight or obese and 16.9% of children were obese.[2] The prevalence of obesity in children has increased 3-fold from the 1960s and 1970s.[3]

Comorbid Conditions

With the increasing prevalence of obesity in children, there has been a concomitant increase in the medical consequences of obesity in children. Overweight and obesity have been associated with orthopedic complications (slipped capital femoral epiphysis and Blount disease), asthma, sleep apnea, diabetes mellitus type 2, dyslipidemia, liver disease, and hypertension.[4] In addition, obese children often become obese adults.[5] Overweight and obese children also incur greater medical costs from more frequent laboratory studies,[6] greater numbers of sick visits, and greater use of mental health services.[7] In terms of psychosocial comorbidities, obese children have reported lower health-related quality of life[8] and had lower self-worth compared with normal-weight children.[9] Studies on depression in obese children are mixed, with some studies linking obesity to depression and some showing no difference when compared with normal-weight peers.[10] Eating disorders may be more frequent among obese youth, with 1 cross-sectional study showing that 30% of severely obese adolescent girls manifested unequivocal binge eating.[11] There may also be higher rates of usage of diet pills, laxatives, and vomiting to control weight.[12]

Nonalcoholic or Metabolic Fatty Liver Disease

Nonalcoholic or metabolic fatty liver disease (NAFLD) has evolved as a key comorbidity associated with obesity.[13] The presentation and severity of NAFLD can vary significantly, from isolated hepatic steatosis (which represents fatty deposition without inflammation) to nonalcoholic steatohepatitis (NASH) (which encompasses steatosis, inflammation, and ballooning degeneration of hepatocytes) to liver fibrosis and end-stage liver disease. Because of increasing rates over the last few decades, NAFLD is now considered to be the most common form of chronic liver disease in most of the Western world, with a prevalence ranging from 20% to 35% in adults and 5% to 17% in children.[14] Children with NAFLD are usually obese and have associated features of metabolic syndrome; insulin resistance, impaired glucose tolerance, and type 2 diabetes may also be present at diagnosis.[15]

EVALUATION OF OBESITY IN CHILDREN

The American Academy of Pediatrics (AAP) recommends yearly evaluation of weight status using BMI measurement and assessment of dietary and exercise patterns to provide opportunities to intervene on poor dietary habits and sedentary behavior.[16] Given that the medical consequences of obesity can involve every organ system, a thorough history and physical examination are paramount in the evaluation of overweight and obese children. Important considerations in the family history include the presence of obesity-related disorders and parental obesity. Genetic factors have a strong influence on the development of conditions such as type 2 diabetes mellitus and cardiovascular disease in childhood.[17] Sleep apnea can occur in severely obese adolescents[18] and usually presents with night-time snoring and daytime somnolence. Obese children should also be questioned on the presence of wheezing and shortness of breath, because asthma seems to be more common in this group as well.[4] The American Diabetes Association recommends that overweight children (≥85th percentile BMI) with any 2 of the following risk factors be screened for type 2 diabetes mellitus: (1) family history of type 2 diabetes, (2) of Native American, African American, Hispanic American, or Asian/South Pacific Islander ethnic background, or (3) have signs of insulin resistance or conditions associated with insulin resistance. Screening should start at age 10 years, or at the onset of puberty if it occurs younger, and should be performed every 2 years.[19] There are no evidence-based guidelines on when and how to best screen for NAFLD in children. However, an AAP expert committee has suggested that aspartate aminotransferase (AST) and alanine aminotransferase (ALT) levels be measured biannually for children with BMI in the 95th percentile or greater and those with BMI in the 85th to 94th percentile with at least 1 other risk factor.[16] Screening for many of the psychological comorbidities of obesity can be accomplished using the HEEADSSS examination, which most pediatricians use in every adolescent visit. This is a series of questions regarding home environment, education and employment, eating, activities, drugs, sexuality, suicide/depression, and safety designed to identify adolescents having difficulties in any of these areas during this high-risk developmental period.[20]

Medical causes of obesity in childhood are rare; however, many pediatricians find themselves needing to address these causes because of parental concern. Hypothyroidism is among the more common causes of weight gain (acquired hypothyroidism has a prevalence of about 1.2% of children in the United States).[21] However, children with this disorder typically have a decrease in their linear growth and a decline in academic performance. Primary Cushing syndrome is another rare cause of obesity in childhood. However, these children also typically have short stature. There are some genetic syndromes associated with obesity, such as Prader-Willi syndrome. These children typically have developmental delay and other medical conditions that precede the obesity.

EVALUATION OF NAFLD IN CHILDREN

The diagnosis of pediatric NAFLD is commonly made after increased serum aminotransferase levels are found during a routine checkup. Many centers have adopted a screening program for NAFLD in high-risk individuals, particularly in those presenting with features of the metabolic syndrome. Liver biopsy, the current gold standard for the diagnosis of NAFLD, is the only way to distinguish between NASH and isolated hepatic steatosis, determine the severity of liver damage and the presence and extent of fibrosis, as well as to rule out other diagnoses, such as autoimmune hepatitis. However, routine noninvasive evaluation (biochemical parameters, imaging tests, and serum biomarkers) are used as the first step to confirm the diagnosis of fatty liver disease, especially in the typical patient with features characteristic of the metabolic syndrome.

Serum Biomarkers

In children with suspected NAFLD or NASH, baseline testing should include levels of AST and ALT, total and direct bilirubin, γ-glutamyltranspeptidase, fasting serum glucose, and insulin, as well as a lipid panel. Aminotransferases may range from normal to 4 to 6 times the upper limit of normal, but mild increases are usually seen, ranging between 1.5 and 2 times the upper limit of normal.[22] Generally, the ratio of AST to ALT is less than 1, but this ratio may increase as fibrosis advances.[23] Circulating levels of aminotransferases may fluctuate over time and may be normal in a large proportion of children with NAFLD and NASH.[15] Furthermore, normal aminotransferase levels do not exclude the presence of fibrosis or even cirrhosis. Given that most patients with NAFLD have some components of the metabolic syndrome, lipid profiles as well as fasting glucose and insulin levels should be verified. Insulin resistance can be determined by fasting insulin levels or by further studies if necessary (glucose challenge or glucose tolerance test). Albumin, bilirubin, and platelet levels are usually normal unless the disease has evolved to cirrhosis. Similar to adults, some children with NAFLD may have positive autoantibodies (antinuclear and anti–smooth muscle antibody) in the absence of autoimmune hepatitis.[24] The significance of this finding is still unclear.

Establishing the diagnosis and disease severity as well as monitoring children over time remains a major challenge for pediatricians taking care of the increasing number of children with NAFLD. A liver biopsy is still considered the goal standard; however, this invasive procedure is not suitable for screening and risk stratification of children with this condition. There is a great need to develop noninvasive, simple, and reliable tests that can replace liver biopsy for these purposes. The currently available noninvasive tests as reviewed earlier have 2 central limitations: the inability to (1) distinguish NASH, from hepatic steatosis and (2) to stage the presence and extent of liver fibrosis. Thus, identifying and validating potential novel noninvasive biomarkers is a central area of research. Diagnostics development in NAFLD have been divided into 2 major groups: those aimed at detecting and quantifying the presence of fibrosis and those aimed at establishing the diagnosis of NASH. Regarding the former, the pediatric NAFLD fibrosis index (PNFI) which is obtained from 3 simple measures (age, waist circumference [WC], and triglycerides [TG]), was recently developed to predict liver fibrosis in children with NAFLD.[25] This index is easy to calculate, with no additional cost to the patient, and it has a good positive predictive value to rule in fibrosis; however, its negative predictive value is suboptimal. These limitations can be overcome when used in a sequential algorithm with the enhanced liver fibrosis (ELF) test. The ELF test uses a combination of 3 extracellular matrix components (hyaluronic acid, amino terminal propeptide of type III collagen, and inhibitor of metalloproteinase 1) and results in an accurate assessment of the presence of liver fibrosis in children.[26] Future studies are still needed to externally cross-validate these findings before the combination of PNFI and ELF can be recommended in children with NAFLD. Moreover, longitudinal studies measuring these panels serially against clinical outcomes will determine if they can be used to measure disease progression and regression.

Hepatocyte apoptosis has been found to be a prominent feature in patients with NASH, making it an interesting focus for biomarker development and for therapeutic intervention.[27] A large body of evidence has shown the usefulness of measuring plasma levels of caspase-generated cytokeratin-18 (CK-18) fragments, a specific by-product of apoptosis in liver cells, in the diagnosis of NASH in adult patients.[28] Recently, Fitzpatrick and colleagues[29] reported that children with biopsy-proven NAFLD also showed considerably increased levels of the CK-18 fragments compared with healthy controls. In addition, those with established NASH showed significantly higher numbers versus those with hepatic steatosis or borderline disease. These findings were further confirmed in a large study including more than 200 children with biopsy-proven NAFLD.[30] Numerous other biomarkers of inflammation, oxidative stress, apoptosis, and fibrosis are under investigation.[31] However, more studies are needed to validate the existing markers and techniques and develop other accurate noninvasive predictors of disease severity.

Imaging Techniques

Several radiologic techniques seem promising for quantifying hepatic steatosis (computed tomography, magnetic resonance imaging, or magnetic resonance spectroscopy) as well as fibrosis (transient elastography). Liver ultrasonography (US) is the most commonly used imaging modality, largely because it is inexpensive, widely available, and user-friendly. Several studies in adults have reported that this technique is highly sensitive and specific for detection of NAFLD.[32,33] Moreover, liver US can provide a good estimate of the degree or extent of hepatic steatosis present based on a series of characteristics, including hepatorenal echo contrast, liver echogenicity, visualization of intrahepatic vessels, and visualization of liver parenchyma and the diaphragm. Based on these characteristics, it was recently shown that liver US is a useful tool for quantifying steatosis in pediatric patients who have suspected NAFLD, with US score strongly correlating with grade of steatosis on liver biopsy.[34] US sensitivity decreases when the liver contains less than 30% of fat. Furthermore, US cannot rule out the presence of steatohepatitis or fibrosis. Both computed tomography and magnetic resonance imaging studies, especially the new technique of magnetic resonance spectroscopy, are more sensitive techniques for the quantification of steatosis. However, they have been mainly used in the research setting, and their clinical usefulness is limited by their cost and the need for sedation in children. None of these imaging tools has sufficient sensitivity and specificity for staging the disease and cannot distinguish between hepatic steatosis and NASH with or without fibrosis.

Several investigators have reported that transient elastography provides a high level of accuracy for detecting significant liver fibrosis, advanced fibrosis, and cirrhosis observed in adult NAFLD.[35] Transient elastography has also been validated to assess liver fibrosis through tissue elasticity measured by US technology in several liver diseases and may be useful in pediatric NAFLD.[36]

Liver Biopsy

Liver biopsy remains the gold standard for establishing the diagnosis of NAFLD and grading and staging the severity,[37] distinguishing steatosis from steatohepatitis, and assessing the degree of fibrosis. Moreover, it is helpful in ruling out alternative causes such as chronic hepatitis C infection, Wilson disease, autoimmune hepatitis, and other metabolic liver disorders. In addition, histology permits the monitoring of disease progression and the response to therapy, because aminotransaminase levels may decrease during the course of the disease, regardless of whether fibrosis progresses or improves. A central limitation for the use of liver biopsy is its invasiveness and the potential for significant complications, such as bleeding. The histologic diagnosis of NASH in pediatric cases may also be challenging, because the features found in liver biopsy often differ from those commonly seen in adults.[38] The typical adult pattern (termed NASH type 1) is characterized by the presence of steatosis (mainly macrovesicular), with ballooning degeneration or perisinusoidal fibrosis (zone 3 lobular involvement), with the portal tracts being relatively spared. Pediatric type NASH (NASH type 2) is described as the presence of steatosis along with portal inflammation or fibrosis in the absence of ballooning degeneration and perisinusoidal fibrosis.[39]

TREATMENT
Goals

For obese children with or without NAFLD, lifestyle and dietary changes with resultant weight loss are the goals.[40] For both conditions, precipitous weight loss is generally not needed, and in the case of NAFLD, this approach can be detrimental. Therefore, the focus should be on instituting healthier behaviors, which over time result in weight loss. It has been shown that 5% reductions in BMI are associated with clinically meaningful changes in WC, and reductions in cholesterol, TG, and insulin resistance levels in children.[41] Also, comparably small changes in weight result in significant improvement of liver enzyme levels in adults.[42] For children with NAFLD, there is an additional focus on treating the liver disease as well as the associated metabolic derangements. Pharmacologic therapy is limited to children with NASH, given that those with isolated hepatic steatosis generally have an excellent prognosis from a liver standpoint.

Interventions for Obesity

Family-based behavioral treatment

Family-based behavioral treatment (FBT) consists of nutrition and exercise education combined with behavior therapy techniques. It is an intensive program, in which the child and parent(s) meet weekly to biweekly over several months for group classes and also receive one-on-one meetings with a behavioral coach for individualized goal setting and problem solving. The behavior therapy curriculum consists of self-monitoring of diet and physical activity, stimulus control, positive reinforcement, parenting skills, goal setting, and relapse prevention.[43,44] Stimulus control focuses on setting up the child's environment to reduce food intake and sedentary activity and increase physical activity. Positive reinforcement includes positive parenting skills (praise) and motivation systems, in which the child earns points for participating in program-related behaviors. Parenting skills includes promotion of authoritative parenting style around eating and exercise and how to model healthy behaviors and set limits. Goal setting refers to contracting for immediate and long-term goals and the disbursement of rewards for achieving these goals (**Fig. 1**). The addition of these components to standard nutrition education has been shown to significantly improve weight loss.[45] The importance of behavioral therapy was also shown in another study comparing a behavioral weight reduction program with the same program plus a short course on general child management skills. Both groups lost weight, but children whose parents received general child management training in addition to the weight reduction program had improved weight maintenance at 1-year follow-up.[46] Golan

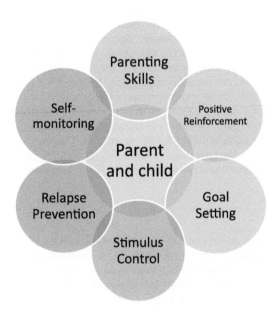

Fig. 1. Components of family-based behavioral therapy.

and colleagues[47] reported that the use of behavioral modification techniques explained 27% of the variance in the child's weight reduction.

One important difference in behavioral therapy for obese children compared with adults is the necessity of involvement of parents. One study compared the effect of targeting behavioral therapy toward the child, the child and parent, or a nonspecific target. Although all groups had similar weight reductions after treatment and at 2-year follow-up, the parent-child group had improved weight outcomes at 10-year follow-up compared with the other groups.[48] In addition, some studies have shown greater reduction in child percent overweight in parent-focused interventions when compared with child-focused interventions.[49,50] More recently, parent-focused programs that require the parent to master weight-control strategies and then teach these strategies to their child without the child attending any treatment sessions themselves have proved to be equally as effective as those including the child in treatment.[51,52]

Several studies have proved FBT an effective treatment of weight loss in children, and FBT is considered the gold standard for the treatment of childhood obesity. Long-term data have shown that 30% of children participating in FBT are normal weight after 10 years.[48] Unique to the treatment of childhood obesity is the need for parent involvement for treatment success.

Dietary

There are few studies of specific dietary approaches to achieve weight loss in children. Many studies of behavioral therapy in children have used the traffic-light diet. This diet categorizes foods into green, yellow, or red, based on the energy density. Green foods are low in energy density and are allowed in unlimited amounts. Yellow foods are moderate in energy density and are to be approached with caution. Red foods are high in fat and simple sugar and should be eaten in limited amounts. Families are instructed to eat few red foods and eat as much green food as possible, but stay within a prescribed calorie range.[53] This diet has been shown to decrease BMI in several studies of behavioral therapy.[45,51,54]

There are few studies of altering carbohydrate content in children. In one of the few studies, a low-carbohydrate, high-protein diet was as effective as a standard portion-controlled diet in 102 children aged 7 to 12 years (ie, both groups had lower BMI z-scores at 12-month follow-up). However, the low-carbohydrate, high-protein diet had lower rates of adherence.[55] Other smaller studies comparing low glycemic index diets with a standard reduced-fat diet in adolescents have shown larger decreases in BMI among the groups with a low glycemic index.[56,57]

Pharmacologic

In adults, 2 appetite-suppressant drugs have been approved by the US Food and Drug Administration (FDA) for weight loss: lorcaserin HCl (Belviq) and phentermine/topiramate (Qsymia). However, the only FDA-approved drug for weight loss in adults and children is orlistat. Orlistat causes weight loss by decreasing fat absorption through inhibition of pancreatic lipase.[58] There have been few trials of this drug in children. A small, short-term study in obese adolescents showed modest reduction of weight (−3.8% ± 4.1% from baseline) when given orlistat in conjunction with a behavioral weight-loss treatment program.[59] In a larger, randomized controlled trial comparing the addition of orlistat or placebo with a diet, exercise, and behavioral therapy program in adolescents, the orlistat group had a mean reduction of BMI by 0.55, whereas the placebo group increased by 0.31. The orlistat group had more gastrointestinal side effects than the placebo group (9% to 50% compared with 1% to 13%).[60]

Interventions for NAFLD

Nonpharmacologic

As described earlier for obese children, gradual weight reduction and physical exercise continue to be the gold standard of treatment of NAFLD in children.[40] Weight reduction has been widely studied in adults and has been shown to improve not only the biochemical parameters but also the liver histology. Based on studies in adults, greater than 5% weight loss was associated with significant improvement in liver histology.[61] The relative efficacy of weight loss and degree of weight loss needed to induce histologic improvement in pediatric NAFLD is unknown, but rapid weight loss is not advised, because it may accelerate inflammation. In the context of evidence-based recommendations for patients with NAFLD, advice is based on the pathologic mechanisms of disease progression, favoring nutrients that have beneficial effects on the metabolic syndrome parameters as well as on inflammation. Consumption of carbohydrates should be limited (especially a high-fructose, high-glucose diet) and foods with a low glycemic index prioritized. Saturated fats are limited in favor of monounsaturated fatty acids as well as polyunsaturated fatty acids (omega-3). Recent pediatric studies evaluating lifestyle dietary changes and weight loss have suggested that in a selective group of children, effective intervention resulting in persistent weight loss is associated with improvement of serum AST and ALT levels and US liver brightness, as well as liver histology.[62]

Pharmacologic

Several drugs that improve insulin sensitivity, such as metformin, or glitazones (rosiglitazone, pioglitazone), lipid-lowering agents, such as clofibrate, or gemfibrozil, hepatoprotective agents, such as ursodeoxycholic acid (UDCA), and antioxidants, such as vitamin E, betaine, or N-acetylcysteine, have been proposed as potential agents for the treatment of NASH in both adults and children (**Table 1**).

Insulin-sensitizing agents Patients with NASH with diabetes are at higher risk of developing more aggressive disease.[63] Insulin-sensitizing agents such as peroxisome proliferator-activated receptor-γ agonists (glitazones) have been tested in adults with NASH, with mixed results.[64] The experience with glitazones in children and adolescence is limited, and there are no studies assessing this medication class in children with NAFLD. Metformin has been shown to be safe and effective in the treatment of diabetes in children and is the only insulin-sensitizing agent thus far evaluated in the treatment of NAFLD in children. Initial small pilot studies in pediatric NAFLD suggested improvement in serum ALT levels and reduction in hepatic steatosis as assessed by radiologic means.[65] However, a recently published large, multicenter, double-blind, randomized controlled trial of metformin or vitamin E in children (the Treatment of nonalcoholic fatty liver disease in children: TONIC trial) showed a complete lack of

Table 1
Various strategies for pharmacologic interventions for NAFLD in children

Strategy	Treatment
Insulin-sensitizing agents	Peroxisome proliferator-activated receptor-γ agonists (thiazolidinedione, rosiglitazone, pioglitazone); metformin
Antioxidants, hepatoprotective	Vitamin E, enteric coated cysteamine, N-acetylcysteine, pentoxifilline, caspase inhibitors
Others	Omega-3-fatty acids, carnitine, lipid-lowering agents

effect of metformin on both serum aminotransferase levels and liver histology.[66] The routine use of these agents in nondiabetic patients with NAFLD should be discouraged outside clinical trials.

Hepatoprotective, antioxidant therapy Several therapeutic agents believed to offer hepatocyte protection have been evaluated. Antioxidants have been hypothesized to decrease the oxidative stress and improve liver damage in NASH. A randomized controlled trial of vitamin E in adults[67] showed improvement in transaminases and fibrosis. Two pediatric studies with a small number of patients with NAFLD and no assessment in histology suggested an improvement of liver enzymes but no changes in liver brightness on US with vitamin E treatment. A large randomized controlled trial of pediatric NASH with changes in liver histology as the primary end point failed to show an additional benefit of vitamin E and C to a successful dietary weight-loss program.[68] Similarly, neither vitamin E nor metformin was superior to placebo in achieving sustained reduction in ALT level or in improving steatosis, lobular inflammation, or fibrosis scores in the TONIC trial. The only histologic feature of NASH that improved with both medications was ballooning. Compared with placebo, only vitamin E significantly improved the NAFLD activity score and was associated with improved resolution of NASH on the repeat liver biopsy (58% vs 28%; *P* value of .006). The investigators suggested that vitamin E should be considered in a subset of children with biopsy-proven NASH and evidence of hepatocellular ballooning degeneration, keeping in mind that the risk of biopsy may outweigh the benefits of therapy.[66]

SUMMARY

Childhood obesity is a serious and widespread problem, with one-third of children in the United States being overweight or obese. All of these children are at risk for a host of medical complications from their condition, including NAFLD. Screening for childhood obesity is important, and weight status should be evaluated via BMI at least yearly for all children. For overweight children, there are guidelines for screening for type 2 diabetes, but no evidence-based recommendations are available for screening for NAFLD and the other comorbidities. Furthermore, diagnosis of NAFLD remains difficult given the lack of reliable biomarkers and impracticality of liver biopsy. The gold standard for childhood weight loss is FBT. Pharmacologic therapy for weight loss in obese children is limited, and for liver disease, is limited to those children with NASH. Even modest weight loss in children can have a significant impact on their overall health.

REFERENCES

1. Kuczmarski R, Ogden C, Grummer-Strawn L. CDC growth charts: United States. Adv Data 2000;324:1–27.
2. Ogden CL, Carroll MD, Kit BK, et al. Prevalence of obesity and trends in body mass index among US children and adolescents, 199-2010. JAMA 2012;207(5): 483–90.
3. Ogden C, Carroll M. Prevalence of obesity among children and adolescents: United States, trends 1963-1965 through 2007-2008. Atlanta (GA): Centers for Disease Control and Prevention, National Center for Health Statistics; 2010. Available at: http://www.cdc.gov/nchs/data/hestat/obesity_child_07_08/obesity_child_07_08.htm.
4. Daniels SR, Arnett DK, Eckel RH, et al. Overweight in children and adolescents: pathophysiology, consequences, prevention, and treatment. Circulation 2005; 111(15):1999–2012.

5. Freedman DS, Khan LK, Serdula MK, et al. The relation of childhood BMI to adult adiposity: the Bogalusa Heart Study. Pediatrics 2005;115:22–7.
6. Hampl SE, Carroll CA, Simon SD, et al. Resource utilization and expenditures for overweight and obese children. Arch Pediatr Adolesc Med 2007; 161:11–4.
7. Estabrooks PA, Shetterly S. The prevalence and health care use of overweight children in an integrated health care system. Arch Pediatr Adolesc Med 2007; 161:222–7.
8. Schwimmer JB, Burwinkle TM, Varni JW. Health-related quality of life of severely obese children and adolescents. JAMA 2003;289:1813–9.
9. Braet C, Mervielde I, Vandereycken W. Psychological aspects of childhood obesity: a controlled study in a clinical and nonclinical sample. J Pediatr Psychol 1997;22(1):59–71.
10. Puhl R, Latner J. Stigma, obesity and the health of the nation's children. Psychol Bull 2007;133(4):557–80.
11. Berkowitz RA, Stunkard J, Stallings VA. Binge-eating disorder in obese adolescent girls. Ann N Y Acad Sci 1993;699:200–6.
12. Boutelle K, Neumark-Sztainer D, Story M, et al. Weight control behaviors among obese, overweight, and nonoverweight adolescents. J Pediatr Psychol 2002; 27(6):531–40.
13. Festi D, Colecchia A, Sacco T, et al. Hepatic steatosis in obese patients: clinical aspects and prognostic significance. Obes Rev 2004;5:27–42.
14. Schwimmer JB, Deutsch R, Kahen T, et al. Prevalence of fatty liver in children and adolescents. Pediatrics 2006;118:1388–93.
15. Feldstein AE, Charatcharoenwitthaya P, Treeprasertsuk S, et al. The natural history of nonalcoholic fatty liver disease in children: a follow-up study for up to 20-years. Gut 2009;58(11):1538–44.
16. Barlow SE. Expert committee and treatment of child and adolescent overweight and obesity: expert committee recommendations regarding the prevention. assessment, Report. Pediatrics 2007;120(Suppl 4):S164–92.
17. Fagot-Campagna A, Pettitt DJ, Engelgau MM, et al. Type 2 diabetes among North American children and adolescents: an epidemiologic review and a public health perspective. J Pediatr 2000;136:664–72.
18. Kalra M, Inge T, Garcia V, et al. Obstructive sleep apnea in extremely overweight adolescents undergoing bariatric surgery. Obes Res 2005;13:1175–9.
19. American Diabetes Association screening for type 2 diabetes. Diabetes Care 2003;26(Suppl 1):521–4.
20. Goldenring JM, Rosen DS. Getting into adolescent heads: an essential update. Contemp Pediatr 2004;21(1):64–92.
21. Rallison ML, Dobyns BM, Keating FR, et al. Occurrence and natural history of chronic lymphocytic thyroiditis in childhood. J Pediatr 1975;86(5):675.
22. Wieckowska A, Feldstein AE. Nonalcoholic fatty liver disease in the pediatric population: a review. Curr Opin Pediatr 2005;17:636–41.
23. Adams LA, Sanderson S, Lindor KD, et al. The histological course of nonalcoholic fatty liver disease: a longitudinal study of 103 patients with sequential liver biopsies. J Hepatol 2005;42:132–8.
24. Vuppalanchi R, Gould RJ, Wilson LA, et al, Nonalcoholic Steatohepatitis Clinical Research Network (NASH CRN). Clinical significance of serum autoantibodies in patients with NAFLD: results from the nonalcoholic steatohepatitis clinical research network. Hepatol Int 2011. [Epub ahead of print].

25. Nobili V, Alisi A, Vania A, et al. The pediatric NAFLD fibrosis index: a predictor of liver fibrosis in children with non-alcoholic fatty liver disease. BMC Med 2009;7:21.
26. Alkhouri N, Carter-Kent C, Lopez R, et al. A combination of the pediatric NAFLD fibrosis index and enhanced liver fibrosis test identifies children with fibrosis. Clin Gastroenterol Hepatol 2011;9(2):150–5.
27. Feldstein AE, Canbay A, Angulo P, et al. Hepatocyte apoptosis and fas expression are prominent features of human nonalcoholic steatohepatitis. Gastroenterology 2003;125(2):437–43.
28. Feldstein AE, Wieckowska A, Lopez AR, et al. Cytokeratin-18 fragment levels as noninvasive biomarkers for nonalcoholic steatohepatitis: a multicenter validation study. Hepatology 2009;50(4):1072–8.
29. Fitzpatrick E, Mitry R, Quaglia A, et al. Serum level of CK18 M30 and leptin are useful predictors of steatohepatitis and fibrosis in paediatric NAFLD. J Pediatr Gastroenterol Nutr 2010;51(4):500–6.
30. Feldstein AE, Alkhouri N, De Vito R, et al. Serum cytokeratin-18 fragment levels are useful biomarkers for nonalcoholic steatohepatitis in children. Am J Gastroenterol 2013;108(9):1526–31.
31. Wieckowska A, Feldstein AE. Diagnosis of nonalcoholic fatty liver disease: invasive versus noninvasive. Semin Liver Dis 2008;28:386–95.
32. Mazhar SM, Shiehmorteza M, Sirlin CB. Noninvasive assessment of hepatic steatosis. Clin Gastroenterol Hepatol 2009;7:135–40.
33. Dasarathy S, Dasarathy J, Khiyami A, et al. Validity of real time ultrasound in the diagnosis of hepatic steatosis: a prospective study. J Hepatol 2009;51:1061–7.
34. Shannon A, Alkhouri N, Carter-Kent C, et al. Ultrasonographic quantitative estimation of hepatic steatosis in children with nonalcoholic fatty liver disease (NAFLD): a prospective study. J Pediatr Gastroenterol Nutr 2011;53(2):190–5.
35. Piscaglia F, Marinelli S, Bota S, et al. The role of ultrasound elastographic techniques in chronic liver disease: current status and future perspectives. Eur J Radiol 2013. http://dx.doi.org/10.1016/j.ejrad.2013.06.009. [Epub ahead of print].
36. Nobili V, Vizzutti F, Arena U, et al. Accuracy and reproducibility of transient elastography for the diagnosis of fibrosis in pediatric nonalcoholic steatohepatitis. Hepatology 2008;48(2):442–8.
37. Adams LA, Feldstein AE. Nonalcoholic steatohepatitis: risk factors and diagnosis. Expert Rev Gastroenterol Hepatol 2010;4(5):623–35.
38. Schwimmer JB, Behling C, Newbury R, et al. Histopathology of pediatric nonalcoholic fatty liver disease. Hepatology 2005;42:641–9.
39. Carter-Kent C, Yerian LM, Brunt EM, et al. Nonalcoholic steatohepatitis in children: a multicenter clinicopathological study. Hepatology 2009;50(4):1113–20.
40. Chalasani N, Younossi Z, Lavine JE, et al. The diagnosis and management of non-alcoholic fatty liver disease: practice guideline by the American Association for the Study of Liver Diseases, American College of Gastroenterology, and the American Gastroenterological Association. Hepatology 2012;55(6):2005–23.
41. Budd G, Hayman L, Crump E, et al. Weight loss in obese African American and Caucasian adolescents: secondary analysis of a randomized clinical trial of behavioral therapy plus sibutramine. J Cardiovasc Nurs 2007;22(4):288–96.
42. St George A, Bauman A, Johnston A, et al. Effects of a lifestyle intervention in patients with abnormal liver enzymes and metabolic risk factors. J Gastroenterol Hepatol 2009;24:399–407.

43. Epstein LH. Family-based behavioural intervention for obese children. Int J Obes Relat Metab Disord 1996;20(Suppl 1):S14–21.
44. Epstein LH, Roemmich JN, Raynor HA. Behavioral therapy in the treatment of pediatric obesity. Pediatr Clin North Am 2001;48(4):981–93.
45. Epstein LH, Wing RR, Koeske R, et al. Child and parent weight loss in family-based behavior modification programs. J Consult Clin Psychol 1981;49:674–85.
46. Israel AC, Stolmaker L, Andrian CA. The effects of training parents in general child management skills on a behavioral weight loss program for children. Behav Ther 1985;16:169–80.
47. Golan M, Fainaru M, Weizman A. Role of behaviour modification in the treatment of childhood obesity with the parents as the exclusive agents of change. Int J Obes Relat Metab Disord 1998;22:1217–24.
48. Epstein LH, Valoski A, Wing RR, et al. Ten-year follow-up of behavioral, family-based treatment for obese children. JAMA 1990;264:2519–23.
49. Golan M, Weizman A, Apter A, et al. Parents as the exclusive agents of change in the treatment of childhood obesity. Am J Clin Nutr 1998;67:1130–5.
50. Golan M, Crow S. Targeting parents exclusively in the treatment of childhood obesity: long-term results. Obes Res 2004;12:357–61.
51. Boutelle KN, Cafri G, Crow SJ. Parent-only treatment for childhood obesity: a randomized controlled trial. Obesity (Silver Spring) 2011;19:574–80.
52. Janicke DM, Sallinen BJ, Perri MG, et al. Comparison of parent-only vs family-based interventions for overweight children in underserved rural settings: outcomes from project story. Arch Pediatr Adolesc Med 2008;162:1119–25.
53. Epstein LH, Wing RR, Penner BC, et al. Effect of diet and controlled exercise on weight loss in obese children. J Pediatr 1985;107(3):358–61.
54. Saelens B, Sallis J, Wilfley D, et al. Behavioral weight control for overweight adolescents initiated in primary care. Obes Res 2002;10(1):22–32.
55. Kirk S, Brehm B, Saelens BE, et al. Role of carbohydrate modification in weight management among obese children: a randomized clinical trial. J Pediatr 2012; 161(2):320–7.
56. Spieth LE, Harnish JD, Lenders CM, et al. A low-glycemic index diet in the treatment of pediatric obesity. Arch Pediatr Adolesc Med 2000;154(9):947–51.
57. Ebbeling CB, Leidig MM, Sinclair KB, et al. A reduced-glycemic load diet in the treatment of adolescent obesity. Arch Pediatr Adolesc Med 2003;157(8):773–9.
58. Heck AM, Yanovski JA, Calis KA. Orlistat, a new lipase inhibitor for the management of obesity. Pharmacotherapy 2000;20(3):270–9.
59. McDuffie JR, Calis KA, Uwaifo GI, et al. Three-month tolerability of orlistat in adolescents with obesity-related comorbid conditions. Obes Res 2002;10(7):642–50.
60. Chanoine JP, Hampl S, Jensen C, et al. Effect of orlistat on weight and body composition in obese adolescents: a randomized controlled trial. JAMA 2005; 293:2873–83.
61. Huang MA, Greenson JK, Chao C, et al. One-year intense nutritional counseling results in histological improvement in patients with nonalcoholic steatohepatitis: a pilot study. Am J Gastroenterol 2005;100:1072–81.
62. Nobili V, Marcellini M, Devito R, et al. NAFLD in children: a prospective clinical-pathological study and effect of lifestyle advice. Hepatology 2006; 44:458–65.
63. Schuppan D, Schattenberg JM. Non-alcoholic steatohepatitis: pathogenesis and novel therapeutic approaches. J Gastroenterol Hepatol 2013;28(Suppl 1): 68–76.

64. Mahady SE, Webster AC, Walker S, et al. The role of thiazolidinediones in non-alcoholic steatohepatitis–a systematic review and meta analysis. J Hepatol 2011;55(6):1383–90.
65. Schwimmer JB, Middleton MS, Deutsch R, et al. A phase 2 clinical trial of metformin as a treatment for non-diabetic paediatric non-alcoholic steatohepatitis. Aliment Pharmacol Ther 2005;21:871–9.
66. Lavine JE, Schwimmer JB, Van Natta ML, et al, Nonalcoholic Steatohepatitis Clinical Research Network. Effect of vitamin E or metformin for treatment of nonalcoholic fatty liver disease in children and adolescents: the TONIC randomized controlled trial. JAMA 2011;305(16):1659–68.
67. Sanyal AJ, Chalasani N, Kowdley KV, et al. Pioglitazone, vitamin E, or placebo for nonalcoholic steatohepatitis. N Engl J Med 2010;362(18):1675–85.
68. Nobili V, Manco M, Devito R, et al. Lifestyle intervention and antioxidant therapy in children with nonalcoholic fatty liver disease: a randomized, controlled trial. Hepatology 2008;48:119–28.

The Interactions of Nonalcoholic Fatty Liver Disease and Cardiovascular Diseases

Hugo Perazzo, MD[a,b], Thierry Poynard, MD, PhD[a,b,c],
Jean-François Dufour, MD[d,e],*

KEYWORDS

- Nonalcoholic fatty liver disease • Liver fibrosis • Cardiovascular disease
- Atherosclerosis • Insulin resistance

KEY POINTS

- Patients with nonalcoholic fatty liver disease present higher overall mortality, and cardiovascular disease is one of the leading causes of death.
- Individuals with fatty liver presented higher carotid and coronary plaques measured by surrogate markers of atherosclerosis.
- NAFLD is associated with new onset of cardiovascular events independently of confounding factors.
- A complex interaction among metabolic factors, adipose tissue lipolysis, insulin resistance, and excessive free fatty acids results in an inflammatory state, hypercoagulability, and endothelial dysfunction, which might explain the association between NAFLD and cardiovascular disease.

Funding Source: This study was supported by the European Union Seventh Framework Programme (FP7/2007-2013) under grant agreement n°Health-F2-2009-241762, for the project FLIP; the Institute of Cardiometabolism and Nutrition (ICAN) funded by MESR 2011-2016 and the Association pour la Recherche sur les Maladies Hépatiques Virales (ARMHV). These sponsors played no role in the interpretation of data.
Conflict of Interest Statement: The authors have nothing to disclose related to this topic.
[a] Hepatology Department, Liver Center, Groupe Hospitalier Pitié-Salpêtrière (GHPS), Assistance Publique Hôpitaux de Paris (APHP), 47-83, Boulevard de l'Hôpital, Paris 75013, France; [b] Pierre et Marie Curie University (Paris 6), Inserm UMR_S 938, Paris, France; [c] Institute of Cardiometabolism and Nutrition (ICAN), Paris, France; [d] University Clinic for Visceral Surgery and Medicine, University of Bern, Inselspital, Freiburgstrasse, Bern 3010, Switzerland; [e] Hepatology, Department of Clinical Research, University of Bern, Bern, Switzerland
* Corresponding author. University Clinic for Visceral Surgery and Medicine, University of Bern, Inselspital, Freiburgstrasse, Bern 3010, Switzerland.
E-mail address: jean-francois.dufour@ikp.unibe.ch

Nonalcoholic fatty liver disease (NAFLD) is one of the most common chronic liver diseases worldwide.[1] This liver disease is characterized by presence of fat accumulation in at least 5% of hepatocytes without others causes of chronic liver disease, including alcohol-induced and drug-induced liver disease, autoimmune or viral hepatitis, and cholestatic or genetic liver disease.[2]

NAFLD presents a large clinical spectrum, ranging from simple steatosis to coexistent hepatocyte injury, nonalcoholic steatohepatitis (NASH), associated with fibrosis and cirrhosis and its complications.[3,4] Simple steatosis usually presents a benign course; however, patients who progress to NASH may develop cirrhosis and suffer from liver-related mortality.[5,6]

Patients with NAFLD usually present metabolic syndrome and its components, common risk factors for cardiovascular disease (CVD).[7] More recently, some studies have reported a close relationship between NAFLD and increased atherosclerosis.[8] This review focuses on the association between NAFLD and CVD, discussing the data linking these major diseases and the likely mechanisms underlying this interaction.

NAFLD AND SURROGATE MARKERS OF ATHEROSCLEROSIS

NAFLD might play an important role in the atherosclerosis complex process, reinforcing the relationship between fatty liver and CVD.[9] Several studies have reported the association of NAFLD with surrogate markers of atherosclerosis as presence of carotid and coronary plaques and cardiac dysfunction.

Cardiac multislice computed tomography accurately assesses coronary plaques.[10] This method calculates the coronary artery calcium (CAC) score, which reflects the underlying total plaque burden that accurately correlates to increased risk of coronary events.[11,12] Individuals with NAFLD presented higher calcified and noncalcified plaques compared with matched controls. In addition, the presence of fatty liver was predictive of coronary artery disease (CAD) after adjustment for confounding factors.[13] Studies have reported a strong relationship between NAFLD and CAC score.[14,15] Increased CAC score was significantly associated with NAFLD independently of metabolic factors, including visceral adiposity.[14] Furthermore, a study reported a strong association between NAFLD and presence of vulnerable plaques, increasing the risk of severe CV outcomes.[16]

Measurement of carotid intima-media thickness (CIMT) and plaque by ultrasonography is a validated method for diagnosing early atherosclerosis and prediction of CVD.[17,18] Several studies have associated carotid with NAFLD independently of components of the metabolic syndrome.[19–22] A systematic review involving 3497 individuals (7 studies) strongly correlated CIMT with fatty liver, showing an increase of up to 13% of CIMT and higher prevalence of plaques in patient with NAFLD.[23] Furthermore, a study reported that severity of histologic features seems to correlates with CIMT, agreeing with the hypothesis that patients with NASH carry a higher risk of CVD than individuals with simple steatosis.[24]

A few studies have reported the relationship between NAFLD and cardiac dysfunction. Increased cardiac left ventricular (LV) mass index and diastolic dysfunction were associated with NAFLD.[25,26] Hallsworth and colleagues[27] described significant changes in cardiac structure and function in NAFLD patients with NAFLD compared with an age-matched, sex-matched, and body mass index (BMI)-matched healthy population. In this study, patients with NAFLD presented thicker LV walls at systole and diastole as well as higher peak whole wall and peak endocardial circumferential strain. Fallo and colleagues[28] also reported a positive correlation between diastolic cardiac dysfunction and severity of fatty liver disease. Yilmaz and colleagues[29] reported a reduced coronary flow reserve, measured by echocardiography, in patients with NAFLD compared with matched controls independently of common metabolic factors. In this study, histologic liver fibrosis was predictive of impaired coronary flow reserve.

Furthermore, NAFLD was also associated with increased risk of cardiac arrhythmia. Targher and colleagues[30,31] reported an increased incidence of atrial fibrillation in type 2 diabetic patients with NAFLD defined by ultrasonography followed for a long-term.

NAFLD AND MORTALITY

Published data have shown that presence of NAFLD seems to be associated with higher mortality than in the general population, mainly as a result of CVD. In a community-based cohort, Adams and colleagues[32] reported that NAFLD increased in 34% of the cohort the risk of overall mortality compared with the general population. Ong and colleagues[33] reported that NAFLD was independently associated with overall and liver-related mortality in a representative sample of the US population. Dunn and colleagues[34] confirmed previous results and showed that presence of NAFLD was associated with cardiovascular (CV)-related death in a subgroup of patients aged from 45 to 54 years. Söderberg and colleagues[35] reported an increase between 70% and 86% on the risk of overall mortality in presence of NAFLD or NASH compared with the general population in a long-term follow-up. In type 2 diabetic patients, Adams and colleagues[36] described NAFLD as a factor independent of overall mortality but not related to specific CV death. However, a recent US, adult population-based prospective cohort study reported no relationship between NAFLD and overall or specific death.[37] Stepenova and Younossi[38] described higher CV-related death in patients with NAFLD compared with patients who did not have NAFLD. However, the presence of NAFLD was not predictive of CV death. The role of noninvasive markers was also evaluated in the prediction of mortality in patients with NAFLD. Fatty liver index (FLI) is a validated surrogate marker of steatosis that uses triglyceride level, BMI, waist circumference, and γ-glutamyltransferase (GGT) to estimate liver steatosis.[39] Despite borderline hazard ratios, NAFLD defined as per the FLI was independently associated with overall, liver-related, and CV-related death.[40] In NAFLD defined by ultrasonography, Kim and colleagues[41] reported no association between NAFLD and overall mortality. However, in this cohort, patients with NAFLD with advanced fibrosis presumed by noninvasive methods, such as NAFLD fibrosis score (NFS),[42] aspartate aminotransferase to platelet ratio index (APRI),[43] and FIB-4[44] score presented higher risk of overall and CV-related death. More recently, Angulo and colleagues[45] confirmed these results in 320 patients with NAFLD proved by biopsy in a multicenter international trial. In this study, patients with advanced fibrosis, estimated by the same noninvasive markers, presented an increased risk for liver-related complications and death. These results confirm that presence of fibrosis should be implicated in increased overall and specific mortality.

CVD was described as one of the leading causes of death in most population-based studies.[32–34,46] Targher and colleagues[47] showed that NAFLD was associated with CV-related death in an Italian population after adjustment for metabolic confounding factors. Rafiq and colleagues[4] reported CVD as the most frequent cause of death in 173 patients with NAFLD proved by biopsy followed for 13 years. In addition, these investigators described higher overall mortality in patients with NASH and those with NAFLD associated with type 2 diabetes mellitus. Despite a similar overall survival of patients with NAFLD compared with an age-matched and gender-matched control group, Ekstedt and colleagues[48] reported a 2-fold higher 14-year risk of CV-related death in patients with NASH. More recently, Stepanova and colleagues[49] described that CVD remains as the leading cause of death among biopsy-proven NAFLD. However, they have not found significant difference in mortality between patients with NASH and those who do not have NASH, suggesting that the presence of hepatic steatosis, rather than the necroinflammatory features, might be the main risk factor of CV death.[49] **Table 1** summarizes the main prospective studies that reported NAFLD and mortality.

Published data on long-term mortality suggest that NAFLD is significantly associated with a higher risk of overall mortality. In addition, CVD is one of the main causes of death in this population. The specific mortality risks attributable to CVD events and to liver-related events are unknown. Further prospective studies should be conducted to establish the real relationship between CV-related death and presence of liver injury features. In NAFLD, the 3 main features are fibrosis, the main cause of liver-related mortality, but also steatosis and necroinflammatory activity.

NAFLD AND CV EVENTS

Type 2 diabetes, insulin resistance (IR), dyslipidemia, and obesity are common risk factors for NAFLD and CVD. Several studies have evaluated whether NAFLD is associated with CVD as a consequence of shared risk factors or whether this disease can actively contribute to CV events independently of these factors (**Table 2**). A second point is whether CVD represents a risk in simple steatosis or whether necroinflammatory liver injury (ie, NASH) must be present to trigger the atherosclerosis process.

The impact of the metabolic syndrome components as confounding factors on ischemic heart disease remains unclear.[50] However, some studies have associated NAFLD and CVD independently of metabolic risk factors.[51,52]

Several studies reported an association between NAFLD and CVD using liver enzymes as fatty liver markers. In a cohort of 163944 Austrian adults, increased GGT levels were associated with CVD mortality. This study also showed a clear dose-response relationship between this liver enzyme and severe CV outcome: CVD death was increased by 66% and 64% per log unit of GGT in men and women, respectively.[53] Lee and colleagues[54,55] reported similar results in the association of high GGT levels with fatal and nonfatal CVD independently of metabolic risk factors and alcohol consumption. A meta-analysis pooling 10 studies[56] confirmed these previous results regarding GGT and CVD. A few studies also reported the association of increased alanine aminotransferase (ALT) levels and CVD.[34,57,58] The major limits of these studies are that GGT and ALT are not specific biomarkers of steatosis, necroinflammatory injury, or fibrosis.

In a community-based cohort of healthy adults,[59] the presence of NAFLD, as per imaging methods, was significantly associated with an increased risk of CV-related events such as myocardial infarction, unstable angina, and ischemic stroke. The presence of NAFLD was also associated with new CV events in type 2 diabetic patients independently of confounding factors.[47] CAD prevalence was higher in patients with NAFLD undergoing coronary angiography compared with the general population, independently of components of the metabolic syndrome.[60] In addition, CAD was more prevalent in NASH-cirrhotic patients compared with patients with cirrhosis from other causes.[61] Wong and colleagues[62] confirmed the relationship between NAFLD and CAD independently of common metabolic factors. However, in this study, fatty liver was not predictive of new CV events in patients with established CVD. More recently Stepanova and Younossi[38] studied a US sample population and showed that CVD was significantly more prevalent in individuals with fatty liver and NAFLD was associated with CV events independently of metabolic risk factors.

Table 1
Main studies that have reported relationship between NAFLD and mortality

Reference	n	Study Population	NAFLD Criteria	CVD Criteria	Design	Main Results (95% Confidence Interval)
Adams et al,[32] 2005	480	Population-based cohort (United States)	Imaging or liver biopsy	Death certificates	Prospective (FU 7.6 y)	CVD second death cause; higher overall mortality (SMR 1.34 [1.003–1.76]; $P = .03$) in patients with NAFLD compared with general population
Adams et al,[36] 2010	337	T2DM population (United States)	Ultrasonography or liver biopsy	Death certificates	Prospective (FU 11 y)	NAFLD increased the risk of overall mortality (HR 2.2 [1.1–4.2]; $P = .03$), but not the CV death (HR 0.9 [0.3–2.4]; $P = .81$)
Ekstedt et al,[48] 2006	129	Patients with NAFLD with ELF (Sweden)	Liver biopsy	Registry of death	Prospective (FU 13.7 y)	Survival similar to a matched population. Mortality was not increased in simple steatosis. Patients with NASH died most from CV and liver
Rafiq et al,[4] 2009	173	Patients with NAFLD (United States)	Liver biopsy	Registry of death	Prospective (FU 13 y)	CVD leading death cause. Similar overall mortality for NASH and non-NASH; liver death was higher in NASH; overall and liver death was higher in patients with NAFLD with T2DM
Soderberg et al,[35] 2010	256	Patients with ELF (Sweden)	Liver biopsy	Registry of death	Prospective (FU 24 y)	CVD leading death cause; NAFLD (SMR 1.69 [1.24–2.25]) and NASH (SMR 1.86 [1.19–2.76]) higher overall mortality compared with matched controls
Lazo et al,[37] 2011	11,371	Population-based cohort (United States)	Ultrasonography	Registry of death	Prospective (FU 14.5 y)	NAFLD was not related to overall (HR 0.92 [(0.67–1.09)], CV (HR 0.86 [0.67–1.12]), or liver mortality (HR 0.64 [0.12–3.59])
Dunn et al,[34] 2008	7574	Population-based cohort (United States)	ELF, imaging, or liver biopsy	Registry of death	Prospective (FU 8.7 y)	NAFLD higher overall mortality (HR 1.37 [0.98–1.91]; $P = .067$); in ages 45–54 y NAFLD related to CV death (HR 8.43 [2.43–22.72])

(continued on next page)

Table 1
(continued)

Reference	n	Study Population	NAFLD Criteria	CVD Criteria	Design	Main Results (95% Confidence Interval)
Ong et al,[33] 2008	11,285	Population-based cohort (United States)	Ultrasonography	Registry of death	Prospective (FU 8.7 y)	NAFLD: higher risk of overall (HR 1.038 [1.036–1.041]; P<.001) and liver death (HR 9.32 [9.21–9.43]; P<.001); CVD top death cause
Calori et al,[40] 2011	2074	Population-based cohort (Italy)	FLI	Registry of death	Prospective (FU 15 y)	NAFLD: higher risk of overall (HR 1.004 [1.001–1.007]; P = .03), CV (HR 1.006 [1.000–1.011]; P = .04), and liver death (HR 1.037 [1.022–1.053]; P<.001)
Kim et al,[41] 2013	11,154	Population-based cohort (United States)	Ultrasonography	Registry of death	Prospective (FU 14.5 y)	NAFLD was not related to overall mortality. HR for NFS: NAFLD with AF as per noninvasive markers associated with overall (1.69 [1.09–2.63]; P = .02) and CV death (HR 3.46 [1.91–6.25]; P<.001)
Stepanova et al,[49] 2013	289	Patients with NAFLD (United States)	Liver biopsy	Registry of death	Prospective (FU 12.5 y)	CVD leading death cause. Overall and CV mortality similar between NASH and non-NASH. NASH (HR 9.16 [2.10–9.88]; P<.001) and T2DM (HR 2.19 [1.00–4.81]; P<.001) higher liver death
Angulo et al,[45] 2013	320	Patients with NAFLD (International)	Liver biopsy	Review of medical records	Prospective (FU 8.8 y)	CVD leading death cause. AF by noninvasive markers represented increased risk of overall death as per NFS (HR 9.8 [2.7–35.3]; P<.001); APRI (HR 3.1 [1.1–8.4]; P = .03) and FIB-4 (HR 6.9 [2.3–20.4]; P = .001)

Abbreviations: AF, advanced fibrosis; ELF, elevated liver function; FU, follow-up; HR, hazard ratio; SMR, standardized mortality ratio; T2DM, type 2 diabetes mellitus.

Data from Refs. [4,32–37,40,41,45,48,49]

Table 2
Main studies associating NAFLD and CV risk

Reference	n	Study Population	NAFLD	CVD Criteria	Design	Outcomes	Main Results (95% Confidence Interval)
Ruttmann et al,[53] 2005	163,944	Population-based cohort (Austria)	GGT	Death certificates	Prospective (FU 11.5 y)	CVD mortality	NAFLD associated with CV death in men (HR 1.64 [1.35–2.0]; $P<.001$) and women (HR 1.51 [1.21–1.89]; $P<.001$); dose-response relationship of GGT and CVD death
Lee et al,[55] 2006	28,838	Population-based cohort (Finland)	GGT	Medical records/ death certificates	Prospective (FU 11.9 y)	Nonfatal MI and fatal-CHD	NAFLD associated with CVD in men (HR 1.57 [1.22–2.01]; $P<.01$) and women (HR 1.44 [1.03–2.02]; $P<.01$)
Schindhelm et al,[57] 2007	1439	Population-based cohort (Netherlands)	ALT	Medical records	Prospective (FU 10 y)	CHD (UA, MI), CHF, stroke	NAFLD associated with CHD (HR 1.88 [1.21–2.92]; $P<.01$)
Hamaguchi et al,[59] 2007	1637	Population-based cohort (Japan)	Ultrasonography	Self-reported questionnaire	Prospective (FU 5 y)	UA; MI; stroke	NAFLD associated with CVD (OR 4.12 [1.58–10.75]; $P=.004$)
Targher et al,[47] 2007	2103	T2DM patients (Italy)	Ultrasonography	No data	Prospective (FU 6.5 y)	Fatal and nonfatal CVD (MI, stroke, coronary bypass)	NAFLD associated with nonfatal and fatal CVD (HR 1.87 [1.2–2.6]; $P<.001$)

(continued on next page)

Table 2
(continued)

Reference	n	Study Population	NAFLD	CVD Criteria	Design	Outcomes	Main Results (95% Confidence Interval)
Arslan et al,[60] 2007	92	Patients undergoing coronary angiography (Turkey)	Ultrasonography	Coronary angiogram	Cross-sectional	CAD	NAFLD was associated with CAD (OR 6.73 [1.14–39.61]; P = .035)
Wong et al,[62] 2011	612	Patients undergoing coronary angiography (Hong Kong)	Ultrasonography	Coronary angiogram; CVD adjudicated	Cross-sectional with posterior FU (87 wk)	CAD; overall mortality; MI and CV death	CAD more prevalent in NAFLD (84.6 vs 61.4%; P<.001). NAFLD associated with CAD (OR 2.31 [1.46–3.64]; P<.001); but not predictive of CV morbidity and mortality in patients with established CVD
Stepanova & Younossi,[38] 2012	2492	Population-based cohort (United States)	Ultrasonography	Self-reported for nonfatal CVD; registry of death	Prospective (FU 14.3 y)	Fatal and nonfatal CVD (MI, stroke, CHF)	CV death 3.76%. CVD was more prevalent in NAFLD (38 vs 29%; P<.05). NAFLD associated with nonfatal CVD (OR 1.23 [1.04–1.44]; P<.001), but not with CV mortality

Abbreviations: ALT, alanine aminotransferase; CAD, coronary artery disease (>50% stenosis major artery); CHD, cardiovascular heart disease; FU, follow-up; HR, hazard ratio; MI, myocardial infarction; OR, odds ratio; SMR, standardized mortality ratio; T2DM, type 2 diabetes mellitus; UA, unstable angina.

Data from Refs.[38,47,53,55,57,59,60,62]

Despite the absence of attributable risk for each liver injury, these studies provide clear evidence that patients with NAFLD have a high risk of CVD. The evidence of this strong association should affect clinical practice, suggesting CV screening of individuals with fatty liver.

POSSIBLE MECHANISMS LINKING NAFLD AND CVD

In IR, adipose and muscle cells oxidize lipids, resulting in increased released of free fatty acids (FFA), which can then be incorporated into triglycerides in the liver, leading to steatosis, representing the first hit. In presence of steatosis, an activation of an inflammatory cascade associated with a complex interaction (ie, multiple second hits) among hepatocytes, stellate, adipose, and Kupffer cells results in progression to apoptosis/necrosis (NASH), fibrosis, and consequently, cirrhosis.[63] The mechanisms linking NAFLD and atherosclerosis might be associated with the multihit process, involving a complex interaction among IR, oxidative stress, and activation of an inflammatory cascade.[64]

IR associated with increased fat content seems to be one of the key features of NAFLD development, NASH progression, and CV outcomes. Hyperinsulinemia results in alteration in cellular FFA transport, leading to fat accumulation away from adipose tissue and toward key metabolic organs, such as skeletal muscle and liver. Impaired insulin metabolism in these organs results in IR exacerbation and consequent cardiometabolic dysfunctional cascade activation.[65] Visceral adipose tissue (VAT) is defined as intra-abdominal fat bounded by parietal peritoneum or transversalis fascia. VAT lipolysis secondary to IR represents a major source of FFA delivered to the liver.[66] Liver fat induces hepatic inflammation through lipotoxicity and increased oxidative stress caused by excess of FFA.[67] The presence of FFA induces an increased CV risk and strongly correlates with liver inflammation and fibrosis in patients with NAFLD.[68–70]

A systemic inflammatory status with proinflammatory and atherogenic molecules, primarily secreted by the liver, may play a decisive role in the relationship between NAFLD and atherosclerosis and CVD. Several studies have reported that patients with NASH presented increased inflammatory cytokines, such as high-sensitive C-reactive protein, tumor necrosis factor α, and interleukin 6, and prothrombotic factors, such as fibrinogen and plasminogen activator inhibitor.[71–73] The complex interaction between higher VAT and IR status leads also to a deranged adipokine profile. Adiponectin acts as a protective adipokine by inhibiting liver gluconeogenesis and suppressing lipogenesis. Patients with fatty liver present higher levels of oxidative stress and inflammation associated with hypoadiponectinemia levels compared with controls.[74,75] In addition, proinflammatory transcription factors might be implicated in this process. Activation of the nuclear factor $\kappa\beta$ (NF-$\kappa\beta$) pathway in the liver of patients with NASH increased the transcription of several proinflammatory genes, amplifying the systemic inflammation.[76] In an experimental model, the presence of hepatic steatosis resulted in upregulation of NF-$\kappa\beta$, which led to hepatic production of proinflammatory cytokines, as well as activation of Kupffer cells and macrophages, worsening hepatic inflammation.[77]

Furthermore, an atherogenic dyslipidemia profile and an endothelial dysfunction that characterize patients with NAFLD should also explain the link between fatty liver and CVD. This atherogenic dyslipidemia profile, defined by high triglyceride levels, low high-density lipoprotein cholesterol and increased low-density lipoprotein (LDL) cholesterol, is strongly associated with severe CV outcomes.[78] Several studies reported that NAFLD, especially in NASH forms, might exacerbate systemic and hepatic IR, leading to development of this atherogenic dyslipidemia.[76,79] Furthermore,

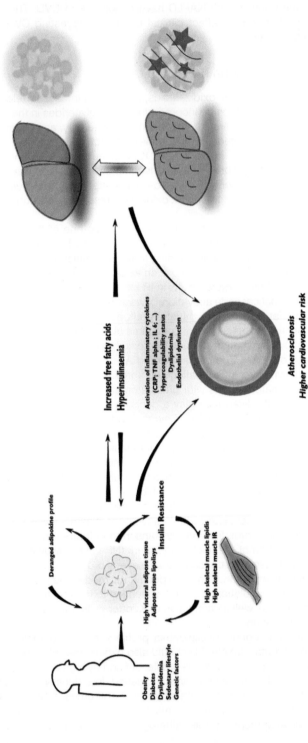

Fig. 1. Complex interrelationship process linking NAFLD and increased CV risk.

endothelial dysfunction plays an important role in atherosclerosis. Studies have described an independent association between impaired endothelium-dependent flow-mediated dilation and NAFLD.[80,81] In addition, more accentuated endothelial dysfunction was observed in patients with NASH than those with simple steatosis, confirming the hypothesis of increased CV risk according to the severity of liver disease in NAFLD.[80]

Fig. 1 summarizes the complex pathologic process linking NAFLD and CV risk. This schematic diagram highlights the role of metabolic factors, IR, FFA, adipokines, and inflammatory cytokines, which may explain the link between fatty liver and CVD.

FRAMINGHAM SCORE TO PREDICT CVD IN PATIENTS WITH NAFLD

The Framingham risk score (FRS) is an accurate tool to predict CVD risk.[82,83] This score is based on gender, age, hypertension, serum total and LDL cholesterol, diabetes, and smoking habits to calculate the risk of development of CV events.[84] FRS can be easily accessed from the Web site http://www.framinghamheartstudy.org/risk/coronary.html.[85] This score stratifies subjects as low (<10%), intermediate (10%–20%), or high CVD risk (>20%).[86] FRS can be used worldwide, despite a potential overestimation of CV risk in some patients, such as the Japanese, Hispanic, and Caribbean-Indian population.[87] Furthermore, this score has already been validated in a European population.[88] This score was validated in patients with NAFLD, showing that the proportion of new onset of coronary heart disease was similar to that predicted at baseline, as per FRS, over 11.5 years of follow-up.[89] Patients with NAFLD and NASH have presented significantly higher 10-year FRS compared with age-matched and gender-matched controls.[21,89,90] FRS can be accurately used to predict CVD in patients with NAFLD.

SUMMARY

NAFLD is a clinicopathologic syndrome characterized by ectopic fat accumulation associated with a chronic inflammatory state, in which IR, abnormal adipose tissue, oxidative stress, and excessive FFAs are the main actors. These complex interactions results in a low-grade chronic inflammation, endothelial dysfunction, and hypercoagulability status that results in potential progression of atherosclerosis and severe CV outcomes.

Major studies have reported that patients with NAFLD are at higher risk of atherosclerosis, CV mortality, and overall mortality compared with the general population, independently of known metabolic factors. This strong association between NAFLD and higher CV risk should be considered in potential screening and surveillance of patients with fatty liver in clinical practice. On the other hand, patients with CVD are possibly at higher risk of liver-related mortality as a result of the risk of cirrhosis and primary liver cancer.

The progress in noninvasive biomarkers of organ injuries should permit better identification of the risk of mortality as a result of cardiovascular or liver diseases. For the liver, specific biomarkers of steatosis, necroinflammatory activity, and fibrosis should also improve the knowledge of possible common pathways.

REFERENCES

1. Williams CD, Stengel J, Asike MI, et al. Prevalence of nonalcoholic fatty liver disease and nonalcoholic steatohepatitis among a largely middle-aged population

utilizing ultrasound and liver biopsy: a prospective study. Gastroenterology 2011;140(1):124–31.

2. Adams LA, Lindor KD. Nonalcoholic fatty liver disease. Ann Epidemiol 2007; 17(11):863–9.

3. Harrison SA, Neuschwander-Tetri BA. Nonalcoholic fatty liver disease and nonalcoholic steatohepatitis. Clin Liver Dis 2004;8(4):861–79, ix.

4. Rafiq N, Bai C, Fang Y, et al. Long-term follow-up of patients with nonalcoholic fatty liver. Clin Gastroenterol Hepatol 2009;7(2):234–8.

5. Edmison J, McCullough AJ. Pathogenesis of non-alcoholic steatohepatitis: human data. Clin Liver Dis 2007;11(1):75–104, ix.

6. Bugianesi E, Leone N, Vanni E, et al. Expanding the natural history of nonalcoholic steatohepatitis: from cryptogenic cirrhosis to hepatocellular carcinoma. Gastroenterology 2002;123(1):134–40.

7. Wong VW, Hui AY, Tsang SW, et al. Metabolic and adipokine profile of Chinese patients with nonalcoholic fatty liver disease. Clin Gastroenterol Hepatol 2006; 4(9):1154–61.

8. Lizardi-Cervera J, Aguilar-Zapata D. Nonalcoholic fatty liver disease and its association with cardiovascular disease. Ann Hepatol 2009;8(Suppl 1):S40–3.

9. Marchesini G, Brizi M, Bianchi G, et al. Nonalcoholic fatty liver disease: a feature of the metabolic syndrome. Diabetes 2001;50(8):1844–50.

10. Budoff MJ, Achenbach S, Blumenthal RS, et al. Assessment of coronary artery disease by cardiac computed tomography: a scientific statement from the American Heart Association Committee on Cardiovascular Imaging and Intervention, Council on Cardiovascular Radiology and Intervention, and Committee on Cardiac Imaging, Council on Clinical Cardiology. Circulation 2006;114(16): 1761–91.

11. Girshman J, Wolff SD. Techniques for quantifying coronary artery calcification. Semin Ultrasound CT MR 2003;24(1):33–8.

12. Wexler L, Brundage B, Crouse J, et al. Coronary artery calcification: pathophysiology, epidemiology, imaging methods, and clinical implications. A statement for health professionals from the American Heart Association. Writing Group. Circulation 1996;94(5):1175–92.

13. Assy N, Djibre A, Farah R, et al. Presence of coronary plaques in patients with nonalcoholic fatty liver disease. Radiology 2010;254(2):393–400.

14. Kim D, Choi SY, Park EH, et al. Nonalcoholic fatty liver disease is associated with coronary artery calcification. Hepatology 2012;56(2):605–13.

15. Chen CH, Nien CK, Yang CC, et al. Association between nonalcoholic fatty liver disease and coronary artery calcification. Dig Dis Sci 2010;55(6):1752–60.

16. Akabame S, Hamaguchi M, Tomiyasu K, et al. Evaluation of vulnerable coronary plaques and non-alcoholic fatty liver disease (NAFLD) by 64-detector multislice computed tomography (MSCT). Circ J 2008;72(4):618–25.

17. Lorenz MW, Markus HS, Bots ML, et al. Prediction of clinical cardiovascular events with carotid intima-media thickness: a systematic review and meta-analysis. Circulation 2007;115(4):459–67.

18. O'Leary DH, Polak JF, Kronmal RA, et al. Carotid-artery intima and media thickness as a risk factor for myocardial infarction and stroke in older adults. Cardiovascular Health Study Collaborative Research Group. N Engl J Med 1999; 340(1):14–22.

19. Caserta CA, Pendino GM, Amante A, et al. Cardiovascular risk factors, nonalcoholic fatty liver disease, and carotid artery intima-media thickness in an adolescent population in southern Italy. Am J Epidemiol 2010;171(11):1195–202.

20. Volzke H, Robinson DM, Kleine V, et al. Hepatic steatosis is associated with an increased risk of carotid atherosclerosis. World J Gastroenterol 2005;11(12): 1848–53.
21. Gastaldelli A, Kozakova M, Hojlund K, et al. Fatty liver is associated with insulin resistance, risk of coronary heart disease, and early atherosclerosis in a large European population. Hepatology 2009;49(5):1537–44.
22. Kozakova M, Palombo C, Eng MP, et al. Fatty liver index, gamma-glutamyltransferase, and early carotid plaques. Hepatology 2012;55(5): 1406–15.
23. Sookoian S, Pirola CJ. Non-alcoholic fatty liver disease is strongly associated with carotid atherosclerosis: a systematic review. J Hepatol 2008;49(4):600–7.
24. Targher G, Bertolini L, Padovani R, et al. Relations between carotid artery wall thickness and liver histology in subjects with nonalcoholic fatty liver disease. Diabetes Care 2006;29(6):1325–30.
25. Goland S, Shimoni S, Zornitzki T, et al. Cardiac abnormalities as a new manifestation of nonalcoholic fatty liver disease: echocardiographic and tissue Doppler imaging assessment. J Clin Gastroenterol 2006;40(10):949–55.
26. Fotbolcu H, Yakar T, Duman D, et al. Impairment of the left ventricular systolic and diastolic function in patients with non-alcoholic fatty liver disease. Cardiol J 2010;17(5):457–63.
27. Hallsworth K, Hollingsworth KG, Thoma C, et al. Cardiac structure and function are altered in adults with non-alcoholic fatty liver disease. J Hepatol 2013;58(4): 757–62.
28. Fallo F, Dalla Pozza A, Sonino N, et al. Non-alcoholic fatty liver disease is associated with left ventricular diastolic dysfunction in essential hypertension. Nutr Metab Cardiovasc Dis 2009;19(9):646–53.
29. Yilmaz Y, Kurt R, Yonal O, et al. Coronary flow reserve is impaired in patients with nonalcoholic fatty liver disease: association with liver fibrosis. Atherosclerosis 2010;211(1):182–6.
30. Targher G, Valbusa F, Bonapace S, et al. Non-alcoholic fatty liver disease is associated with an increased incidence of atrial fibrillation in patients with type 2 diabetes. PLoS One 2013;8(2):e57183.
31. Targher G, Mantovani A, Pichiri I, et al. Non-alcoholic fatty liver disease is associated with an increased prevalence of atrial fibrillation in hospitalized patients with type 2 diabetes. Clin Sci (Lond) 2013;125(6):301–9.
32. Adams LA, Lymp JF, St Sauver J, et al. The natural history of nonalcoholic fatty liver disease: a population-based cohort study. Gastroenterology 2005;129(1): 113–21.
33. Ong JP, Pitts A, Younossi ZM. Increased overall mortality and liver-related mortality in non-alcoholic fatty liver disease. J Hepatol 2008;49(4):608–12.
34. Dunn W, Xu R, Wingard DL, et al. Suspected nonalcoholic fatty liver disease and mortality risk in a population-based cohort study. Am J Gastroenterol 2008; 103(9):2263–71.
35. Söderberg C, Stal P, Askling J, et al. Decreased survival of subjects with elevated liver function tests during a 28-year follow-up. Hepatology 2010; 51(2):595–602.
36. Adams LA, Harmsen S, St Sauver JL, et al. Nonalcoholic fatty liver disease increases risk of death among patients with diabetes: a community-based cohort study. Am J Gastroenterol 2010;105(7):1567–73.
37. Lazo M, Hernaez R, Bonekamp S, et al. Non-alcoholic fatty liver disease and mortality among US adults: prospective cohort study. BMJ 2011;343:d6891.

38. Stepanova M, Younossi ZM. Independent association between nonalcoholic fatty liver disease and cardiovascular disease in the US population. Clin Gastroenterol Hepatol 2012;10(6):646–50.
39. Bedogni G, Bellentani S, Miglioli L, et al. The Fatty Liver Index: a simple and accurate predictor of hepatic steatosis in the general population. BMC Gastroenterol 2006;6:33.
40. Calori G, Lattuada G, Ragogna F, et al. Fatty liver index and mortality: the Cremona study in the 15th year of follow-up. Hepatology 2011;54(1):145–52.
41. Kim D, Kim WR, Kim HJ, et al. Association between noninvasive fibrosis markers and mortality among adults with nonalcoholic fatty liver disease in the United States. Hepatology 2013;57(4):1357–65.
42. Angulo P, Hui JM, Marchesini G, et al. The NAFLD fibrosis score: a noninvasive system that identifies liver fibrosis in patients with NAFLD. Hepatology 2007; 45(4):846–54.
43. Wai CT, Greenson JK, Fontana RJ, et al. A simple noninvasive index can predict both significant fibrosis and cirrhosis in patients with chronic hepatitis C. Hepatology 2003;38(2):518–26.
44. Shah AG, Lydecker A, Murray K, et al. Comparison of noninvasive markers of fibrosis in patients with nonalcoholic fatty liver disease. Clin Gastroenterol Hepatol 2009;7(10):1104–12.
45. Angulo P, Bugianesi E, Bjornsson ES, et al. Simple non-invasive systems predict long-term outcomes of patients with nonalcoholic fatty liver disease. Gastroenterology 2013;145:782–9.
46. Dam-Larsen S, Becker U, Franzmann MB, et al. Final results of a long-term, clinical follow-up in fatty liver patients. Scand J Gastroenterol 2009;44(10):1236–43.
47. Targher G, Bertolini L, Rodella S, et al. Nonalcoholic fatty liver disease is independently associated with an increased incidence of cardiovascular events in type 2 diabetic patients. Diabetes Care 2007;30(8):2119–21.
48. Ekstedt M, Franzen LE, Mathiesen UL, et al. Long-term follow-up of patients with NAFLD and elevated liver enzymes. Hepatology 2006;44(4):865–73.
49. Stepanova M, Rafiq N, Makhlouf H, et al. Predictors of all-cause mortality and liver-related mortality in patients with non-alcoholic fatty liver disease (NAFLD). Dig Dis Sci 2013;58:3017–23.
50. Zhao XQ, Krasuski RA, Baer J, et al. Effects of combination lipid therapy on coronary stenosis progression and clinical cardiovascular events in coronary disease patients with metabolic syndrome: a combined analysis of the Familial Atherosclerosis Treatment Study (FATS), the HDL-Atherosclerosis Treatment Study (HATS), and the Armed Forces Regression Study (AFREGS). Am J Cardiol 2009;104(11):1457–64.
51. Bhatia LS, Curzen NP, Calder PC, et al. Non-alcoholic fatty liver disease: a new and important cardiovascular risk factor? Eur Heart J 2012;33(10): 1190–200.
52. Targher G, Marra F, Marchesini G. Increased risk of cardiovascular disease in non-alcoholic fatty liver disease: causal effect or epiphenomenon? Diabetologia 2008;51(11):1947–53.
53. Ruttmann E, Brant LJ, Concin H, et al. Gamma-glutamyltransferase as a risk factor for cardiovascular disease mortality: an epidemiological investigation in a cohort of 163,944 Austrian adults. Circulation 2005;112(14):2130–7.
54. Lee DS, Evans JC, Robins SJ, et al. Gamma glutamyl transferase and metabolic syndrome, cardiovascular disease, and mortality risk: the Framingham Heart Study. Arterioscler Thromb Vasc Biol 2007;27(1):127–33.

55. Lee DH, Silventoinen K, Hu G, et al. Serum gamma-glutamyltransferase predicts non-fatal myocardial infarction and fatal coronary heart disease among 28,838 middle-aged men and women. Eur Heart J 2006;27(18):2170–6.
56. Fraser A, Harris R, Sattar N, et al. Gamma-glutamyltransferase is associated with incident vascular events independently of alcohol intake: analysis of the British Women's Heart and Health Study and Meta-Analysis. Arterioscler Thromb Vasc Biol 2007;27(12):2729–35.
57. Schindhelm RK, Dekker JM, Nijpels G, et al. Alanine aminotransferase predicts coronary heart disease events: a 10-year follow-up of the Hoorn Study. Atherosclerosis 2007;191(2):391–6.
58. Yun KE, Shin CY, Yoon YS, et al. Elevated alanine aminotransferase levels predict mortality from cardiovascular disease and diabetes in Koreans. Atherosclerosis 2009;205(2):533–7.
59. Hamaguchi M, Kojima T, Takeda N, et al. Nonalcoholic fatty liver disease is a novel predictor of cardiovascular disease. World J Gastroenterol 2007;13(10): 1579–84.
60. Arslan U, Turkoglu S, Balcioglu S, et al. Association between nonalcoholic fatty liver disease and coronary artery disease. Coron Artery Dis 2007;18(6):433–6.
61. Kadayifci A, Tan V, Ursell PC, et al. Clinical and pathologic risk factors for atherosclerosis in cirrhosis: a comparison between NASH-related cirrhosis and cirrhosis due to other aetiologies. J Hepatol 2008;49(4):595–9.
62. Wong VW, Wong GL, Yip GW, et al. Coronary artery disease and cardiovascular outcomes in patients with non-alcoholic fatty liver disease. Gut 2011;60(12):1721–7.
63. Day CP, James OF. Steatohepatitis: a tale of two "hits"? Gastroenterology 1998; 114(4):842–5.
64. Kotronen A, Juurinen L, Tiikkainen M, et al. Increased liver fat, impaired insulin clearance, and hepatic and adipose tissue insulin resistance in type 2 diabetes. Gastroenterology 2008;135(1):122–30.
65. Fabbrini E, Magkos F, Mohammed BS, et al. Intrahepatic fat, not visceral fat, is linked with metabolic complications of obesity. Proc Natl Acad Sci U S A 2009; 106(36):15430–5.
66. Bjorntorp P. "Portal" adipose tissue as a generator of risk factors for cardiovascular disease and diabetes. Arteriosclerosis 1990;10(4):493–6.
67. Shoelson SE, Lee J, Goldfine AB. Inflammation and insulin resistance. J Clin Invest 2006;116(7):1793–801.
68. Kotronen A, Westerbacka J, Bergholm R, et al. Liver fat in the metabolic syndrome. J Clin Endocrinol Metab 2007;92(9):3490–7.
69. Despres JP, Lemieux I, Bergeron J, et al. Abdominal obesity and the metabolic syndrome: contribution to global cardiometabolic risk. Arterioscler Thromb Vasc Biol 2008;28(6):1039–49.
70. van der Poorten D, Milner KL, Hui J, et al. Visceral fat: a key mediator of steatohepatitis in metabolic liver disease. Hepatology 2008;48(2):449–57.
71. Lavie CJ, Milani RV, Verma A, et al. C-reactive protein and cardiovascular diseases–is it ready for primetime? Am J Med Sci 2009;338(6):486–92.
72. Dowman JK, Tomlinson JW, Newsome PN. Pathogenesis of non-alcoholic fatty liver disease. QJM 2010;103(2):71–83.
73. Videla LA, Tapia G, Rodrigo R, et al. Liver NF-kappaB and AP-1 DNA binding in obese patients. Obesity (Silver Spring) 2009;17(5):973–9.
74. McKimmie RL, Daniel KR, Carr JJ, et al. Hepatic steatosis and subclinical cardiovascular disease in a cohort enriched for type 2 diabetes: the Diabetes Heart Study. Am J Gastroenterol 2008;103(12):3029–35.

75. Otsuka F, Sugiyama S, Kojima S, et al. Hypoadiponectinemia is associated with impaired glucose tolerance and coronary artery disease in non-diabetic men. Circ J 2007;71(11):1703–9.
76. Stefan N, Kantartzis K, Haring HU. Causes and metabolic consequences of fatty liver. Endocr Rev 2008;29(7):939–60.
77. Cai D, Yuan M, Frantz DF, et al. Local and systemic insulin resistance resulting from hepatic activation of IKK-beta and NF-kappaB. Nat Med 2005;11(2): 183–90.
78. Gaziano JM, Hennekens CH, O'Donnell CJ, et al. Fasting triglycerides, high-density lipoprotein, and risk of myocardial infarction. Circulation 1997;96(8): 2520–5.
79. Shoelson SE, Herrero L, Naaz A. Obesity, inflammation, and insulin resistance. Gastroenterology 2007;132(6):2169–80.
80. Villanova N, Moscatiello S, Ramilli S, et al. Endothelial dysfunction and cardio-vascular risk profile in nonalcoholic fatty liver disease. Hepatology 2005;42(2): 473–80.
81. Schindhelm RK, Diamant M, Bakker SJ, et al. Liver alanine aminotransferase, in-sulin resistance and endothelial dysfunction in normotriglyceridaemic subjects with type 2 diabetes mellitus. Eur J Clin Invest 2005;35(6):369–74.
82. Kannel WB, McGee D, Gordon T. A general cardiovascular risk profile: the Fra-mingham Study. Am J Cardiol 1976;38(1):46–51.
83. Framingham Heart Study Bibliography. Available at: http://www. framinghamheartstudy.org/biblio/index.html. Accessed June 6, 2013.
84. Wilson PW, D'Agostino RB, Levy D, et al. Prediction of coronary heart disease using risk factor categories. Circulation 1998;97(18):1837–47.
85. Cosin Aguilar J, Hernandiz Martinez A, Rodriguez Padial L, et al. Assessment of cardiovascular risk in population groups. Comparison of Score system and Framingham in hypertensive patients. Rev Clin Esp 2006;206(4):182–7 [in Spanish].
86. Ford ES, Giles WH, Mokdad AH. The distribution of 10-year risk for coronary heart disease among US adults: findings from the National Health and Nutrition Examination Survey III. J Am Coll Cardiol 2004;43(10):1791–6.
87. Jaquet A, Deloumeaux J, Dumoulin M, et al. Metabolic syndrome and Framing-ham risk score for prediction of cardiovascular events in Caribbean Indian pa-tients with blood glucose abnormalities. Diabetes Metab 2008;34(2):177–81.
88. Brindle P, Emberson J, Lampe F, et al. Predictive accuracy of the Framingham coronary risk score in British men: prospective cohort study. BMJ 2003; 327(7426):1267.
89. Treeprasertsuk S, Leverage S, Adams LA, et al. The Framingham risk score and heart disease in nonalcoholic fatty liver disease. Liver Int 2012;32(6):945–50.
90. Sung KC, Ryan MC, Wilson AM. The severity of nonalcoholic fatty liver disease is associated with increased cardiovascular risk in a large cohort of non-obese Asian subjects. Atherosclerosis 2009;203(2):581–6.

Host Genetic Variants in Obesity-Related Nonalcoholic Fatty Liver Disease

Rohini Mehta, PhD[a], Aybike Birerdinc, PhD[a,b],
Zobair M. Younossi, MD, MPH, AGAF[a,c],*

KEYWORDS

• SNP • GWAS • Polymorphism • Steatosis

KEY POINTS

• Identifying genetic associations with nonalcoholic fatty liver disease (NAFLD) may offer insights into the mechanisms of disease pathogenesis, provide new diagnostic tools, and identify new therapeutic targets.

• Single-nucleotide polymorphisms (SNPs) or polymorphisms are single nucleotide substitutions in DNA that may result in the altered expression of a particular gene or altered function of the expressed protein.

• SNPs may be used in combination panels to better predict disease susceptibility and subsequent resolution.

• Future directions in genome-wide association studies need to include studies of SNPs from major regulatory genes in large cohorts of multiethnic populations to fully illustrate the combinatorial effects of these changes.

INTRODUCTION

Nonalcoholic fatty liver disease (NAFLD) is the leading cause of chronic liver disease over the last 3 decades.[1,2] NAFLD is a spectrum of disorders characterized by the deposition of fat in the liver, steatosis, which is not caused by significant alcohol consumption. Steatosis may progress to nonalcoholic steatohepatitis (NASH) in which there is inflammation, with a 20% risk of progressing to fibrosis and cirrhosis (**Fig. 1**).[3] Despite numerous lines of research on NAFLD, the epidemiology and natural history of NAFLD

The authors have nothing to disclose.
[a] Betty and Guy Beatty Center for Integrated Research, Center for Liver Disease, Inova Health System, Claude Moore Building, 3300 Gallows Road, Falls Church, VA 22042, USA; [b] Center for the Study of Chronic Metabolic Diseases, School of Systems Biology, George Mason University, 4400 University Drive, Fairfax, VA 22030 USA; [c] Department of Medicine, Center for Liver Disease, VCU-Inova Campus, Inova Fairfax Hospital, Claude Moore Building, 3300 Gallows Road, Falls Church, VA 22042, USA
* Corresponding author. Department of Medicine, VCU-Inova Campus, Inova Fairfax Hospital, Inova Health System, Falls Church, VA.
E-mail address: Zobair.Younossi@inova.org

Clin Liver Dis 18 (2014) 249–267
http://dx.doi.org/10.1016/j.cld.2013.09.017
1089-3261/14/$ – see front matter © 2014 Elsevier Inc. All rights reserved.

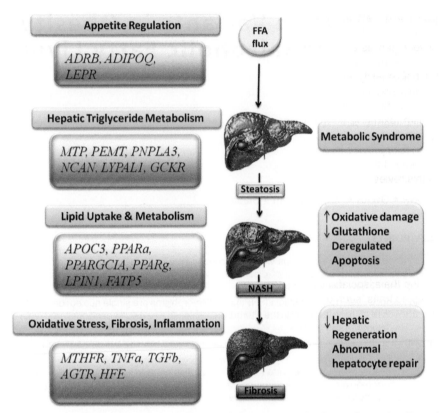

Fig. 1. Sequential steps of NAFLD pathology and the genes involved in pathways implicated in NAFLD. FFA, free fatty acids.

remain incompletely understood.[1] NAFLD is estimated to affect more than 35 million people in the United States and 28 million people worldwide.[4] Unfortunately, the prevalence of NAFLD in the general population is often underreported, largely because of a lack of symptoms in the early stages and, therefore, varies widely, ranging from 19% to 45%.[4] This variability may also be attributed to the inherent sensitivities of the different tools used in the diagnosis of NAFLD, such as liver enzymes (alanine transaminase [ALT]), ultrasound, magnetic resonance spectroscopy, biopsy, and so forth.[1] In Spain, a multicenter cross-sectional study shows the prevalence of NAFLD to be at 26% of the general population.[5] Another study reported a 42% prevalence of biopsy-proven NASH in Bangladesh, similar to reports from Western countries.[6] The overall prevalence of NAFLD in the participants of the Dallas Heart Study, a multiethnic population-based study in Dallas County, Texas, was 34% using magnetic resonance spectroscopy for hepatic triglyceride quantitation.[7] Although the prevalence of NAFLD based on elevated aminotransferases (ALT and aspartate transaminase [AST]) alone is between 7% and 11%, this is most likely an underestimation because numerous studies using biopsy as the diagnostic tool have shown that aminotransferases can be normal in individuals with NAFLD. As expected, liver biopsy of potential living donors for liver transplantation estimated the prevalence of steatosis as 20%.[8]

NAFLD is a complex disease with interplay between environmental and genetic factors contributing to the considerable variability of the natural history of the disease. A possible genetic involvement in NAFLD development was initially suggested based on studies that showed the coexistence of NASH and/or cryptogenic cirrhosis within several families.[9] Further support came from the observed ethnic differences in NAFLD prevalence, which are only partially explained by differences in the risk factors, such as obesity, insulin resistance, and dyslipidemia.[6,7,10,11] Importantly, there is substantial evidence that genetic polymorphisms underlying diabetes mellitus and obesity may predispose individuals to NAFLD by influencing insulin signaling, lipid metabolism, oxidative stress, fibrogenesis, and inflammation (see **Fig. 1**).[12,13] Identifying genetic associations with NAFLD may offer insights into mechanisms of disease pathogenesis, provide new diagnostic tools, and identify new therapeutic targets.

Some of the genetic variants and their biologic implications in NAFLD are discussed in this review.

GENETIC ASSOCIATION STUDIES

Genetic association studies can be divided into 2 broad categories: (1) family based versus population based and (2) candidate gene studies versus genome-wide association studies (GWAS). GWAS is a powerful, hypothesis-free method for systematically testing the association between all common variants in the human genome and polymorphic traits, such as disease, drug response, drug toxicity, and others.[13,14] GWAS are only able to identify a region within the genome that is associated with a phenotype. The identification of the causal or functional polymorphism needs to be followed up with additional studies. A good GWAS requires a stringent threshold for statistical significance; correction for multiple testing; and large, well-characterized cohorts to have enough power to detect real associations.[14]

Candidate gene studies, on the other hand, are selected for examination by their putative or known role in the pathogenesis of the disease or are based on the results of genomic and proteomic studies. The selection of a candidate gene is followed by the performance of a case-control SNP association study.[15] The limited number of SNPs selected in candidate gene studies minimizes the cost. The threshold for statistical significance is lower, although correction for multiple testing should still be performed. Unfortunately, such statistical vigilance has not always been the case. Another limitation of these targeted studies is the difficulty of correcting for population stratification; invalid associations can be created by systematic differences because of the shared ancestry between subgroups of study subjects. Panels of ancestry markers, or informative markers extracted from genome-wide genotyping data, can be used to address this issue.[16]

GENETIC VARIANTS ASSOCIATED WITH NAFLD
Polymorphisms in Genes Involved in the Synthesis, Storage, and Export of Hepatic Triglyceride

One of the features of the NAFLD spectrum of disease is the accumulation of triglycerides (TG) within hepatocytes. Genes that affect hepatic fat storage and mobilization as well as variants of transcription factors controlling lipid metabolism in the liver and adipose are, therefore, likely candidates in the development and progression of NAFLD. Two important GWAS identified polymorphisms in Patatin-like phospholipase domain-containing protein 3 (*PNPLA3*), neurocan (*NCAN*), and protein phosphatase 1, regulatory subunit 3B (*PPP1R3B*) as being associated with hepatic and serum TG levels, respectively.[17,18] Several candidate gene studies have also identified additional polymorphisms.

Microsomal triglyceride transport protein

The human microsomal triglyceride transport protein (MTP) is a heterodimer of a large and unique 97-kDa subunit and a 55-kDa protein disulfide isomerase.[19] MTP catalyzes the transfer of neutral lipids to nascent apolipoprotein B and plays a pivotal role in incorporating hepatic TG into very-low-density lipoproteins (VLDL) for lipid export from the liver.[20] Given the role of MTP in lipid cycling, several studies have explored the association of MTP variants and the accumulation of lipids in the liver. An SNP in the promoter region of MTP-rs1800804 (−164 T/C) has been shown to regulate the basal transcription of the gene.[21] The minor allele (−164 C) resulted in lower transcription of the MTP gene both in vivo and in vitro, which resulted in a relative decrease in MTP activity and, consequently, decreased VLDL assembly.[22] Thus, the presence of the C allele may contribute to intrahepatocyte TG accumulation by inhibiting TG export from the liver.

Additionally, the rs1800804 polymorphism has been demonstrated to be associated with an increased risk of ischemic heart disease, higher body mass index (BMI), and higher plasma insulin levels.[22,23] Peng and colleagues[24] and Ledmyr and colleagues[23] show the minor allele (−164 C) to be associated with decreased levels of plasma TG as compared with carriers of the common alleles. As compared with the patients with the TT homozygous allele, carriers of the heterozygous TC and homozygous CC alleles had a significantly increased risk of NAFLD (adjusted odds ratio [OR] 1.44, 95% confidence interval [CI] 1.07–1.92 for TC genotype; adjusted OR 1.87, 95% CI 1.01–3.47 for GG genotype) in an allelic dose–response manner (adjusted P_{Trend} = 0.004).[24]

The rs1800804 polymorphism lies in a putative consensus sequence (−174 to −163), which is homologous to the human LDL receptor promoter sterol response element.[25] Sterol response element binding protein (SREBP)-1a binds with a relatively higher strength to the MTP promoter region bearing the −164 T allele.[26] SREBPs play a central role in hepatic lipid metabolism, regulating the synthesis and uptake of cholesterol and fatty acids. It can, thus, be speculated that the presence of the −164 minor allele interferes with SREBPs mediated lipogenesis and uptake of free fatty acids (FFA).

Another polymorphism reported in the promoter region of MTP is rs1800591 (−493 G/T). The −493 G/T SNP is common and has been described as functional, with the G allele promoting less transcriptional activity than the T allele.[27,28] Unfortunately, the studies on the association of this SNP with NAFLD are inconsistent. The G-allele frequency was significantly higher in Japanese patients with biopsy-proven NASH, and the GG genotype in patients with NASH predicted more severe steatosis.[29] A relatively small study from Italy demonstrated that the −493 G/G genotype was found to have more severe liver disease and a more atherogenic postprandial lipoprotein profile.[30] However, Peng and colleagues[24] did not find any significant association between rs1800591 and the risk for NAFLD in the Chinese Han population. This result was similar to a recent study by Oliveira and colleagues[31] that reported an absence of an association between 493 G/T polymorphism and NAFLD in the Brazilian population. In patients with type 2 diabetes, the −493 G/T MTP gene polymorphism was associated independently with elevated serum ALT levels, which is a surrogate marker for NAFLD.[28] The variability seen in these studies raises the possibility that there may be geographic differences in the genes responsible for susceptibility to NAFLD. Based on the evidence thus far, further studies in larger samples of different populations are required to elucidate the participation of rs1800591 MTP polymorphism in NAFLD susceptibility.

Phosphatidylethanolamine N-methyltransferase

Another protein involved in the regulation of lipid export from hepatocytes is phosphatidylethanolamine N-methyltransferase (PEMT). PEMT catalyzes the major pathway of de novo synthesis of phosphatidylcholine in the liver.[32] Phosphatidylcholine molecules are essential for VLDL formation; when they are not available, fat droplets accumulate in the cytosol of hepatocytes. PEMT is, thus, involved in the flux of lipid between the liver and plasma and the delivery of essential fatty acids to blood and peripheral tissues via the liver-derived lipoproteins.[33] Song and colleagues[34] identified an SNP in the PEMT gene (523 G–>A), which results in a loss-of-function valine to methionine (V175M) substitution in the encoded protein. This loss-of-function variant was found to occur 1.7 fold more frequently in patients with biopsy-proven NAFLD as compared with controls.[34] Similarly, Dong and colleagues[35] found that a Val175Met variant was significantly more frequent in Japanese patients with biopsy-proven NASH than in 150 healthy volunteers and also found that nonobese carriers of the Val175Met variant were at an increased risk of NASH. In contrast, Romeo and colleagues[36] did not find an association between the V175M allele and hepatic triglyceride content in the Dallas Heart Study multiethnic cohort of 2349 individuals.

Patatin-like phospholipase domain-containing 3
The patatin-like phospholipase domain-containing 3 gene (PNPLA3) encodes a protein of 481 amino acids with triacylglycerol lipase activity, which mediates triacylglycerol hydrolysis. It is expressed mainly on the surface of lipid droplets in hepatocytes and adipocytes and is regulated by insulin through a signaling cascade that includes Liver X receptor (LXR) and SREBP-1c.[37] Two SNPs have been evaluated with regard to NAFLD: (1) a G-to-C change leading to the substitution of isoleucine with methionine at codon 148 (I148M, rs738409) and (2) a G-to-T change leading to the substitution of serine with isoleucine at codon 453 (S453I, rs6006460).

Romeo and colleagues[17] first identified the missense mutation rs738409 by GWAS. GWAS has found this variant to be the strongest genetic determinant of liver fat and ALT levels.[17,38,39] Valenti and colleagues[40] found rs738409 to be associated with higher ALT ($P = .0007$) in a dose-dependent manner in the Italian and UK population. This variant was found to influence liver fat independent of insulin resistance, dyslipidemia, and body mass.[17,39] The rs738409 variant occurs in higher frequency in the Hispanic population, who are known to be at an increased risk for NASH and cryptogenic cirrhosis.[17]

In a study in an Italian and UK population, the rs738409 SNP influenced both the presence of NASH and the severity of fibrosis in patients with NAFLD with histologic evaluation of liver damage, independent of body mass, diabetes, and NASH.[40] The occurrence of the GG genotype was similar in the Italian and UK population. The frequency distribution of the mutant G allele was significantly higher in Italian patients with NAFLD than in geographically-matched, age-matched, and sex-matched healthy controls with normal liver enzymes and metabolic parameters and a normal fatty liver index (OR 3.29, 95% CI 1.8–6.9). The GG genotype was associated with a higher LDL in both of the populations. The CG and GG genotypes were associated with lower high-density lipoprotein cholesterol (HDL-C) only in the Italian population.[40] The investigators also found the G allele to be an independent predictor of the presence of grade 2/3 steatosis similar to previous studies.[17,39,41,42]

Despite the plethora of published genetic association studies in NAFLD and NASH, this mutation remains the only robust and convincing association between a single SNP and the presence of hepatic steatosis.[15]

Other gene variants
A recent GWAS identified 3 additional gene variants associated with the severity of steatosis and other aspects of the NAFLD phenotype.[18] The neurocan (NCAN)

rs2228603 variant, glucokinase regulator (GCKR) rs780094 variant, and lysophospholipase-like 1 (LYPLAL1) rs12137855 variant were associated with both increasing hepatic steatosis and histologic NAFLD. A previously reported locus *PNPLA3* was also confirmed to be associated with both increasing hepatic steatosis and histologic NAFLD.[18] GCKR, a regulator of glucose metabolism and LYPLAL1, which exerts a complementary function to the PNPLA3 protein in triglyceride breakdown, was also associated with histologically assessed lobular inflammation and/or fibrosis. The rs780094 GCKR polymorphism was in strong linkage disequilibrium with another GCKR variant rs1260326 (P446L), which influences the ability of GCKR to inhibit glucokinase in response to fructose-6-phosphate, thereby resulting in a constant increase in hepatic glucokinase activity and glucose uptake by the liver.[43]

Polymorphism in Genes Influencing Lipid Metabolism

Apolipoproteins influence serum lipid metabolism. They associate with lipids and form lipoproteins. Variants of apolipoproteins may influence serum lipoprotein accumulation and may, thus, influence NAFLD.

Apolipoprotein C-III

Apolipoprotein C-III (APOC3) encodes a 79 amino acid lipid-binding glycoprotein. It also inhibits the function of lipoprotein lipase and interferes with the hepatic uptake of lipoproteins. Studies have suggested that 2 SNPs in the gene encoding *APOC3* may be associated with hypertriglyceridemia. The 2 SNPs in *APOC3*-rs2854116 (T455C) and rs2854117 (C482T) are located in the promoter region and are in strong linkage disequilibrium. These variant alleles interfere with the insulin-mediated regulation of APOC3 and, thus, are associated with higher APOC3 expression in vitro than the respective wild-type alleles.[44] These variants are associated with lipid metabolism, insulin signaling, metabolic syndrome (MetS), and hypertriglyceridaemia.[45] Further confirmation of this association comes from a meta-analysis indicating that the functional rs2854116 promoter polymorphism in *APOC3* was associated with an approximately 2-fold increased risk in MetS.[46] Additional research suggests that these variants predispose Indian men to liver fat accumulation by altering lipid metabolism and insulin resistance (IR).[47] This association is, however, absent in the Caucasian population.[48]

Peroxisome proliferator-activated receptor-alpha

Peroxisome proliferator-activated receptor-alpha (PPARα) is a member of the nuclear hormone receptor superfamily. It is expressed in cells with high catabolic rates of fatty acids, such as liver and skeletal muscle, and high peroxisome-dependent activities. Under conditions of increased hepatic fatty acid influx or decreased fatty acid efflux, PPARα activation prevents the accumulation of TG by increasing the expression of genes involved in fatty acid catabolism.[49] This response is associated with increased mitochondrial reactive oxygen species.[50] Dysfunctions of PPARα are expected to influence the normal metabolism of fatty acid and thus cause steatohepatitis. In fact, Chen and colleagues[49] reported significant differences in the allele frequency of PPARa between NAFLD and the control subjects. The frequency of the TT genotype (Val227Val) was 93.67% in patients with NAFLD compared with 79.37% in control subjects. The frequency of the CC/CT genotype (Ala227Ala and Val227Ala) was 6.33% in patients with NAFLD compared with 20.63% (13 of 63) in control subjects.[49] The investigators hypothesized that the differences among the variants may be caused by different activity levels. In fact, the Val227 isoform has lower activity than the Ala227 isoform; the presence of the Val227 isoform results in reduced lipid catabolism and an increased risk for NAFLD.[49] Studies examining other PPARa variants found that the Leu162Val PPARα loss-of-function polymorphism did not influence the risk of NAFLD in Italian patients, where it was associated with IR but not with histologically assessed NAFLD severity.[51,52] This finding suggests that the risk related to increased insulin resistance may be balanced by the protective effect of decreased oxidative stress.

Peroxisome proliferator-activated receptor g coactivator 1-alpha

Peroxisome proliferator-activated receptor g coactivator 1-alpha (PPARGC1A) is an important cofactor involved in the regulation of genes of the glucose and lipid metabolism pathway. Yoneda and colleagues[53] examined 15 SNPs in PPARGC1A in the Japanese population; rs2290602 was found to be closely associated with NASH, and the T allele frequency was higher in patients with NASH. The OR (95% CI) was 2.73 (1.48–5.06) for T allele; thus, the relative risk of developing NAFLD for these patients was 2.73 fold higher than among the patients without the T allele. Serum AST and ALT values of the patients with NAFLD with the TT allele were significantly higher than those of the patients with NAFLD and NASH with the GT or GG allele at SNP rs2290602. It is plausible that the TT allele may interfere with the transcription rate or stability of the mRNA of PPARGC1A because mRNA expression was significantly lower in the TT group than in the GG or GT group at SNP rs2290602 (T171G). However, the mechanism of underlying transcriptional reduction is yet to be demonstrated. A study among the Chinese Han people did not find any association between rs2290602 and NAFLD in the Chinese Han people.[54]

Peroxisome proliferator-activated receptor-gamma

Peroxisome proliferator-activated receptor-gamma (PPARγ) is highly expressed in adipose tissue and regulates adipocyte differentiation, FFA uptake, and storage. Pharmacologic activation of PPARγ improves insulin resistance in diabetes and has been reported to decrease liver damage in NAFLD by restoring adipose tissue insulin sensitivity and decreasing FFA flux to the liver. The Pro12Ala loss-of-function SNP in PPARγ2 is thought to induce a modest impairment of transcriptional activation because of decreased DNA-binding affinity.[52] Dongiovanni and colleagues[52] assessed the association of biopsy-proven NAFLD and this common variant in the Italian population and found that the 12Ala allele was not associated with NAFLD susceptibility, liver damage, or IR in 212 Italian patients with NAFLD. Rey[55] similarly found no association between the 12Ala allele and the progression of liver disease in patients with NAFLD. C161T is another polymorphism in PPARγ reported to have a correlation with lower plasma levels of adiponectin and increased susceptibility to NAFLD in the Chinese Han population.[54] These polymorphisms need further verification in independent multiethnic studies, and the functional role of these SNPs needs to be verified with additional molecular studies.

Lipin1

Another interesting candidate is Lipin1 (LPIN1), a phosphatidate phosphatase that is highly expressed in adipose tissue. LPIN1 has dual enzymatic-coactivator activity and is involved in the metabolism of phospholipids and triacylglycerol, is required for adipogenesis and normal metabolic flux between adipose tissue and liver.[56] LPIN1 mRNA expression in the liver and adipose tissue has been positively associated with body mass and IR. To date, only one study has reported the association of LPIN1 variants with NAFLD. The LPIN1 rs13412852 C>T polymorphism was associated with NASH and fibrosis in pediatric Italian patients with NAFLD, finding that the TT genotype was underrepresented in the pediatric patients but not in the adult patients with NAFLD. Furthermore, the TT genotype was associated with less severe dyslipidemia, and children with this genotype had a trend for a lower prevalence of NASH and significantly less severe liver damage independently of the *PNPLA3* genotype and other risk factors.[57] Although independent validation of these results is required, these data suggest that the *LPIN1* genotype may predispose patients to progressive NASH at an early age by influencing lipogenesis and core lipid metabolism.

Fatty Acid Transport Protein 5

Fatty Acid Transport Protein (FATP) proteins are involved in the hepatic uptake of fat.[58] Thus, gain-of function polymorphism may result in hepatic steatosis. A FATP5 promoter polymorphism rs56225452 (−1324G>A) was investigated with parameters of fasting and postprandial lipid and glucose metabolism in 2 cohorts. One cohort was the Metabolic Intervention Cohort Kiel (MICK) comprising 716 patients, and the second cohort included 103 patients with histologically proven NAFLD.[59] An in silico analysis has shown the G->A change to result in an allele-specific binding of GATA-2 and GATA-3.[60,61] In the MICK cohort, ALT levels, postprandial insulin levels, and TG concentrations were higher in patients carrying the rare A-allele than in GG homozygotes. In the A variant carriers, the insulin sensitivity index was also lower. Male patients with NAFLD carrying allele A had a significantly higher ALT activity ($P = .03$) with no difference in BMI, fasting TG, glucose, and insulin. The degree of steatosis within A-allele carriers was significantly associated with BMI ($P = .01$). Patients with NAFLD carrying the allele A also presented with higher ALT activity.[59] This study is the only known study exploring liver-specific FATP polymorphism in NAFLD. However, a major drawback is that the prevalence of NAFLD in the MICK cohort is unknown, which may result in false associations; independent studies verifying the association of this polymorphism with NAFLD are needed.

Beta-adrenergic receptor

Patients with NAFLD are often obese and have insulin resistance; thus, it is logical to examine gene polymorphisms that increase predisposition to obesity and IR as underlying risk factors for NAFLD. One such family of genes is β-adrenergic receptors (ADRB), which plays an important role in regulating energy expenditure, in part, by stimulating lipid mobilization through lipolysis. Several polymorphisms have been detected in ADRB genes with influence on energy mobilization.[62]

One of the nonsynonymous polymorphisms studied was W64R codon substitution in the β3-adrenergic receptor gene (ADRB3). The frequency of the polymorphism resulting in a W/R substitution was determined in 63 patients with biopsy-proven NASH. The R allele frequency in patients with NASH was significantly higher as compared with that in the control subjects (OR 1.97, $P = .01$), and the R(R/W and R/R) genotype frequency in patients with NASH was significantly higher in comparison with that in the control subjects (OR 2.38, $P = .01$).[63] This study is, however, limited to a small Japanese population.

Additional studies examined 2 nonsynonymous polymorphisms in another ADRB gene, β2-adrenergic receptor gene (ADRB2), on the premise that genetic predisposition to obesity is a risk factor for the development of NAFLD.[64,65] In a small cohort, the 2 polymorphisms examined were Gln27Glu and Arg16Gly.

Gln27Glu is a common mutation resulting in the substitution of an amino acid in the extracellular domain of the receptor, the functional implication of which is as yet unknown. The allelic frequency of the ADRB2 gene mutation in codons 16 and 27 did not differ between obese patients (BMI >25.0 kg/m^2, n = 151) and nonobese patients (BMI ≤25.0 kg/m^2, n = 100) in the Japanese population.[64]

In the Japanese population, glycine at codon 16 was associated with lower HDL-C levels as compared with arginine homozygotes.[64] The Gly16 homozygotes had a lower

HDL-C level than the Arg16 homozygotes (1.50 ± 0.4 vs 1.32 ± 0.3 mmol/L, $P = .014$). However, no significant association with fatty liver was observed in the Gly16 allele frequency. The Gln27Glu heterozygotes showed higher concentrations of serum TG than the Gln27Gln homozygotes (1.62 ± 0.93 vs 2.21 ± 1.67 mmol/L, $P = .013$). This correlation was also observed in all patients regardless of weight classification. Univariate analysis indicated that patients with the heterozygous Gln27Glu mutant alleles had a significantly higher prevalence of fatty liver as compared with those without the mutation (Glu27 allele frequency 0.07 vs 0.12, $P = .047$; OR 1.92, 95% CI 1.01–3.68). However, multivariate logistic regression models showed the prevalence of fatty liver to be significantly related to the homeostasis model assessment (HOMA) index, BMI, TG, and HDL-C.[64] This trend was not seen in the Saudi population.[65] The investigators did not see a significant association between the allelic frequency of Glu27 polymorphism among the groups based on BMI normal, overweight, and obese groups, although the Glu27 homozygote (Glu/Glu) was seen more frequently in obese patients and had higher concentrations of TG, leptin, and insulin as compared with the Gln27 heterozygotes and Gln/Gln homozygotes.[65] The conflicting results from these candidate gene studies may be better addressed with additional studies in other ethnic groups and multiethnic studies.

Polymorphisms in Genes Involved in Adipogenesis, Appetite Regulation, Fibrosis, Oxidative Load, and Inflammation

Genes involved in fibrogenesis in the liver are obvious candidates for their role in NAFLD, particularly NASH and fibrosis. Some of the candidate genes implicated in fibrogenesis are transforming growth factor (TGF)-β1; connective tissue growth factor (CTGF); matrix metalloproteinase 3; PPARγ; and some fibrogenic adipocytokines, including leptin and angiotensin II.[66] The role of FFA oxidation in the pathogenesis of NAFLD is complex because the reactive oxygen species generated may initiate and perpetuate fibrosis.[66] Appropriate fat oxidation is required to prevent fat accumulation in the liver.[67] It can be speculated that gain-of-function mutations in peroxisomal and microsomal fat oxidation genes would predispose individuals to higher levels of Reactive Oxygen Species (ROS) and, therefore, susceptibility to NASH. Alternatively, loss-of-function polymorphisms may protect against mitochondrial overload during times of excessive FFA supply, thus predisposing patients to steatosis and NASH.[67]

Methylenetetrahydrofolate reductase

DNA methylation is an important epigenetic mechanism of gene expression regulation and is directly correlated with cellular folate status. Methylenetetrahydrofolate reductase (MTHFR) catalyzes the conversion of the 5,10-methylenetetrahydrofolate into 5-methytetrahydofolate, which is then used for methylation of homocysteine. Thus, loss of function polymorphisms in methylenetetrahydrofolate reductase (MTHFR) may result in low levels of methylation and an aberrant gene expression pattern. Sazci and colleagues,[68] investigated C677T and A1298C polymorphisms of the MTHFR gene in a subgroup of the Turkish population and its association with NASH. They found that the MTHFR 1298C allele was significantly associated with NASH (OR 2.4, 95% CI 1.28–4.78, chi-square [chi.sq] = 7.7, $df = 1$, $P = .006$). The MTHFR C677C/A1298C compound genotype (OR 2.2, 95% CI 1.003–4.9, chi.sq = 3.9, $df = 1$; $P = .046$) in men, MTHFR C1298C genotype (OR 2.9, 95% CI 1.02–8.6, chi.sq = 4.3, $df = 1$, $P = .037$) and C677C/C1298C compound genotype in women were significantly associated with NASH. In contrast, the MTHFR A1298A genotype (OR 0.4, 95% CI 0.2–0.7, chi.sq = 7.7, $df = 1$, $P = .006$) in the total cohort (OR 0.3, 95% CI 0.1–0.9, chi.sq = 4.4, $df = 1$, $P = .035$) conferred protection toward NASH. A similar study was carried out in a Brazilian population[69] whereby the investigators found a higher frequency of 677TT homozygous polymorphism in patients with NAFLD (17.14%) as compared with controls (4.44%), although the difference was nonsignificant (P>.05). The A1298C polymorphism also did not differ significantly between groups.[69] Much more detailed work needs to be done in this area, with specific considerations such as race and gender.

Tumor necrosis factor α

Tumor necrosis factor α (TNF-α) cytokine plays a role in fatty liver disease as well as progression to an advanced stage of liver disease.[70] Four polymorphisms have been reported in the promoter region of the TNF-α gene.[71] Two of the promoter polymorphisms in TNF-α have been associated with the susceptibility of NAFLD: one at position −308 (called TNF2 allele) and another at position −238 (TNFA allele). The TNF2 allele leads to high TNF-α production and is associated with insulin-dependent diabetes mellitus. Valenti and colleagues[72] investigated the relationship between −238 and −308 TNF-α promoter polymorphisms and insulin resistance and the occurrence of NAFLD known to be associated with an increased release of this cytokine. The prevalence of the −238 TNF-α polymorphism was higher in Italian patients with NAFLD than controls, and patients with these polymorphisms had higher insulin resistance indices. Tokushige and colleagues[73] determined the prevalence of several TNF-α promoter region polymorphisms (positions −1031, −863, −857, −308, and −238) in a group of Japanese patients with NAFLD and control subjects. Surprisingly, there were no significant differences in the allele frequencies of any of the 6 polymorphisms among the Japanese patients with NAFLD and the control group.[73] The −238 polymorphism previously reported to be associated with NAFLD in Italian patients[72] was not significantly associated in the Japanese population with NAFLD. The frequency of the −238 polymorphism was, however, much lower in the Japanese population.[73] Tokushige and colleagues[73] found the frequency of the −1031C and −863A polymorphisms to be significantly higher in the NASH group compared with the simple steatosis group. These two polymorphisms were also associated with higher levels of insulin resistance measured by HOMA-IR. In another study by Wong and colleagues, in a Chinese population, no significant difference was found in TNFA polymorphisms between NAFLD and the control group. This finding could be attributed to the small population size, which would reduce the strength of the association. In a recent meta analysis by Wang and colleagues,[74] significant differences were found in TNFA −238 genotype distribution between NAFLD and the control, regardless of races (GA/AA vs GG, OR 2.06, 95% CI 1.58–2.69, P<.0001).

Transforming growth factor beta 1 and angiotensin II

Dixon and colleagues[75] investigated the relationship between the presence of advanced fibrosis and the 2 functional polymorphisms of TGF-B1, which resulted in higher levels of expression (angiotensinogen G-6A polymorphism and TGF-B1 Pro25Arg polymorphism) in a group of severely obese patients. The investigators found a positive association of angiotensin II −6 A/A polymorphism and advanced grade 3 or 4 fibrosis (chi-square, OR 3.6, 95% CI 1.05–12.8, P = .033); however, this association disappeared when corrected for gender. However, patients who inherited both high angiotensin and TGF-β1 producing polymorphisms had a higher risk of advanced fibrosis (OR 4.9, 95% CI 1.1–22, P = .037).[75] In another study, none of the 5 variants of the Angiotensin II Receptor, Type 1 gene (rs3772622, rs3772627, rs3772630, rs3772633, and rs2276736) were associated with susceptibility to NAFLD and NASH in a cohort composed of Malayan, Indian, and Chinese populations. However, after ethnic stratification, in the Indian ethnic subgroup, the rs2276736, rs3772630, and rs3772627 were found to be protective against NAFLD (OR 0.40, 95% CI 0.20–0.81, $P = $ .010; OR 0.43, 95% CI 0.22–0.86, $P = $ .016; and OR 0.46, 95% CI 0.23–0.91, $P = $ .026, respectively). In the Indian ethnic subgroup, the 3 SNPs (rs2276736, rs3772630, and rs3772627) were also protective against NASH (OR 0.42, 95% CI 0.21–0.86, $P = $ .017; OR 0.46, 95% CI 0.22–0.92, $P = $ .029; and OR 0.49, 95% CI 0.24–0.98, $P = $ .045, respectively).[76] This finding is in contrast to a study in a Japanese population whereby 5 SNPs (rs3772622, rs3772633, rs2276736, rs3772630, and rs3772627) were significantly associated with NAFLD.[77] AGTR1 is shown to be an important regulator of hepatic steatosis[78]; thus, additional studies examining polymorphisms and their functional implications may help develop prognosis/diagnostic tools.

Leptin receptor

Leptin is an adipocytokine whose main role is the regulation of food intake via interaction with its receptor leptin receptor (LEPR). The LEPR 3057 variant may contribute to the onset of NAFLD by regulating lipid metabolism and insulin sensitivity in Chinese patients through interference with LEPR signaling.[79] A recent study by Zain and colleagues[80] examined the association between nonsynonymous polymorphisms in LEPR and NAFLD across different ethnic groups (Malayan, Indian, Chinese). LEPR rs1137100 (G/A) and rs1137101 were associated with susceptibility to NAFLD (OR 1.64, 95% CI 1.18–2.28, $P = $ .003; and OR 1.61, 95% CI 1.11–2.34, $P = $ .013, respectively) and to NASH (OR 1.49, 95% CI 1.05–2.12, $P = $ .026; and OR 1.57, 95% CI 1.05–2.35, $P = $ .029, respectively). The G allele of rs1137100 is associated with a less severe form of liver disease. The LEPR rs1137100 is also associated with simple steatosis (OR 2.27, 95% CI 1.27–4.08, $P = $ .006). The analysis of gene-gene interaction revealed a strong interaction between the LEPR and PNPLA3 genes (empiric $P = $ .001). The joint effect of LEPR and PNPLA3 greatly exacerbated the risk of NAFLD (OR 3.73, 95% CI 1.84–7.55, $P<$.0001). The G allele of rs1137100 was also associated with a lower fibrosis score (OR 0.47, 95% CI 0.28–0.78, $P = $ .001).[80] Another polymorphism examined by Aller and colleagues[81] was Lys656Asn. The investigators found that this polymorphism was associated with obesity parameters, insulin resistance, and glucose levels in patients with NAFLD. Thus, LEPR variants may set the stage for progressive NAFLD by influencing insulin sensitivity and lipid metabolism. Several polymorphisms in the LEPR gene have been studied in the context of obesity, but additional studies are needed to delineate the role of these polymorphisms in NAFLD.

Adiponectin

Adiponectin (ADIPOQ) is an abundant adipocyte-derived cytokine with important roles in mobilization, transport, and oxidation of FFA. It has also been implicated in NAFLD and hepatic fibrogenesis in combination with leptin.[66,82] ADIPOQ has a protective effect; it decreases hepatic and systematic IR and attenuates liver inflammation and fibrosis. ADIPOQ generally predicts the steatosis grade and severity of NAFLD, but the mechanism remains unclear.[82–85] A study in the Chinese population analyzed T45G and G276T polymorphisms, finding no correlation between SNP +45 or SNP +276 in NAFLD or patients with NAFLD with MetS. Patients carrying the G allele of SNP +45 showed higher levels of TG, fasting blood sugar, HOMA, BMI, ALT, and lower plasma adiponectin levels. In the normal-weight group of SNP276, patients carrying the G allele showed a higher HOMA and patients carrying the T allele showed a lower BMI.[86] In another study involving the Chinese population, the polymorphisms of adiponectin −C11377G, −G11391A, +T45G, and +G276T were analyzed. Wong and colleagues[84] obtained similar results with no significant differences in allelic frequencies among all adiponectin gene polymorphisms between patients with NAFLD and the controls. Tokushige and colleagues[83] found the G allele of +45 SNP to be significantly higher in the severe fibrosis group than that in the mild fibrosis group, whereas the +G276T allele was not statistically different. This study had a larger cohort as compared with the other studies. Musso and colleagues[85] reported that the ADIPOQ SNPs 45TT and 276GT/TT were more prevalent in Italian patients with NAFLD than in the general population; these polymorphisms independently predicted the severity of liver disease in NASH and exhibited a blunted postprandial adiponectin response and higher postprandial TG levels.

Human hemochromatosis protein

The liver is the major organ for iron and lipid metabolism. Iron is an integral part of some enzymes and transporters involved in lipid metabolism. It, thus, exerts a direct effect on hepatic lipid load, intrahepatic metabolic pathways, and hepatic lipid secretion. Iron in its ferrous form may indirectly affect lipid metabolism through its ability to induce oxidative stress and inflammation.[87,88] Although the mechanism is debated, it is possible that iron overload may serve as the second hit in the progression of NAFLD in a proinflammatory setting.

Human hemochromatosis protein (HFE) plays a crucial role in the control of cellular iron homeostasis.[87] HFE interacts with cell surface transferrin receptors to modulate cellular iron uptake and signal the control of the expression of hepcidin, the master regulator of body iron homeostasis. The central role of HFE in iron regulation has led to several studies investigating mutations in *HFE* as a risk factor for NAFLD. Feder and colleagues[89] identified a cysteine-to-tyrosine substitution at the amino acid 282 (C282Y) and the histidine-to-aspartate change at the amino acid 63 (H63D) variants of the *HFE* gene. These variants are responsible for most cases of hereditary hemochromatosis and are most common in Caucasians (6.2% and 15.1%, respectively).[90] Compared with other genotypes, C282Y homozygotes are at a greater risk of iron overload, followed by compound heterozygotes with one C282Y mutant allele and one H63D mutant allele; simple heterozygotes for both C282Y and H63D may also develop increased serum iron markers but to a lesser extent.[91] S65C is considered to be a neutral polymorphism.[92] In combination with C282Y (C282Y/S65C), the penetrance of this polymorphism is low.[93] The S65C substitution is in close proximity to the position of the H63D substitution in the HFE protein sequence. For H63D, the histidine-to-aspartic acid substitution in the $\alpha 1$ domain is predicted to disrupt a salt bridge with a neighboring aspartic acid residue, leading to a local rearrangement in the protein secondary structure. It is not clear whether the serine-to-cysteine substitution of S65C causes a conformational change in the protein, affecting HFE function.[92]

The prevalence of HFE gene mutations (C282Y, H63D, and S65C) in patients with NAFLD has been variable, depending on the population studied, and their relevance remains largely unknown. The first report of the association between *HFE* gene mutations and NAFLD showed a positive correlation between levels of serum ferritin, iron, and transferrin saturation and the presence of the mutated allele as well as between C282Y mutation and more severe fibrosis in a North American population[94,95] support these findings; but subsequent larger studies have not confirmed such an association. Although Chitturi and colleagues[96] question the link between hepatic iron and liver fibrogenesis, Lee and colleagues[97] found the presence of H63D mutations to be an independent factor associated with NAFLD in the Korean population. The prevalence of the H63D mutation was higher in the NAFLD group (14.4%) than in the controls (7.2%) (P = .032). The prevalence of the H63D mutation was significantly higher in the men with NAFLD than in the male control group (OR 5.51, P = .007). Raszeja-Wyszomirska,[98] on the other hand, did not find any association between HFE polymorphisms and NAFLD in a Polish population. In a meta-analysis, Hernaez and colleagues[91] found no associations between iron-overloading HFE mutations (C282Y/C282Y, C282Y/H63D) and NAFLD. The investigators report a nonsignificant OR for NAFLD among Caucasians carrying the *HFE* mutations (C282Y or H63D) as compared with controls (OR 1.03, 95% CI 0.90, 1.17). Among non-Caucasians, there was a significant association between *HFE* mutations (C282Y or H63D) as compared with controls (OR 1.64, 95% CI 1.20, 2.24). The small non-Caucasian population limits the reliability of this association.

SUMMARY

There are methodological limitations to some of the association studies described, including limited phenotypic characterization, use of surrogate markers (eg, ALT) for NAFLD, different diagnostic techniques (biopsy, ultrasound), inadequate sample size, referral and ascertainment biases, different ethnic backgrounds, lack of mediators' adjustment, or publication bias and the lack of validation studies in independent populations. In addition, studied SNPs may be in linkage disequilibrium with true functional SNPs, and SNPs may interact with each other. These variables have more than likely resulted in inconsistent reports on variants and their association with NAFLD.

SNPs or polymorphisms are single nucleotide substitutions in DNA that may result in the altered expression of a particular gene or altered function of the expressed protein. The increased risk of any given disease being related to a single SNP, however, is generally small; it is much more likely that multiple SNPs may influence the phenotypic expression the disease.[99] In fact, the studies surveyed earlier suggest a much more nuanced and geographically parsed impact of SNPs on disease status and outcomes. It is very probable that SNPs, much like biomarkers, may be used in combination panels to better predict disease susceptibility and subsequent resolution. Future directions in GWAS need to include studies of SNPs from major regulatory genes in large cohorts of multiethnic populations to fully illustrate the combinatorial effects of these changes.

REFERENCES

1. Vernon G, Baranova A, Younossi ZM. Systematic review: the epidemiology and natural history of non-alcoholic fatty liver disease and non-alcoholic steatohepatitis in adults. Aliment Pharmacol Ther 2011;34(3):274–85. http://dx.doi.org/10.1111/j.1365-2036.2011.04724.x.
2. Charlton MR, Burns JM, Pedersen RA, et al. Frequency and outcomes of liver transplantation for nonalcoholic steatohepatitis in the United States. Gastroenterology 2011;141(4):1249–53. http://dx.doi.org/10.1053/j.gastro.2011.06.061.
3. Mehta R, Younossi ZM. Natural history of nonalcoholic fatty liver disease. Clin Liver Dis 2012;1(4):111–2. http://dx.doi.org/10.1002/cld.27.
4. Lazo M, Hernaez R, Eberhardt MS, et al. Prevalence of nonalcoholic fatty liver disease in the United States: the Third National Health and Nutrition Examination Survey, 1988-1994. Am J Epidemiol 2013. http://dx.doi.org/10.1093/aje/kws448.
5. Caballería L, Pera G, Auladell MA, et al. Prevalence and factors associated with the presence of nonalcoholic fatty liver disease in an adult population in Spain. Eur J Gastroenterol Hepatol 2010;22(1):24–32. http://dx.doi.org/10.1097/MEG.0b013e32832fcdf0.
6. Alam S, Noor-E-Alam SM, Chowdhury ZR, et al. Nonalcoholic steatohepatitis in nonalcoholic fatty liver disease patients of Bangladesh. World J Hepatol 2013;5(5):281–7. http://dx.doi.org/10.4254/wjh.v5.i5.281.

7. Browning JD, Szczepaniak LS, Dobbins R, et al. Prevalence of hepatic steatosis in an urban population in the United States: impact of ethnicity. Hepatology 2004;40(6):1387–95. http://dx.doi.org/10.1002/hep.20466.

8. Marcos A, Fisher RA, Ham JM, et al. Selection and outcome of living donors for adult to adult right lobe transplantation. Transplantation 2000;69(11):2410–5.

9. Duvnjak M, Barsic N, Tomasic V, et al. Genetic polymorphisms in non-alcoholic fatty liver disease: clues to pathogenesis and disease progression. World J Gastroenterol 2009;15(48):6023–7. http://dx.doi.org/10.3748/wjg.15.6023.

10. Amarapurkar D, Kamani P, Patel N, et al. Prevalence of non-alcoholic fatty liver disease: population based study. Ann Hepatol 2007;6(3):161–3.

11. Lee JY, Kim KM, Lee SG, et al. Prevalence and risk factors of non-alcoholic fatty liver disease in potential living liver donors in Korea: a review of 589 consecutive liver biopsies in a single center. J Hepatol 2007;47(2):239–44. http://dx.doi.org/10.1016/j.jhep.2007.02.007.

12. Hooper AJ, Adams LA, Burnett JR. Genetic determinants of hepatic steatosis in man. J Lipid Res 2011;52(4):593–617. http://dx.doi.org/10.1194/jlr.R008896.

13. Adams LA, White SW, Marsh JA, et al. Association between liver-specific gene polymorphisms and their expression levels with nonalcoholic fatty liver disease. Hepatology 2013;57(2):590–600. http://dx.doi.org/10.1002/hep.26184.

14. Lewis CM, Knight J. Introduction to Genetic Association Studies. Cold Spring Harb Protoc 2012;2012(3). http://dx.doi.org/10.1101/pdb.top068163. pdb.top068163.

15. Hernaez R. Genetic factors associated with the presence and progression of nonalcoholic fatty liver disease: a narrative review. Gastroenterol Hepatol 2012;35(1):32–41. http://dx.doi.org/10.1016/j.gastrohep.2011.08.002.

16. McHutchison JG. The role of genetic markers in hepatitis C virus therapy: a major step for individualized care. Liver Int 2011;31:29–35. http://dx.doi.org/10.1111/j.1478-3231.2010.02389.x.

17. Romeo S, Kozlitina J, Xing C, et al. Genetic variation in PNPLA3 confers susceptibility to nonalcoholic fatty liver disease. Nat Genet 2008;40(12):1461–5. http://dx.doi.org/10.1038/ng.257.

18. Speliotes EK, Yerges-Armstrong LM, Wu J, et al. Genome-wide association analysis identifies variants associated with nonalcoholic fatty liver disease that have distinct effects on metabolic traits. PLoS Genet 2011;7(3):e1001324.

19. Sharp D, Ricci B, Kienzle B, et al. Human microsomal triglyceride transfer protein large subunit gene structure. Biochemistry 1994;33(31):9057–61.

20. Lehner R, Lian J, Quiroga AD. Lumenal lipid metabolism implications for lipoprotein assembly. Arterioscler Thromb Vasc Biol 2012;32(5):1087–93. http://dx.doi.org/10.1161/ATVBAHA.111.241497.

21. Hagan DL, Kienzle B, Jamil H, et al. Transcriptional regulation of human and hamster microsomal triglyceride transfer protein genes. Cell type-specific expression and response to metabolic regulators. J Biol Chem 1994;269(46):28737–44.

22. Aminoff A, Ledmyr H, Thulin P, et al. Allele-specific regulation of MTTP expression influences the risk of ischemic heart disease. J Lipid Res 2010;51(1):103–11. http://dx.doi.org/10.1194/jlr.M900195-JLR200.

23. Ledmyr H, Karpe F, Lundahl B, et al. Variants of the microsomal triglyceride transfer protein gene are associated with plasma cholesterol levels and body mass index. J Lipid Res 2002;43(1):51–8.

24. Peng XE, Wu YL, Lu QQ, et al. MTTP polymorphisms and susceptibility to nonalcoholic fatty liver disease in a Han Chinese population. Liver Int 2013. http://dx.doi.org/10.1111/liv.12220.

25. Briggs MR, Yokoyama C, Wang X, et al. Nuclear protein that binds sterol regulatory element of low density lipoprotein receptor promoter. I. Identification of the protein and delineation of its target nucleotide sequence. J Biol Chem 1993; 268(19):14490–6.

26. Rubin D, Schneider-Muntau A, Klapper M, et al. Functional analysis of promoter variants in the microsomal triglyceride transfer protein (MTTP) gene. Hum Mutat 2008;29(1):123–9. http://dx.doi.org/10.1002/humu.20615.

27. Karpe F, Lundahl B, Ehrenborg E, et al. A common functional polymorphism in the promoter region of the microsomal triglyceride transfer protein gene influences plasma LDL levels. Arterioscler Thromb Vasc Biol 1998;18(5):756–61.

28. Bernard S, Touzet S, Personne I, et al. Association between microsomal triglyceride transfer protein gene polymorphism and the biological features of liver steatosis in patients with type II diabetes. Diabetologia 2000;43(8):995–9. http://dx.doi.org/10.1007/s001250051481.

29. Namikawa C, Shu-Ping Z, Vyselaar JR, et al. Polymorphisms of microsomal triglyceride transfer protein gene and manganese superoxide dismutase gene in non-alcoholic steatohepatitis. J Hepatol 2004;40(5):781–6. http://dx.doi.org/10.1016/j.jhep.2004.01.028.

30. Gambino R, Cassader M, Pagano G, et al. Polymorphism in microsomal triglyceride transfer protein: a link between liver disease and atherogenic postprandial lipid profile in NASH? Hepatology 2007;45(5):1097–107. http://dx.doi.org/10.1002/hep.21631.

31. Oliveira CP, Stefano JT, Cavaleiro AM, et al. Association of polymorphisms of glutamate-cystein ligase and microsomal triglyceride transfer protein genes in non-alcoholic fatty liver disease. J Gastroenterol Hepatol 2010;25(2):357–61. http://dx.doi.org/10.1111/j.1440-1746.2009.06001.x.

32. Corbin KD, Zeisel SH. Choline metabolism provides novel insights into nonalcoholic fatty liver disease and its progression. Curr Opin Gastroenterol 2012;28(2): 159–65. http://dx.doi.org/10.1097/MOG.0b013e32834e7b4b.

33. Watkins SM, Zhu X, Zeisel SH. Phosphatidylethanolamine-N-methyltransferase activity and dietary choline regulate liver-plasma lipid flux and essential fatty acid metabolism in mice. J Nutr 2003;133(11):3386–91.

34. Song J, da Costa KA, Fischer LM, et al. Polymorphism of the PEMT gene and susceptibility to nonalcoholic fatty liver disease (NAFLD). FASEB J 2005; 19(10):1266–71. http://dx.doi.org/10.1096/fj.04-3580com.

35. Dong H, Wang J, Li C, et al. The phosphatidylethanolamine N-methyltransferase gene V175M single nucleotide polymorphism confers the susceptibility to NASH in Japanese population. J Hepatol 2007;46(5):915–20. http://dx.doi.org/10.1016/j.jhep.2006.12.012.

36. Romeo S, Cohen JC, Hobbs HH. No association between polymorphism in PEMT (V175M) and hepatic triglyceride content in the Dallas Heart Study. FASEB J 2006;20(12):2180. http://dx.doi.org/10.1096/fj.06-1004ufm [author reply: 2181–2].

37. Duseja A, Aggarwal R. APOC3 and PNPLA3 in non-alcoholic fatty liver disease: need to clear the air. J Gastroenterol Hepatol 2012;27(5):848–51. http://dx.doi.org/10.1111/j.1440-1746.2012.07103.x.

38. Yuan X, Waterworth D, Perry JR, et al. Population-based genome-wide association studies reveal six loci influencing plasma levels of liver enzymes. Am J Hum Genet 2008;83(4):520–8. http://dx.doi.org/10.1016/j.ajhg.2008.09.012.

39. Romeo S, Sentinelli F, Dash S, et al. Morbid obesity exposes the association between PNPLA3 I148M (rs738409) and indices of hepatic injury in individuals of

European descent. Int J Obes 2010;34(1):190–4. http://dx.doi.org/10.1038/ijo. 2009.216.

40. Valenti L, Al-Serri A, Daly AK, et al. Homozygosity for the PNPLA3/adiponutrin I148 M polymorphism influences liver fibrosis in patients with nonalcoholic fatty liver disease. Hepatology 2010;51:1209–17.

41. Sookoian S, Pirola CJ. Meta-analysis of the influence of I148M variant of patatin-like phospholipase domain containing 3 gene (PNPLA3) on the susceptibility and histological severity of nonalcoholic fatty liver disease. Hepatology 2011; 53(6):1883–94. http://dx.doi.org/10.1002/hep.24283.

42. Kotronen A, Johansson LE, Johansson LM, et al. A common variant in PNPLA3, which encodes adiponutrin, is associated with liver fat content in humans. Diabetologia 2009;52(6):1056–60. http://dx.doi.org/10.1007/s00125-009-1285-z.

43. Beer NL, Tribble ND, McCulloch LJ, et al. The P446L variant in GCKR associated with fasting plasma glucose and triglyceride levels exerts its effect through increased glucokinase activity in liver. Hum Mol Genet 2009;18(21):4081–8. http://dx.doi.org/10.1093/hmg/ddp357.

44. Li WW, Dammerman MM, Smith JD, et al. Common genetic variation in the promoter of the human apo CIII gene abolishes regulation by insulin and may contribute to hypertriglyceridemia. J Clin Invest 1995;96(6):2601–5. http://dx.doi.org/10.1172/JCI118324.

45. Miller M, Rhyne J, Chen H, et al. APOC3 promoter polymorphisms C-482T and T-455C are associated with the metabolic syndrome. Arch Med Res 2007;38(4): 444–51. http://dx.doi.org/10.1016/j.arcmed.2006.10.013.

46. Pollex RL, Ban MR, Young TK, et al. Association between the -455T>C promoter polymorphism of the APOC3 gene and the metabolic syndrome in a multi-ethnic sample. BMC Med Genet 2007;8(1):80. http://dx.doi.org/10.1186/1471-2350-8-80.

47. Petersen KF, Dufour S, Hariri A, et al. Apolipoprotein C3 gene variants in nonalcoholic fatty liver disease. N Engl J Med 2010;362(12):1082–9. http://dx.doi.org/10.1056/NEJMoa0907295.

48. Valenti L, Nobili V, Al-Serri A, et al. The APOC3 T-455C and C-482T promoter region polymorphisms are not associated with the severity of liver damage independently of PNPLA3 I148M genotype in patients with nonalcoholic fatty liver. J Hepatol 2011;55(6):1409–14. http://dx.doi.org/10.1016/j.jhep.2011.03.035.

49. Chen S, Li Y, Li S, et al. A Val227Ala substitution in the peroxisome proliferator activated receptor alpha (PPAR alpha) gene associated with non-alcoholic fatty liver disease and decreased waist circumference and waist-to-hip ratio. J Gastroenterol Hepatol 2008;23(9):1415–8. http://dx.doi.org/10.1111/j.1440-1746.2008.05523.x.

50. Rosca MG, Vazquez EJ, Chen Q, et al. Oxidation of fatty acids is the source of increased mitochondrial reactive oxygen species production in kidney cortical tubules in early diabetes. Diabetes 2012;61(8):2074–83. http://dx.doi.org/10.2337/db11-1437.

51. Sparsø T, Hussain MS, Andersen G, et al. Relationships between the functional PPARα Leu162Val polymorphism and obesity, type 2 diabetes, dyslipidaemia, and related quantitative traits in studies of 5799 middle-aged white people. Mol Genet Metab 2007;90(2):205–9. http://dx.doi.org/10.1016/j.ymgme.2006.10.007.

52. Dongiovanni P, Rametta R, Fracanzani A, et al. Lack of association between peroxisome proliferator-activated receptors alpha and gamma2 polymorphisms and progressive liver damage in patients with non-alcoholic fatty liver disease: a case control study. BMC Gastroenterol 2010;10(1):102.

53. Yoneda M, Hotta K, Nozaki Y, et al. Association between PPARGC1A polymorphisms and the occurrence of nonalcoholic fatty liver disease (NAFLD). BMC Gastroenterol 2008;8:27. http://dx.doi.org/10.1186/1471-230X-8-27.

54. Hui Y, Yu-Yuan L, Yu-Qiang N, et al. Effect of peroxisome proliferator-activated receptors-γ and co-activator-1α genetic polymorphisms on plasma adiponectin levels and susceptibility of non-alcoholic fatty liver disease in Chinese people. Liver Int 2008;28(3):385–92. http://dx.doi.org/10.1111/j.1478-3231.2007.01623.x.

55. Rey JW. Pro12Ala polymorphism of the peroxisome proliferator-activated receptor γ2 in patients with fatty liver diseases. World J Gastroenterol 2010;16(46): 5830. http://dx.doi.org/10.3748/wjg.v16.i46.5830.

56. Reue K, Zhang P. The lipin protein family: dual roles in lipid biosynthesis and gene expression. FEBS Lett 2008;582(1):90–6. http://dx.doi.org/10.1016/j.febslet.2007.11.014.

57. Valenti L, Motta BM, Alisi A, et al. LPIN1 rs13412852 polymorphism in pediatric nonalcoholic fatty liver disease. J Pediatr Gastroenterol Nutr 2012;54(5):588–93. http://dx.doi.org/10.1097/MPG.0b013e3182442a55.

58. Doege H, Grimm D, Falcon A, et al. Silencing of hepatic fatty acid transporter protein 5 in vivo reverses diet-induced non-alcoholic fatty liver disease and improves hyperglycemia. J Biol Chem 2008;283(32):22186–92. http://dx.doi.org/10.1074/jbc.M803510200.

59. Auinger A, Valenti L, Pfeuffer M, et al. A promoter polymorphism in the liver-specific fatty acid transport protein 5 is associated with features of the metabolic syndrome and steatosis. Horm Metab Res 2010;42(12):854–9. http://dx.doi.org/10.1055/s-0030-1267186.

60. Merika M, Orkin SH. DNA-binding specificity of GATA family transcription factors. Mol Cell Biol 1993;13(7):3999–4010.

61. Wingender E, Dietze P, Karas H, et al. TRANSFAC: a database on transcription factors and their DNA binding sites. Nucleic Acids Res 1996;24(1):238–41.

62. Liggett SB. Pharmacogenetics of beta-1- and beta-2-adrenergic receptors. Pharmacology 2000;61(3):167–73. doi:28397.

63. Nozaki Y, Saibara T, Nemoto Y, et al. Polymorphisms of interleukin-1 beta and beta 3-adrenergic receptor in Japanese patients with nonalcoholic steatohepatitis. Alcohol Clin Exp Res 2004;28(8 Suppl Proceedings):106S–10S.

64. Iwamoto N, Ogawa Y, Kajihara S, et al. Gln27Glu β2-adrenergic receptor variant is associated with hypertriglyceridemia and the development of fatty liver. Clin Chim Acta 2001;314(1–2):85–91. http://dx.doi.org/10.1016/S0009-8981(01) 00633-7.

65. Daghestani MH, Warsy A, Daghestani MH, et al. The Gln27Glu polymorphism in β2-adrenergic receptor gene is linked to hypertriglyceridemia, hyperinsulinemia and hyperleptinemia in Saudis. Lipids Health Dis 2010;9(1):90. http://dx.doi.org/10.1186/1476-511X-9-90.

66. Lee UE, Friedman SL. Mechanisms of hepatic fibrogenesis. Best Pract Res Clin Gastroenterol 2011;25(2):195–206. http://dx.doi.org/10.1016/j.bpg.2011.02.005.

67. Day CP. Genes or environment to determine alcoholic liver disease and non-alcoholic fatty liver disease. Liver Int 2006;26(9):1021–8. http://dx.doi.org/10.1111/j.1478-3231.2006.01323.x.

68. Sazci A, Ergul E, Aygun C, et al. Methylenetetrahydrofolate reductase gene polymorphisms in patients with nonalcoholic steatohepatitis (NASH). Cell Biochem Funct 2008;26(3):291–6. http://dx.doi.org/10.1002/cbf.1424.

69. Siqueira ER, Oliveira CP, Muniz MT, et al. Methylenetetrahydrofolate reductase (MTHFR) C677T polymorphism and high plasma homocysteine in chronic

hepatitis C (CHC) infected patients from the northeast of Brazil. Nutr J 2011; 10(1):86. http://dx.doi.org/10.1186/1475-2891-10-86.

70. Tilg H. The role of cytokines in non-alcoholic fatty liver disease. Dig Dis 2010; 28(1):179–85. http://dx.doi.org/10.1159/000282083.

71. Frigerio S, Ciusani E, Pozzi A, et al. Tumor necrosis factor microsatellite polymorphisms in Italian glioblastoma patients. Cancer Genet Cytogenet 1999;109(2): 172–4.

72. Valenti L, Fracanzani AL, Dongiovanni P, et al. Tumor necrosis factor alpha promoter polymorphisms and insulin resistance in nonalcoholic fatty liver disease. Gastroenterology 2002;122(2):274–80.

73. Tokushige K, Takakura M, Tsuchiya-Matsushita N, et al. Influence of TNF gene polymorphisms in Japanese patients with NASH and simple steatosis. J Hepatol 2007;46(6):1104–10. http://dx.doi.org/10.1016/j.jhep.2007.01.028.

74. Wang J, Feng Z, Li Y, et al. Association of tumor necrosis factor-α gene promoter polymorphism at sites -308 and -238 with non-alcoholic fatty liver disease: a meta-analysis. J Gastroenterol Hepatol 2012;27(4):670–6. http://dx.doi.org/10. 1111/j.1440-1746.2011.06978.x.

75. Dixon JB, Bhathal PS, Jonsson JR, et al. Pro-fibrotic polymorphisms predictive of advanced liver fibrosis in the severely obese. J Hepatol 2003;39(6):967–71.

76. Zain SM, Mohamed Z, Mahadeva S, et al. Susceptibility and gene interaction study of the angiotensin ii type 1 receptor (AGTR1) gene polymorphisms with non-alcoholic fatty liver disease in a multi-ethnic population. PLoS One 2013; 8(3):e58538. http://dx.doi.org/10.1371/journal.pone.0058538.

77. Yoneda M, Hotta K, Nozaki Y, et al. Association between angiotensin II type 1 receptor polymorphisms and the occurrence of nonalcoholic fatty liver disease. Liver Int 2009;29(7):1078–85. http://dx.doi.org/10.1111/j.1478-3231.2009. 01988.x.

78. Nabeshima Y, Tazuma S, Kanno K, et al. Deletion of angiotensin II type I receptor reduces hepatic steatosis. J Hepatol 2009;50(6):1226–35. http://dx.doi.org/ 10.1016/j.jhep.2009.01.018.

79. Lu H, Sun J, Sun L, et al. Polymorphism of human leptin receptor gene is associated with type 2 diabetic patients complicated with non-alcoholic fatty liver disease in China. J Gastroenterol Hepatol 2009;24(2):228–32. http://dx.doi. org/10.1111/j.1440-1746.2008.05544.x.

80. Zain SM, Mohamed Z, Mahadeva S, et al. Impact of leptin receptor gene variants on risk of non-alcoholic fatty liver disease and its interaction with adiponutrin gene. J Gastroenterol Hepatol 2013;28(5):873–9. http://dx.doi.org/10.1111/ jgh.12104.

81. Aller R, De Luis DA, Izaola O, et al. Lys656Asn polymorphism of leptin receptor, leptin levels and insulin resistance in patients with non alcoholic fatty liver disease. Eur Rev Med Pharmacol Sci 2012;16(3):335–41.

82. Polyzos SA, Kountouras J, Zavos C, et al. The role of adiponectin in the pathogenesis and treatment of non-alcoholic fatty liver disease. Diabetes Obes Metab 2010;12(5):365–83. http://dx.doi.org/10.1111/j.1463-1326.2009.01176.x.

83. Tokushige K, Hashimoto E, Noto H, et al. Influence of adiponectin gene polymorphisms in Japanese patients with non-alcoholic fatty liver disease. J Gastroenterol 2009;44(9):976–82. http://dx.doi.org/10.1007/s00535-009-0085-z.

84. Wong VW, Wong GL, Tsang SW, et al. Genetic polymorphisms of adiponectin and tumor necrosis factor-alpha and nonalcoholic fatty liver disease in Chinese people. J Gastroenterol Hepatol 2008;23(6):914–21. http://dx.doi.org/10.1111/j. 1440-1746.2008.05344.x.

85. Musso G, Gambino R, De Michieli F, et al. Adiponectin gene polymorphisms modulate acute adiponectin response to dietary fat: possible pathogenetic role in NASH. Hepatology 2008;47(4):1167–77. http://dx.doi.org/10.1002/hep.22142.
86. Wang ZL, Xia B, Shrestha U, et al. Correlation between adiponectin polymorphisms and non-alcoholic fatty liver disease with or without metabolic syndrome in Chinese population. J Endocrinol Invest 2008;31(12):1086–91.
87. Guyader D, Deugnier Y. Steatosis, iron and HFE genes. J Hepatol 2008;48(3):514–5. http://dx.doi.org/10.1016/j.jhep.2007.12.002.
88. Ahmed U, Latham PS, Oates PS. Interactions between hepatic iron and lipid metabolism with possible relevance to steatohepatitis. World J Gastroenterol 2012;18(34):4651–8. http://dx.doi.org/10.3748/wjg.v18.i34.4651.
89. Feder JN, Gnirke A, Thomas W, et al. A novel MHC class I–like gene is mutated in patients with hereditary haemochromatosis. Nat Genet 1996;13(4):399–408. http://dx.doi.org/10.1038/ng0896-399.
90. Scott JD, Garland N. Chronic liver disease in aboriginal North Americans. World J Gastroenterol 2008;14(29):4607–15. http://dx.doi.org/10.3748/wjg.14.4607.
91. Hernaez R, Yeung E, Clark JM, et al. Hemochromatosis gene and nonalcoholic fatty liver disease: a systematic review and meta-analysis. J Hepatol 2011;55(5):1079–85. http://dx.doi.org/10.1016/j.jhep.2011.02.013.
92. Mura C, Raguenes O, Férec C. HFE mutations analysis in 711 hemochromatosis probands: evidence for S65C implication in mild form of hemochromatosis. Blood 1999;93(8):2502–5.
93. Wallace DF, Walker AP, Pietrangelo A, et al. Frequency of the S65C mutation of HFE and iron overload in 309 subjects heterozygous for C282Y. J Hepatol 2002;36(4):474–9.
94. Bonkovsky HL, Jawaid Q, Tortorelli K, et al. Non-alcoholic steatohepatitis and iron: increased prevalence of mutations of the HFE gene in non-alcoholic steatohepatitis. J Hepatol 1999;31(3):421–9. http://dx.doi.org/10.1016/S0168-8278(99)80032-4.
95. George DK, Goldwurm S, MacDonald GA, et al. Increased hepatic iron concentration in nonalcoholic steatohepatitis is associated with increased fibrosis. Gastroenterology 1998;114(2):311–8.
96. Chitturi S, Weltman M, Farrell GC, et al. HFE mutations, hepatic iron, and fibrosis: ethnic-specific association of NASH with C282Y but not with fibrotic severity. Hepatology 2002;36(1):142–9. http://dx.doi.org/10.1053/jhep.2002.33892.
97. Lee SH, Jeong S-H, Lee D, et al. An epidemiologic study on the incidence and significance of HFE mutations in a Korean cohort with nonalcoholic fatty liver disease. J Clin Gastroenterol 2010;44(7):e154–61. http://dx.doi.org/10.1097/MCG.0b013e3181d347d9.
98. Raszeja-Wyszomirska J, Kurzawski G, Lawniczak M, et al. Nonalcoholic fatty liver disease and HFE gene mutations: a Polish study. World J Gastroenterol 2010;16(20):2531–6. http://dx.doi.org/10.3748/wjg.v16.i20.2531.
99. Lvovs D, Favorova OO, Favorov AV. A polygenic approach to the study of polygenic diseases. Acta Naturae 2012;4(3):59–71.

Index

Note: Page numbers of article titles are in **boldface** type.

Absorption
  impaired, 181
Acetaminophen
  liver injury related to, 172–173
Activity
  defined, 114
Adenoma(s)
  hepatocellular, 38
Adipokine(s)
  from visceral fat
    obesity effects on, 44–45
Adiponectin
  polymorphisms in
    in obesity-associated NAFLD, 259–260
Adipose tissue
  as endocrine organ, **41–58**
    introduction, 41–42
    visceral fat composition, 42–44
Alcohol
  HCC effects of, 160
Alcoholic liver disease (ALD)
  epidemiology of, 157
  mortality related to
    obesity and metabolic syndrome effects on, 159–160
  obesity and metabolic syndrome effects on, **157–163**
    clinical management of, 160–162
    future directions in, 160–162
    mortality-related, 159–160
    progression-related, 158–159
  progression of
    diabetes mellitus effects on, 160
    obesity effects on, 158–159
  spectrum of, 158
ALD. *See* Alcoholic liver disease (ALD)
Anesthesia/anesthetics
  liver injury related to, 173
Antibiotics
  in obesity-associated NAFLD, 66–67
Antioxidants
  in NAFLD management, 77–80, 101–105

Clin Liver Dis 18 (2014) 269–280
http://dx.doi.org/10.1016/S1089-3261(13)00106-2
1089-3261/14/$ – see front matter © 2014 Elsevier Inc. All rights reserved.

liver.theclinics.com

Moving?

Make sure your subscription moves with you!

To notify us of your new address, find your **Clinics Account Number** (located on your mailing label above your name), and contact customer service at:

Email: **journalscustomerservice-usa@elsevier.com**

800-654-2452 (subscribers in the U.S. & Canada)
314-447-8871 (subscribers outside of the U.S. & Canada)

Fax number: 314-447-8029

Elsevier Health Sciences Division
Subscription Customer Service
3251 Riverport Lane
Maryland Heights, MO 63043

*To ensure uninterrupted delivery of your subscription, please notify us at least 4 weeks in advance of move.

Printed and bound by CPI Group (UK) Ltd, Croydon, CR0 4YY

03/10/2024

01040478-0011